NEOPLASIA
IN
CHILDHOOD

Proceedings of the Annual Clinical Conferences on Cancer sponsored by The University of Texas M. D. Anderson Hospital and Tumor Institute at Houston, and published by Year Book Medical Publishers, Inc.

TUMORS OF THE SKIN

TUMORS OF BONE AND SOFT TISSUE

RECENT ADVANCES IN THE DIAGNOSIS OF CANCER

CANCER OF THE GASTROINTESTINAL TRACT

CANCER OF THE UTERUS AND OVARY

NEOPLASIA IN CHILDHOOD

NEOPLASIA

IN

CHILDHOOD

A Collection of Papers Presented at the
Twelfth Annual Clinical Conference on Cancer, 1967
at The University of Texas M. D. Anderson Hospital
and Tumor Institute at Houston, Houston, Texas

YEAR BOOK MEDICAL PUBLISHERS, INC.

35 EAST WACKER DRIVE, CHICAGO

Library of Congress Catalog Card Number: 75-97245

8151-0205-4

Table of Contents

Acknowledgments

THE STAFF of The University of Texas M. D. Anderson Hospital and Tumor Institute at Houston gratefully acknowledges the assistance of the Texas Division of The American Cancer Society; the Division of Continuing Education of The University of Texas Graduate School of Biomedical Sciences at Houston; and a training grant from the National Center for Chronic Disease Control, Cancer Control Program, United States Public Health Service, all of which helped make possible both the Twelfth Annual Clinical Conference and the publication of this volume.

The staff of this institution owes a special debt of thanks to the program committee's chairman, Grant Taylor, and co-chairman, Wataru W. Sutow, and to the members of the committee: James J. Butler, Lillian M. Fuller, Myron R. Karon, Richard G. Martin, and Margaret P. Sullivan.

This volume was prepared for publication by the following members of the Department of Publications at The University of Texas M. D. Anderson Hospital and Tumor Institute at Houston: Russell W. Cumley, Joan McCay, Wendelyn White, Jan Devereaux, Judith James, and Gail Arnold. Assisting with the editing were: Pamela Bornmueller, Lynda Burgner, Carol Dimopoulos, Janina Ely, and Carol Thompson.

Most of the illustrations in this volume were prepared by members of the Department of Medical Communications.

Introduction
to
The Twelfth
Annual Clinical Conference

R. LEE CLARK, M.D., M.Sc., D.Sc. (Hon.)

President, The University of Texas
M. D. Anderson Hospital and Tumor Institute at Houston,
Houston, Texas

THE ANNUAL CLINICAL CONFERENCE ON CANCER was established 12 years ago to provide a forum for reporting the analysis and evaluation of methods used at The University of Texas M. D. Anderson Hospital and Tumor Institute at Houston for the diagnosis and treatment of patients with carcinomas of specific anatomic sites. This is the first year in which the subject of the clinical conference has encompassed a spectrum of neoplasms unique to a specific age group.

A personal facet is invariably present in the treatment of pediatric cancer patients which generally is not encountered in the treatment of adult cancer patients. Furthermore, all of us are especially hopeful, even optimistic, that we can attain success in curing or controlling cancer in these children. Because of this personal intangible, the choice by the program committee of "Neoplasia in Childhood" as the subject for this year's clinical conference on cancer is of particular significance.

Cancer usually is regarded as a disease of the elderly in the minds of both laymen and physicians. Admittedly rare in children, cancer is nonetheless the second leading cause of death in children between birth and 15 years of age in this country. Only accidents cause more deaths in children of this age group. At the turn of the century, the contagious or communicable infectious diseases were the leading causes of mortality in children, but with the control of these diseases, cancer has become one of the foremost challenges in pediatric medicine.

Cancers in children differ biologically from those which occur in adults, and in addition, differ in relation to specific ages. Thus, we are confronted with a spectrum of tumors which is not like that characteristic for adults. In children, as in adults, neoplasia may occur in nearly every part of the body. Excluding the leukemias and lymphomas, the most common sites of malignant neoplasms in children are the soft tissues, the central nervous system, kidney, bone, and skin.

Data on childhood cancer from widely separated geographic areas show consistent trends in percentage rates of tumor type and incidence; the variations are negligible. The specialty or specialties peculiar to a specific institution may frequently produce incidence rates which are higher than normally expected. For example, a medical center with a strong department of neurology will tend to report a preponderance of brain tumors; those with strong departments of urology will report a greater percentage of genitourinary tract tumors. Obviously, this factor has no scientific relevance to actual incidence or the concurrent implication of geographic, environmental, or ethnic influences on cancer etiology.

Incidence and type percentages of childhood neoplasias at Anderson Hospital are consistent with most data reported from other institutions and areas. Children afflicted with the leukemias and lymphomas constitute 40 per cent of our pediatric cancer patient load. Soft tissue sarcomas (predominantly rhabdomyosarcomas) are the second most frequently occurring neoplasia of children; in our experience at Anderson Hospital, these occur in almost 15 per cent of our young patients.

Epidemiologic studies of three diverse areas of Texas (El Paso, Travis County, and Abilene) have been carried out by the Anderson Hospital Department of Epidemiology for the past 15 years. One or more cases of pediatric carcinoma occurring in the buccal cavity, thyroid, stomach, lung, intestines, liver, bladder, and male and female genital tracts, and metastatic cancer with no primary discovered have been reported in this study.

Other factors emerging from this study provoke strong speculation about the possible etiologic significance of environment, demography, and heredity in the development of cancer. A calculation of annual average age-specific incidence rates per 100,000 population for these three Texas areas (with further division of the incidence in El Paso into Latin-American and Anglo-American groups of children) demonstrated significant differences in incidence rates. Cancer occurred in 15.0 per 100,000 Anglo-American children in the 10- to 19-year-old age group living in the El Paso area; the incidence for this same age-specific group in Abilene was only 8.0 per 100,000 children. Comparative incidence rates for these two areas in children from birth to nine years of age were not statistically significant; the rate was 17.0 per 100,000 population in El Paso Anglo-American children compared to 13.5 per 100,000 children in Abilene. These results raise the question of possible epidemiologic influences in the etiology of childhood neoplasia.

The concepts of therapy for children with cancer are changing rapidly and the parameters for care are expanding at an equal pace. We can see definite progress when we review the papers presented at the 1960 post-graduate course titled "Management of Children with Cancer." Their recommendations regarding the management of malignant neoplasms in children would not be considered adequate therapy today. Chemotherapy, then limited almost exclusively to the management of leukemia and lymphoma, is assuming a major role as an important adjuvant, and sometimes as a primary, therapy for solid tumors of children. We are witnessing the eclipse of the surgeon and radiotherapist in treating children who have cancer and the assumption of this key role by the chemotherapist-pediatrician. I am not suggesting that the surgeon and the radiotherapist are being retired. Patients with Wilms' tumor, for example, can be cured by using surgical therapy alone in a substantial number of children.

The same statement can be made about retinoblastomas and rhabdomyosarcomas. We do effect cures in children afflicted with these tumors by using standard surgical and/or irradiation therapy alone. However, with the addition of chemotherapy, we save children now who would not have been saved with standard therapy alone.

The role of chemotherapy today in pediatric oncology is, hopefully, (1) to increase the per cent of survival in children with the leukemias and lymphomas, (2) to save those children with solid tumors who might die without this added therapy, and (3) to provide long-term survival or palliation in children with metastatic disease.

The use of chemotherapeutic drugs in the management of Wilms' tumor has produced the best results yet attained with this modality. Sidney Farber, recipient of this year's Heath Award, pioneered the use of actinomycin D (now referred to as Dactinomycin) in the therapy for Wilms' tumor. Dactinomycin still remains one of the two most effective agents for control of this tumor—vincristine being the other.

In children with metastatic involvement on diagnosis, for whom radiation alone does not control the disease, we now find that chemotherapy may effect complete cure in some. I hasten to add that we report this with caution.

Although results thus far with the use of chemotherapy in the treatment for other solid tumors of children have not been as dramatic as those for

Wilms' tumors, there are positive indications that three of the other solid tumors have varying sensitivities to chemotherapy. Cyclophosphamide seems to be an effective agent for the control of neuroblastomas. Therapeutic effects of drugs have been noted in children with rhabdomyosarcomas. Chemotherapy has definitely contributed to the improved results in therapy for retinoblastomas. Enucleation of the involved orbit followed with irradiation was and still is the standard therapy in children with unilateral retinoblastoma. In children with advanced bilateral involvement, however, the addition of triethylene melamine to the regimen may improve the over-all survival picture and, in some children, may make possible the saving of the eye which is less involved.

Cancer in a child exacts in multiple and varying degrees a toll from each member of the child's family including both parents and normal siblings. Consideration of the economical, physical, and psychological effects that prolongation of life in the child with cancer imposes on family members places an extra burden on the attendant physicians. In effect, we are producing problem by-products in our realization of increased survival. Is the prolongation of the sick child's life worthwhile in the face of possible deprivation of essential needs of the normal siblings?

Hopefully, the papers today will present substantiating evidence that the encouraging improvement in the over-all picture for children with cancer is worth the price. I share the hopes of the program committee that the papers will bring out the concepts of therapy and the philosophies behind these concepts, and will emphasize the increased role of chemotherapy in the treatment of childhood neoplasms.

Epidemiology of Childhood Neoplasia

ROBERT W. MILLER, M.D.

Epidemiology Branch, National Cancer Institute
Bethesda, Maryland

EPIDEMIOLOGIC STUDIES have helped to identify a variety of environmental agents which are oncogenic in man (Doll, 1967), but only one of these —ionizing radiation—has induced cancer in children (Sutow and Conard, 1965). In part, this difference is caused by the much smaller exposure of children to oncogenic agents which adults encounter in occupations or by habit. The scope of epidemiologic studies of childhood cancer is nevertheless immense. It encompasses studies of disease frequency by such variables as age, sex, race, and socioeconomic status; clustering in time and space; familial aggregation; concordance rates in twins; associations with specific congenital defects; and other delineations of high-risk groups. It also includes international comparisons and tests of hypotheses about etiology—cell type by cell type. In this presentation, only the major areas will be discussed and emphasis will be given to etiological clues derived from descriptive studies and from the association between certain cancers and congenital defects.

Neoplasms with Mortality Peaks in Children under Five Years of Age

Mortality rates in children with specific forms of cancer exhibit dynamic changes with every year of age. These variations must reflect important etiological influences. Among four-year-old Caucasian children in the United States, the mortality rate for those with leukemia exhibits a huge peak which is absent among nonwhite children (Court Brown and Doll, 1961). There is no such peak for children with acute myelogenous leukemia. Thus, there must be racial differences in exposure or susceptibility to some agent which induces acute lymphocytic leukemia but not acute myelogenous leukemia.

13

In children about four years of age, there are also peaks in mortality from renal neoplasms (principally Wilms' tumor) and neuroblastomas (Ederer, Miller, and Scotto, 1965; Miller, Fraumeni, and Hill, 1968)— cancers whose intrauterine origins are suggested by their occurrence in very young patients and by the high frequency with which they are found in situ (microscopically) at autopsy in patients younger than three months of age, but not thereafter (Beckwith and Perrin, 1963; unpublished data). The same age pattern is exhibited for primary liver cancers and perhaps for adrenocortical neoplasia (Fraumeni, Miller, and Hill, 1968; Fraumeni and Miller, 1967a). These tumors may be linked with or distinguished from one another by the specific congenital defects with which they are associated. Leukemia is not like the other neoplasms of childhood because it occurs excessively in Down's syndrome, Bloom's syndrome, and Fanconi's aplastic anemia (Miller, 1967). Common to these observations and to other groups with an exceptionally high risk for leukemia are special genetic or chromosomal features, summarized in Table 1. The probability of developing leukemia in these groups is greater than one in 100, in contrast with the usual risk among Caucasian children in the United States of about one in 2,800 during the first 10 years of life.

Three of the childhood tumors with early age peaks occur excessively with congenital hemihypertrophy—Wilms' tumor, primary liver cancer, and adrenocortical neoplasia (Miller, Fraumeni, and Manning, 1964; Fraumeni, Miller, and Hill, 1968; Fraumeni and Miller, 1967a). Hemihypertrophy also is associated with two other forms of growth excess

TABLE 1.—PERSONS WITH EXCEPTIONALLY HIGH RISK FOR LEUKEMIA

CHARACTERISTIC	RISK	INTERVAL	EXCEPTIONAL GENETIC FEATURE
1. Identical twins of leukemic children	1:5*	Weeks or months	Identical genes
2. Polycythemia vera. Treatment: x-ray and/or p32	1:6	12 years	Aneuploidy before treatment; chromosomal breaks subsequently
3. Bloom's syndrome (and probably Fanconi's aplastic anemia)	1:8†	< 30 years of age	Chromosomal fragility on culture
4. Hiroshima survivors who had been within 1,000 m of the atomic bomb	1:60	12 years	Chromosomal breakage
5. Down's syndrome	1:95	< 10 years of age	Trisomy 21

*Among 22 identical twins with childhood leukemia, the co-twin was affected in five instances (MacMahon and Levy, 1964).

†Three patients with leukemia among 23 persons with Bloom's syndrome (Sawitsky, Bloom, and German, 1966).

(Fig. 1): the visceral cytomegaly syndrome (Beckwith, in press) and hamartomas (pigmented or vascular nevi) (Gesell, 1927). Hamartomas are, in turn, associated with Wilms' tumor and adrenocortical carcinoma (Fraumeni and Miller, 1967a) and may undergo neoplastic change, *e.g.,* multiple neurofibromatosis to neurofibrosarcoma, glioma, or pheochromocytoma (Crowe, Schull, and Neel, 1956). The relationship among these four forms of growth excess is shown in Figure 1. It is noteworthy that when two of these growth excesses occur in the same individual, they need not be anatomically linked. Thus, hemihypertrophy may occur contralateral to vascular nevi or Wilms' tumor (Gesell, 1927; Miller, Fraumeni, and Manning, 1964). It is of particular interest that visceral cytomegaly affects the three organs (kidney, adrenal cortex, and liver) in which neoplasms occur in association with hemihypertrophy (Beckwith, in press). Although sharing the epidemiological and pathological characteristics of neoplasms associated with hemihypertrophy, neuroblastoma does not occur excessively with this or with any other congenital defect (Miller, Fraumeni, and Hill, 1968). Thus, neuroblastoma does not belong in the pattern shown in Figure 1.

Wilms' tumor is associated with hemihypertrophy, and also with aniridia (congenital absence of the iris of the eye) (Miller, Fraumeni, and Manning, 1964). Since this association was first described (in 1964), additional cases have been observed in the United States (Miller, 1966a)

Fig. 1.—Diagrammatic representation of the relationship among four forms of growth excess. Arrows point away from pre-existent disease.

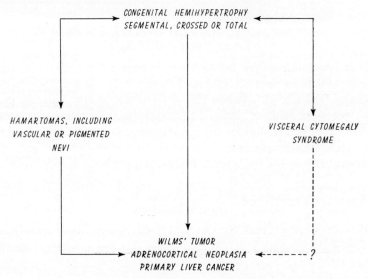

and in France (Schweisguth, Campinchi, Pivoteau, and Lemerle, 1967). A syndrome is now apparent which consists of Wilms' tumor; congenital aniridia, usually with secondary cataracts and often with microcephaly, facial dysostosis, and mental retardation; malformation of the upper auditory pinna; and anomalies of the genitourinary tract. Aniridia is usually caused by the action of a dominant gene; on the average, two of three affected children have an affected parent, but in the Wilms' tumor-aniridia syndrome, the parents characteristically are unaffected (Miller, 1966a). Thus, the occurrence of the eye defect with Wilms' tumor must represent either a mutation or the effect of an environmental agent which mimics the action of a gene. Aniridia has not been described with congenital hemihypertrophy, so each of these anomalies is independently associated with Wilms' tumor.

In consequence of these observations, one might say that Wilms' tumor, primary liver cancer, and adrenocortical neoplasia may be induced by an agent which is not only oncogenic but also teratogenic, whereas neuroblastoma represents an oncogenic response which is not accompanied excessively by teratogenesis.

There is a possibility that a screening test developed through study of abnormalities associated with a high risk of certain forms of cancer might be of use in predicting the occurrence of these tumors in the absence of congenital defects. Recognition of high-risk groups also provides the opportunity to perform more frequent clinical examinations than usual in an effort to detect as early as possible the development of a tumor, whose removal might be lifesaving.

Other Neoplasms with Peak Occurrence in Children under Five Years of Age

It is impossible at present to separate by cell type the coded death-certificate data on several childhood tumors (filed at the National Vital Statistics Division, U.S. Public Health Service). In consequence, studies have not been made of national mortality rates for these neoplasms, a circumstance which impedes the epidemiological search for clues to their etiology. Clinical experience, however, indicates an increased rate of occurrence early in life for several of these neoplasms.

BRAIN TUMORS

Hospital charts reveal that the peak age at diagnosis of ependymoma and medulloblastoma is in children under five years, whereas glioma is diagnosed at a relatively constant rate in those from one through 11 years of age (Miller, unpublished data). No study has been made of congenital defects associated with ependymoma. The risk of glioma, however, is very much increased in tuberous sclerosis and multiple neurofibromatosis (Paulson and Lyle, 1966). There is a possibility that, even in subclinical form, these genetically induced hamartomatous syndromes may predispose to glioma and may account for excessive family aggregation such as that found in the large case-control study of van der Wiel (1960).

Apparently in the same category is the basal cell nevus syndrome. Recently this disease has been reported in several families in which young children have been observed with medulloblastomas with or without signs of the syndrome (Aita, 1967). In two instances, the brain tumor was the first manifestation of the syndrome, a fact which indicates the importance of the family history not only with respect to brain tumors, but also with respect to characteristics of syndromes in which such neoplasia may be found.

It appears that brain tumors also occur excessively in children with other primary neoplasms. Two cases of astrocytoma have been described among 62 children with adrenocortical neoplasia (Fraumeni and Miller, 1967a). Of 150 children in western New York State who had cancer and underwent autopsy, three had brain tumors which were synchronous with primary lesions elsewhere: neuroastrocytoma with adenocarcinoma of the colon, neuroastrocytoma with acute lymphocytic leukemia, and glioblastoma multiforme with hepatocarcinoma (Regelson, Bross, Hananian, and Nigogosyan, 1965).

In two instances, brain tumors have been reported in children with severe, genetically induced, immunologic impairments which carry an increased risk of lymphoreticular neoplasia: Wiskott-Aldrich syndrome with astrocytoma (Amiet, 1963) and ataxia-telangiectasia with medulloblastoma (Shuster et al., 1966).

Van der Wiel (1960), in his large study of relatives of persons with glioma, found 29 people with major congenital defects of the spine or skull (anencephalia, spina bifida, or hydrocephalus) as compared with only one among the controls. It would be of interest to confirm this finding in a study focusing more sharply on these particular anomalies.

OTHER NEOPLASMS

Other neoplasms with peak frequency in diagnosis among children under five years of age include retinoblastoma, rhabdomyosarcoma, and teratoma. The lineal transmission of retinoblastoma has been well studied, but its other epidemiological characteristics have not, in part because of its rarity. Rhabdomyosarcoma and teratoma have received even less epidemiological attention.

Neoplasms without A Mortality Peak in Children under Five Years of Age

It has been noted that an age peak in mortality in children under five years of age does not necessarily signify that neoplasms occur excessively with specific congenital defects; neuroblastoma is an example. Similarly, absence of an early peak in mortality does not signify the absence of an association between the neoplasm and congenital defects.

GONADOBLASTOMA

At present, gonadoblastoma is the only neoplasm for which a congenital defect—gonadal dysgenesis—is known to be a prerequisite (Melicow, 1966). In Poland, the occurrence of gonadal tumors was studied in 25 patients with Turner's syndrome and in 26 other patients whose legal sex was female and who had gonadal dysgenesis with primary amenorrhea. The results are summarized in Table 2. Exploratory laparotomy, mostly elective, revealed the presence of seven unsuspected gonadal tumors in addition to the three that were diagnosed preoperatively. Four classes of tumor were described, and the tumor frequency appeared to be greater among the patients who did not have Turner's syndrome.

LYMPHOMA

Mortality rates for children in the United States with lymphoma do not show significant variation by single year of age (Ederer, Miller, and Scotto, 1965). Nevertheless, various forms of lymphoma do occur exces-

---

TABLE 2.—FREQUENCY OF TUMORS IN PATIENTS WITH GONADAL DYSGENESIS

HABITUS	NUMBER STUDIED*	KARYOTYPE	TUMORS
Turner's syndrome	25	XO/XY	1 Gonadoblastoma
		—	1 Interstitial hilar cell tumor
Other gonadal dysgenesis	26	XY	2 Gonadoblastomas (1 in situ)
		XY	5 Seminomas
		XY	1 Brenner tumor

*Mainly elective surgical treatment; female, legal sex; primary amenorrhea. Seven of the 10 tumors were not diagnosed preoperatively. (After Teter and Boczkowski, 1967.)

sively with specific inherited anomalies which are characterized by an immunologic deficiency, namely, the Bruton (X-linked) type of congenital agammaglobulinemia, ataxia-telangiectasia, the Wiskott-Aldrich syndrome, and the Chédiak-Higashi syndrome (Fraumeni and Miller, 1967b). These genetic disorders, which are associated with lymphoma, are not associated with any leukemias except the acute lymphocytic type. Conversely, whether the predisposing characteristic is inherited, as in mongolism, or acquired, as from ionizing radiation, persons with a high risk for leukemia (Table 1) do not also have a high risk for lymphoma. Thus, leukemia and lymphoma appear to be etiologically dissimilar.

Mortality patterns for patients with Hodgkin's disease display several peculiarities which are presumably of etiological significance (Miller, 1966b). First, there are very few deaths from this disease in children under five years of age (only 22 in the entire United States, 1960-64); this may be an indication of a delay in exposure or susceptibility to oncogenic influences. Second, the sex ratio (M/F) is a static 3.0 in children from five to 11 years of age and then falls steadily to the level of 1.5 in

Fig. 2.—Mortality from Hodgkin's disease among white children in the United States, 1950–59; sex ratio (M/F) as related to death rate by single year of age and sex (Miller, 1966b).

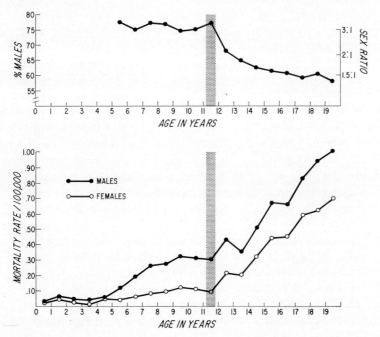

adults. This fall occurs because of a climb in mortality rates which begins at 11 years of age and prevents the maintenance of the high sex ratio (Fig. 2). Since the average survival time among children with Hodgkin's disease is about 2.7 years (Evans and Nyhan, 1964), the rise in rate at 11 years of age must reflect an increase in exposure or susceptibility before eight years. There is no evidence for suspecting one environmental agent rather than another at present. As to susceptibility, perhaps the largest physiological change at about eight years of age is a tremendous involution of the lymphatic tissue (*e.g.,* tonsils and adenoids). This involution, if faulty, might predispose to Hodgkin's disease, an ailment in which a substantial number of immunologic abnormalities has been found (Aisenberg, 1966).

Another epidemiological characteristic which provides an etiological clue is the bimodality of mortality from Hodgkin's disease in all countries studied except Japan (MacMahon, 1966). Mortality rates begin to rise at 11 years of age, reach a peak at 25-29 years, and then drop before another climb to a second peak late in life. In Japan, the mortality patterns clearly reveal the absence of the first peak. Thus, as MacMahon has indicated, the usual bimodality represents the presence of two age distributions, an epidemiological feature which suggests that two different sets of etiological factors are operative.

BONE NEOPLASIA

Study of bone sarcoma in dogs strongly suggests that the occurrence of this neoplasm is closely related to bone growth. The relative risk among giant breeds of dogs, such as the Saint Bernard and Great Dane, is about 200 times that for small- or medium-sized breeds (Tjalma, 1966). This observation is consistent with the similarity in man between patterns of growth (stature) and mortality rates from bone cancer. The average height by single year of age for boys and girls rises progressively and is virtually identical until 13 years of age when boys grow taller than girls. Mortality rates from bone cancer are virtually identical for both sexes until precisely the same age, 13 years, when the rates for boys first exceed those for girls (Ederer, Miller, and Scotto, 1965). It is to be expected, then, that children with bone cancer will be taller than average. Finding data collected in the past to test this hypothesis is difficult. In the one study that has been made of stature *after* tumor development, the affected children were significantly taller than average (Fraumeni, 1967). The absolute differences in height, however, were small.

From studies of radium-dial painters, there is no doubt that radioisotopes in sufficient dosage can induce osteogenic sarcoma in man (Aub, Evans, Hempelmann, and Martland, 1952). The neoplasm also can be induced by doses of external radiation in excess of 3,000 r (United Nations, 1964).

THYROID CANCER

Although thyroid cancer is a rare cause of death in childhood, there is little doubt that it was induced relatively easily in the past by therapeutic irradiation of the thymus in infancy (Hempelmann, Pifer, Burke, Terry, and Ames, 1967). Benign tumors of the thyroid have been induced by the same treatment procedure (Pincus, Reichlin, and Hempelmann, 1967) by the I^{131} in the fallout to which children on the Marshall Islands were exposed (Robbins, Rall, and Conard, 1967), and perhaps by the atomic bomb exposure in Japan (Socolow, Hashizume, Neriishi, and Niitani, 1963).

The Viral Etiology of Childhood Cancer

As enthusiasm has grown for the viral etiological explanation of childhood leukemia, epidemiologists have attempted to respond by using their devices to evaluate the applicability in man of concepts developed in the laboratory and elsewhere. The results of epidemiological studies can be very helpful in determining the nature of agents which induce leukemia in human beings.

CLUSTERING OF CASES

A most important, but little appreciated, development in cancer research has been the invention of statistical techniques for determining dispassionately whether the frequency with which a rare event clusters in time and space exceeds normal expectation (Stark and Mantel, 1967; Mantel, 1967). There is no doubt that, after examining the distribution of cases on a scatter map, epidemiologists can identify individual clusters of rare diseases by inspection and can draw tight boundaries around them. The question is not "Do rare events cluster?" but "Do they cluster excessively?" To date, the application of new statistical procedures in studies of leukemia has provided no solid evidence of an excess suggesting an infectious mode of spread (Fraumeni and Miller, 1967b). In contrast, the application of one of these techniques to data for Burkitt's lymphoma in the West Nile District of Uganda has shown considerable evidence of clustering (Pike, Williams, and Wright, 1967). For this reason, among others, an infectious origin seems more likely for African lymphoma than for leukemia.

Similar studies of other childhood neoplasms are in progress. Thus far, it has been found that mortality from neuroblastoma among white children in the United States, 1960-64, exhibited year-to-year fluctuations which were statistically significant in three of the nine geographic divisions of the United States (Miller, Fraumeni, and Hill, 1968). This observation suggests the possibility of an environmental oncogenic influence in these areas during certain years.

TESTING HYPOTHESES

In studies of the origins of neoplasia, one of the greatest uses of the epidemiological approach is in the testing of hypotheses developed in the laboratory, at the bedside, or through other epidemiological studies. A great variety of ideas concerning the viral origin of leukemia has been tested in this way, but none has suggested a viral mode of spread in man (Fraumeni and Miller, 1967b; Miller and Fraumeni, 1967; Miller, 1968). This observation does not exclude the possibility of a viral role in leukemogenesis. It does indicate that, if viruses are involved, other methods will have to be devised to reveal their presence.

Conclusions

Clues to the etiology of the various forms of childhood neoplasia can be derived from contrasts and similarities in patterns of distribution and among persons at exceptionally high risk. From such studies, certain tumors which seem unrelated may be suspected of having a common origin (*e.g.,* Wilms' tumor, adrenocortical neoplasia, and primary liver cancer, all of which are associated with congenital hemihypertrophy). In a similar fashion, other neoplasms which are thought to have a common origin—such as acute leukemia and lymphoma—may be etiologically separable. Finally, by determining the pre-existent disorders which carry a high risk of a certain type of cancer, one may open new avenues of research, for the origins of the neoplasm then can be studied in terms of what is known about the disease with which it is associated.

REFERENCES

Aisenberg, A. C.: Manifestations of immunologic unresponsiveness in Hodgkin's disease. *Cancer Research,* 26:1152-1160, June 1966.
Aita, J. A.: Genetic aspects of tumors in the nervous system. In Lynch, H. T., Ed.:

Hereditary Factors in Carcinoma, Vol. 12 in *Recent Results in Cancer Research.* New York. New York, Springer-Verlag, 1967, pp. 86-110.

Amiet, A.: Aldrich-syndrom. Beobachtung zweier Fälle. *Annales Paediatrici*, 201: 315-335, No. 4, 1963.

Aub, J. C., Evans, R. D., Hempelmann, L. H., and Martland, H. S.: The late effects of internally-deposited radioactive materials in man. *Medicine*, 31:221-329, September 1952

Beckwith, J. B.: Macroglossia, omphalocele, adrenal cytomegaly, gigantism and hyperplastic visceromegaly. In McKusick, V. A., Ed.: *Proceedings of the First Conference on Birth Defects.* (In press.)

Beckwith, J. B., and Perrin, E. V.: In situ neuroblastomas: A contribution to the natural history of neural crest tumors. *American Journal of Pathology*, 43:1089-1104, December 1963.

————: Unpublished data.

Court Brown, W. M., and Doll, R.: Leukaemia in childhood and young adult life. Trends in mortality in relation to aetiology. *British Medical Journal*, 1:981-988, April 8, 1961.

Crowe, F. W., Schull, W. J., and Neel, J. V.: *A Clinical, Pathological and Genetic Study of Multiple Neurofibromatosis.* Springfield, Illinois, Charles C Thomas, 1956, 181 pp.

Doll, R.: *Prevention of Cancer. Pointers from Epidemiology.* London, England, Whitefriars Press Ltd., 1967, 143 pp.

Ederer, F., Miller, R. W., and Scotto, J.: U S childhood cancer mortality patterns, 1950-1959. Etiologic implications. *Journal of the American Medical Association*, 192:593-596, May 17, 1965.

Evans, H. E., and Nyhan, W. L.: Hodgkin's disease in children. *Bulletin of the Johns Hopkins Hospital*, 114:237-248, April 1964.

Fraumeni, J. F., Jr.: Stature and malignant tumors of bone in childhood and adolescence. *Cancer*, 20:967-973, June 1967.

Fraumeni, J. F., Jr., and Miller, R. W.: Adrenocortical neoplasms with hemihypertrophy, brain tumors and other disorders. *Journal of Pediatrics*, 70:129-138, January 1967a.

————: Epidemiology of human leukemia: Recent observations. *Journal of the National Cancer Institute*, 38:593-605, April 1967b.

Fraumeni, J. F., Jr., Miller, R. W., and Hill, J. A.: Primary carcinoma of the liver in childhood: An epidemiologic study. *Journal of the National Cancer Institute*, 40:1087-1099, May 1968.

Gesell, A.: Hemihypertrophy and twinning. A further study of the nature of hemihypertrophy with report of a new case. *The American Journal of the Medical Sciences*, 173:542-555, April 1927.

Hempelmann, L. H., Pifer, J. W., Burke, G. J., Terry, R., and Ames, W. R.: Neoplasms in persons treated with X rays in infancy for thymic enlargement. A report of the third follow-up survey. *Journal of the National Cancer Institute*, 38:317-341, March 1967.

MacMahon, B.: Epidemiology of Hodgkin's disease. *Cancer Research*, 26:1189-1200, June 1966.

MacMahon, B., and Levy, M. A.: Prenatal origin of childhood leukemia. Evidence from twins. *New England Journal of Medicine*, 270:1082-1085, May 21, 1964.

Mantel, N.: The detection of disease clustering and a generalized regression approach. *Cancer Research*, 27:209-220, February 1967.

Melicow, M. M.: Tumors of dysgenetic gonads in intersexes: Case reports and discussion regarding their place in gonadal oncology. *Bulletin of New York Academy of Medicine*, 42:3-20, January 1966.

Miller, R. W.: Relation between cancer and congenital defects in man. *New England Journal of Medicine,* 275:87-93, July 14, 1966a.

———: Mortality in childhood Hodgkin's disease. *Journal of the American Medical Association,* 198:1216-1217, December 12, 1966b.

———: Persons at exceptionally high risk of leukemia. *Cancer Research,* 27 Part I: 2420-2423, December 1967.

———: The viral etiology of leukemia: An epidemiologic evaluation. In Zarafonetis, C. J. D.: *Proceedings of the International Conference on Leukemia-Lymphoma.* Philadelphia, Pennsylvania, Lea & Febiger, 1968.

———: Unpublished data.

Miller, R. W., and Fraumeni, J. F., Jr.: "Leukemia houses." *Annals of Internal Medicine,* 67:674-676, September 1967.

Miller, R. W., Fraumeni, J. F., Jr., and Hill, J. A.: Neuroblastoma: Epidemiologic approach to its origins. *American Journal of Diseases of Children,* 115:253-261, February 1968.

Miller, R. W., Fraumeni, J. F., Jr., and Manning, M. D.: Association of Wilms's tumor with aniridia, hemihypertrophy and other congenital malformation. *New England Journal of Medicine,* 270:922-927, April 30, 1964.

Paulson, G. W., and Lyle, C. B.: Tuberous sclerosis. *Developmental Medicine and Child Neurology,* 8:571-586, October 1966.

Pike, M. C., Williams, E. H., and Wright, B.: Burkitt's tumour in the West Nile District of Uganda 1961-5. *British Medical Journal,* 2:395-399, May 13, 1967.

Pincus, R. A., Reichlin, S., and Hempelmann, L. H.: Thyroid abnormalities after radiation exposure in infancy. *Annals of Internal Medicine,* 66:1154-1164, June 1967.

Regelson, W., Bross, I. D. J., Hananian, J., and Nigogosyan, G.: Incidence of second primary tumors in children with cancer and leukemia. A seven-year survey of 150 consecutive autopsied cases. *Cancer,* 18:58-72, January 1965.

Robbins, J., Rall, J. E., and Conard, R. A.: Late effects of radioactive iodine in fallout. Combined clinical staff conference at the National Institutes of Health. *Annals of Internal Medicine,* 66:1214-1242, June 1967.

Sawitsky, A., Bloom, D., and German, J.: Chromosomal breakage and acute leukemia in congenital telangiectatic erythema and stunted growth. *Annals of Internal Medicine,* 65:487-495, September 1966.

Schweisguth, O., Campinchi, R., Pivoteau, B., and Lemberle, J.: L'association aniridie-tumeur du rein chez l'enfant. A propos de 4 cas. *Bulletin des Sociétés d'Ophtalmologie de France,* 57:1099-1107, December 1967.

Shuster, J., Hart, Z., Stimson, C. W., Brough, A. J., and Poulik, M. D.: Ataxia telangiectasia with cerebellar tumor. *Pediatrics,* 37:776-786, May 1966.

Socolow, E. L., Hashizume, A., Neriishi, S., and Niitani, R.: Thyroid carcinoma in man after exposure to ionizing radiation. *New England Journal of Medicine,* 268: 406-410, February 21, 1963.

Stark, C. R., and Mantel, N.: Lack of seasonal- or temporal-spatial clustering of Down's syndrome births in Michigan. *American Journal of Epidemiology,* 86:199-213, July 1967.

Sutow, W. W., and Conard, R. A.: Effects of ionizing radiation in children. *Journal of Pediatrics,* 67:658-673, October 1965.

Teter, J., and Boczkowski, K.: Occurrence of tumors in dysgenetic gonads. *Cancer,* 20:1301-1310, August 1967.

Tjalma, R. A.: Canine bone sarcoma: Estimation of relative risk as a function of body size. *Journal of the National Cancer Institute,* 36:1137-1150, June 1966.

Van der Wiel, H. J.: Inheritance of glioma. *The Genetic Aspects of Cerebral Glioma and Its Relation to Status Dysraphicus.* Amsterdam, The Netherlands, Elsevier Publishing Company, 1960, 275 pp.

Background and Current Status of the Search for Etiological Agents in Leukemia and Lymphoma in Man

FRANK J. RAUSCHER, JR., PH.D.

Viral Oncology Area, Etiology,
National Cancer Institute, Bethesda, Maryland

THE PRIMARY PURPOSE of this paper is to present a brief review of recent background and current facts and leads emerging from studies on the detection and characterization of viruses and viruslike particles in leukemia and lymphoma materials from human beings. The biological agents, antigens, and antibodies most frequently detected or isolated from leukemia and lymphoma patients to 1967 include the following: herpes-type virus, type "C" viruslike particles, *Mycoplasma,* cytomegalovirus, herpes simplex viruses, reovirus 3, and simian adenovirus, type 7.

Of these, the unidentified herpes-type virus, type C particles, reoviruses, and *Mycoplasma* are those which are detected most frequently by means of present technology; they consequently have received the attention of most investigators seeking to determine whether viruses similar to (or different from) those known to be associated with the induction of leukemia and lymphoma in laboratory and domestic animals also are involved in the etiology of leukemia and lymphoma in man.

Type C Particles

In 1957, Dmochowski and Grey demonstrated the presence of viruslike particles in thin sections of a biopsy specimen from a lymph node of a patient with acute lymphocytic leukemia. Since then these investigators have demonstrated the presence of similar particles in biopsy specimens from lymph nodes of other patients with acute lymphocytic leukemia and from those with acute myelocytic leukemia, malignant lymphoma, and

25

Hodgkin's disease (Dmochowski, 1961; Dmochowski and Grey, 1958; Dmochowski et al., 1965). Part of this work was done at a time when techniques for preservation of material for thin sectioning were not as good as they are today. In addition, much more is now known about the morphology and mode of formation of viruses of the avian leukosis (Haguenau and Beard, 1962; Haguenau, Febvre, and Arnoult, 1962; Heine, de Thé, Ishiguro, and Beard, 1962) and murine leukemia (Bernhard, 1960; Dalton, Law, Moloney, and Manaker, 1961; de Harven and Friend, 1960; Dmochowski, Padgett, and Gross, 1964; Feldman and Gross, 1964; Okano, Kunii, and Furth, 1963) groups, as well as of polyoma virus (Howatson and Almeida, 1960; Howatson et al., 1960).

It appears that the particles described by Dmochowski and co-workers bear a closer resemblance to those associated with avian leukosis and murine leukemia than to any others. They are similar to the type C particles of Bernhard (1960) and are found most frequently in an extracellular position or within cytoplasmic vacuoles. Mature particles possess a centrally located, electron dense nucleoid, which is separated by an electron lucent space from an outer smooth-surfaced coat. Several instances of "budding" of particles from plasma membranes also were noted in this material.

The similarity in morphology and mode of formation between these particles and particles known to be related etiologically to avian leukosis and murine leukemia may have real significance. Conversely, the findings may represent the purely coincidental presence of particles with similar morphology, but without the same biological activity. Particles with the same morphology as those capable of inducing murine leukemia have been demonstrated in tissue cultures of strain "L" cells (Dales and Howatson, 1961). To date, these particles have not been shown to possess leukemogenic activity. It also should be noted that in another laboratory no viruslike particles were observed in biopsy specimens of lymph nodes from a series of patients with lymphoid malignancies (Bernhard and Leplus, 1964). Thus, no conclusions can be drawn from the evidence presented to date, but it is clear that the studies of Dmochowski and co-workers, as difficult and time-consuming as they have been, should be expanded and reviewed for possible confirmation in other laboratories.

Plasma pellets from patients with leukemia were examined in several laboratories in recent years (Burger et al., 1964; Dmochowski, 1965, Porter, Dalton, Moloney, and Mitchell, 1964; Smith, Benyesh-Melnick, and Fernbach, 1964). These studies were carried out, at least in part, because typical murine leukemia virus particles could be readily detected in and concentrated from the plasma of rats with induced murine leukemia (Dalton and Moloney, 1962). Viruslike particles similar in morphology to murine leukemia virus were observed in this material, by the use of both the negative staining technique (Burger *et al.,* 1964; Smith, Benyesh-Melnick, and Fernbach, 1964) and thin sections (Dalton *et al.,* 1964; Dmochowski, 1965; Porter, Dalton, Moloney, and Mitchell, 1964). Some investigators believe that these viruslike particles are produced during the process of disintegration of blood cells and platelets (Prince and Adams, 1965). Others believe that this is not always the case (Dalton and Mitchell, 1966; Dalton *et al.,* 1964). In any event, the significance of the presence of viruslike particles in any given material can be determined only by bioassay.

The fluorescent antibody technique of Coons and Kaplan (1950) is directly applicable to the detection of antigens associated with many of the necrotizing viruses and certain of the tumor viruses (Fink and Malmgren, 1963), including the Friend leukemia agent, but not with other strains of the animal leukemia viruses. Fink and Malmgren introduced modifications of the procedure which enabled them to detect specific antigens associated with a strain of mouse leukemia virus (Rauscher), and they and their associates have applied the modified method to the study of leukemia in human beings (Fink, Malmgren, Karon, and Orr, 1965; Fink *et al.,* 1964).

The applicability of immunological methods for the detection of a virus or its specific antibody depends upon the availability of the complementary diagnostic reagent, *i.e.,* viral antibody or viral antigen, respectively. In their approach to the problem in human beings, Fink, Malmgren, and their associates (1965) employed material containing type C particles derived from leukemic plasma for the induction of antibodies in heterologous hosts (rabbits and monkeys). The antibody was absorbed exhaustively and then conjugated with fluorescein isothiocyanate and used as a specific stain for the detection of antigen in cells in the buffy coat, bone marrow, and biopsy specimens, or tissue culture explants thereof, derived from patients with leukemia and lymphoma.

Of 72 leukemic patients tested by Fink and Malmgren (1963), 49 (68 per cent) showed reaction with the antihuman leukemic fluorescent antibody. Eight of them also showed positive reactions to the anti-Rauscher virus fluorescent antibody, as did eight other patients who failed to react positively with the antihuman leukemic reagent. None of the specimens tested against other control sera showed positive reactions, nor did any of the antigen-control specimens react positively with the antihuman leukemia fluorescent antibody.

Cells in tissue culture derived from biopsies of nine patients with Burkitt lymphoma and leukocyte cell lines derived from six patients with leukemia also were tested against the antihuman leukemic fluorescent antibody. All showed positive fluorescent reactions and herpeslike viral particles when examined by electron microscopy.

Fink and Malmgren (1963) interpret their findings to support the thesis that the antigen detected by immunofluorescence with the antihuman leukemia antibody "is concerned with the leukemic process." Although these data are concerned with the hypothesis of a viral etiology of human leukemia, whether the antigen detected is of viral origin remains to be determined.

Of considerable interest is the report (Yohn and Grace, 1966) that pooled normal marrow in human beings is capable of completely absorbing the Fink-type immunofluorescent antibody prepared against human type C viruslike particles. This finding suggests at least two alternatives for consideration: (1) prior to absorption with bone marrow, the immunofluorescent antibody is capable of detecting an antigen of immature leukocytes which rarely appears in the peripheral blood under ordinary conditions, or (2) a virus or viral antigen related to viruslike particles recovered from leukemic plasma of human beings was present in the pool of adult bone marrow. The second consideration is based, of course, on the reasonable assumption that while less than one per cent of the population can be expected to develop leukemia, the vast majority of people is infected with a virus(es) which may be capable of inducing leukemia. This assumption is based on the known relationship between infection and disease with polio and other necrotizing viruses.

If this relationship between infection and disease with necrotizing viruses is characteristic of leukemia viruses, then it would be reasonable to expect that the bone marrow might be the site for latent retention of virus and/or viral antigen. This hypothesis, while attractive, does not appear to be supported by Fink and Malmgren (1963), who have failed to detect immunofluorescent antigens in the bone marrow of normal individuals or patients with diseases other than leukemia or lymphoma. One would expect that if sufficient antigen were present in bone marrow to allow complete absorption of immunofluorescent antibody, there also should be enough antigen to be detectable with the unabsorbed immunofluorescent antibody.

Other type C or myxolike particles in human beings are being studied by investigators at Baylor University College of Medicine, Houston, Texas. Benyesh-Melnick, Fernbach, and Lewis (1963) reported the long-term propagation in tissue culture of bone marrow cells from children with acute lymphoid leukemia or infectious mononucleosis and from nondiseased controls. A spontaneous lymphoblastoid transformation occurred in some of the fibroblastic cultures. The transformed cultures consisted of fibroblastic and lymphoblastoid cells; the latter strongly resembled immature cells seen in the bone marrow of children with acute leukemia.

More recently, Benyesh-Melnick and Melnick (personal communication) reported that 10 per cent of fibroblastic bone marrow cultures derived from children with leukemia and 57 per cent of those derived from children with infectious mononucleosis underwent a spontaneous "lymphoblastoid transformation" which resulted in mixed populations of lymphoblastoid and fibroblastic cells. During a four-year period, 584 long-term bone marrow cultures derived from diseased and normal children were studied to establish the frequency of lymphoblastoid transformation. Fifty cultures underwent this change. Of these, 15 were derived from nine of 92 children with acute leukemia, 25 were derived from 25 of 43 children with infectious mononucleosis, and 10 were derived from 10 children with presumptive infectious mononucleosis. None of the cultures from 152 children with various other disorders and from 12 normal children revealed such transformations. Of importance is the apparent replication in the cultures of large quantities of myxovirus-like particles, morphologically similar to the viruses of avian myeloblastosis and Moloney murine leukemia (Benyesh-Melnick, Smith, and Fernbach, 1964). These particles were morphologically identical to those found and quantitated by Smith, Benyesh-Melnick, and Fernbach (1964). These two studies showed such particles in the plasma and sera of 79 per cent (18 of 23) of leukemia patients, 100 per cent (8 of 8) of infectious mononucleosis patients, and 22 per cent (7 of 32) of normal children. These latter authors recommended that these observations be interpreted cautiously since strikingly similar particles, although fewer in number, can be released into the plasma experimentally during prolonged storage of normal whole blood.

Electron microscopy remains the chief method used in the search for type C viruses in human beings with leukemia and lymphoma. Since relatively high concentrations of virus particles, *e.g.* 10^6 or more per milliliter in a fluid suspension, are necessary to give a reasonable chance for their detection, this method is less sensitive and therefore less likely to detect small quantities of mature virus (such as those that might be present in primary specimens containing virus in a carrier state) than one of the immunological methods. Conversely, immunological methods cannot be applied in a systematic search for new viruses, since either the viral antigen or its antibody must be available in advance as a diagnostic reagent.

The fluorescent antibody method of Fink and Malmgren appears to detect a leukemia-associated antigen, which could be viral in origin. However, it should be emphasized that the plasma fractions which were pooled to provide the antigen for producing the fluorescent-antibody diagnostic reagent were selected by means of electron microscopy, and that only those specimens in which viruslike particles were seen were used. Without this preselection, it is doubtful whether sufficient amounts of specific antigen would have been present, in a random pool, for example, for the production of a useful antibody reagent. The electron microscope therefore remains the primary tool, even for the application of this immunological method.

Mycoplasma

In the search for viruslike particles in unknown material, it has become increasingly clear that depending solely on the use of the negative staining technique with phosphotungstate is not advisable. Viruses with known surface structure can be readily classified into groups with this technique; but the viruses of avian leukosis and murine leukemia that possess smooth outer coats and no clear-cut internal structures cannot be identified with certainty. In this kind of search, it is essential that both negative staining and thin sectioning techniques be employed (Bryan *et al.*, 1965). Even under these circumstances, difficulties may be encountered in distinguishing the virus particles from certain cell components and from *Mycoplasma* (pleuropneumonia-like organisms) (Anderson, 1965). *Mycoplasma* frequently exhibit an extreme degree of pleomorphism, in terms of both size (30 mμ to 1 μ) and structure (Anderson, 1965; Anderson and Barile, 1965; Dmochowski *et al.*, 1964; Hayflick, 1965; Hummeler, Tomassini, and Hayflick, 1965). Some forms are filterable (Laidlaw and Elford, 1936) and undoubtedly have been confused with viruses on occasion. They have been isolated indirectly (Dmochowski *et al.*, 1965; Grist and Fallon, 1964; Murphy and Furtado, 1963; Negroni, 1964) and directly (Barile *et al.*, 1966; Hayflick and Koprowski, 1965) from bone marrow and plasma of patients with leukemia.

Mycoplasma thus form a group of organisms which, for several reasons, are important to those studying the etiology of leukemia in human beings. First, by their presence they may complicate attempts to isolate viruses by means of tissue culture. Second, because of their pleomorphism and filtrability, they may be confused with viruses both morphologically and biologically. Third, because of their frequent occurrence in leukemic material, their possible role in the etiology of leukemia—either as inciting agents or as adjuvants to other presently unknown agents—cannot be completely ruled out.

There is, however, a growing body of information which cautions against the consideration of *Mycoplasma* as primary etiologic agents of neoplasia. This information includes the following facts: (1) no apparent differences exist between the amount and kind of *Mycoplasma* associated with cancer patients and patients with nonneoplastic diseases. (2) *Mycoplasma* were often present in laboratory-passaged specimens as adventitious contaminants derived from aerosols, from laboratory animals and people, and from trypsin and sera used for tissue cultures. (3) Murine leukemia and Rous sarcoma viruses known to be free of *Mycoplasma* will, after inoculation into specific-pathogen-free or germfree mice, and chickens, respectively, which are known to be free of *Mycoplasma*—induce typical progressive leukemia or sarcoma. (4) Viruses free of *Mycoplasma* are recoverable from these induced diseases (Reyniers and Sacksteder, personal communication). Because of these findings and because of the apparent role of *Mycoplasma* as ubiquitous contaminants, it may be justifiable, in studies of cancer etiology, to limit work on these organisms to the monitoring of leukemic materials which are to be used in attempts to isolate virus.

The Herpes-type Virus

Epstein, Achong, and Barr (1964) reported successful tissue culture propagation of cells from several Burkitt's lymphoma biopsy specimens. Almost concurrently, Iwakata and Grace (1964) were able to culture cells derived from the peripheral blood of a patient with chronic myeloid leukemia. Both patient sources yielded cell lines in which particles with the morphology and characteristics of herpes-type viruses were detected. Over 125 cell lines from cancer and noncancer patients have been established by investigators in laboratories in England, Australia, New Guinea, Japan, Sweden, Africa, and the United States (*e.g.* Dalton and Manaker, 1967; Epstein, Achong, and Barr, 1964; Epstein *et al.,* 1966; Epstein, Achong, and Pope, 1967; Epstein, Barr, and Achong, 1964, 1965, 1966; Epstein, Henle, Achong, and Barr, 1965; Foley *et al.,* 1965; Hinuma and Grace, 1967; Iwakata and Grace, 1964; Jensen, Korol, Dittmar, and Medrek, 1967; Landon, Ellis, Zeve, and Fabrizio, in press; Minowada *et al.,* 1967; Moore, Gerner, and Minowada, 1968; O'Connor and Rabson, 1965; Pulvertaft, 1965; Rabson *et al.,* 1966; Stewart, Lovelace, Whang, and Ngu, 1965; Yamaguchi, Hinuma, and Grace, 1967; Zeve, Lucas, and Manaker, 1966; Clarkson, personal communication). Table 1

TABLE 1.—SUMMARY: CELL LINES FROM HUMAN BEINGS AND HERPES-TYPE VIRUS

CATEGORY	CULTURES FROM PATIENTS PATIENTS ATTEMPTED*		PATIENTS HTV+† CULTURES FROM PATIENTS		LINES HTV+† LINES CULTURED	
	No.	Per cent	No.	Per cent	No.	Per cent
Lymphoma	31/61	51%	19/31	61%	23/41	56%
Lymphoid leukemia	15/111	14%	4/15	27%	4/17	24%
Myeloid leukemia	34/138	25%	14/34	41%	23/100	23%
Sarcoma-carcinoma	25/54	46%	7/25	28%	11/46	24%
Total (cancer)	105/364	29%	44/105	42%	61/204	30%
Other diseases	5/54	9%	1/5	20%	1/5	20%
Normal	14/81	17%	3/14	21%	4/20	20%
Total (noncancer)	19/135	14%	4/19	21%	5/25	20%

Abbreviation: HTV, herpes-type virus (prototype = Epstein's EB1).
*Approximate. Successful attempts understandably are nearly always reported; unsuccessful attempts usually are not.
†These numerators are not identical because (1) several positive lines have been started from the same patient, and (2) up to six lines have been started from the same patient, of which only one or two are positive.

presents data which approximate the number of lines which were established as of July 1967 according to disease and nondisease categories and according to the presence or absence of a herpes-type virus. Viruses other than the herpes-type have not been reported in these lines. It is important to note that the numbers and percentages of the table are approximate. The data were provided by investigators throughout the world, especially those who were doing work within the scope of the Special Virus-Leukemia Program of the National Cancer Institute. The cells of nearly all of these cultures are large and mononucleated and resemble lymphoblasts. They usually do not attach to the surface of the tissue culture vessel and appear to grow best in static suspension cultures. However, Moore at Roswell Park Memorial Institute, Buffalo, New York, has had considerable success in growing large quantities of some cell lines in spinner cultures (Moore, Gerner, and Minowada, 1968).

Comparative immunofluorescent and electron microscopy studies have shown that only one to five per cent of the cells of most of these lines is positive at any one time for the antigen and the virus particle, respectively (Fink, Malmgren, Karon, and Orr, 1965; Fink, Manaker, Dalton, and Cranford, 1966; Henle and Henle, 1966, in press; Levy and Henle, 1966). This apparently low incidence of infected cells has made it extremely difficult to extract and purify adequate quantities of virus for further characterization. Faced with these and other problems imposed by relatively small numbers of apparently infected cells, investigators at Roswell Park Memorial Institute attempted to increase virus production by selecting clones of more heavily infected cells (Hinuma and Grace, 1967). Using a cloning technique in semisolid agar, they derived 49 sublines from the P3J Burkitt's lymphoma line. One of these sublines, designated P3HR-1 showed 15 to 40 per cent of the cells to be infected after four months of propagation. When the cells were incubated at 35°C or 32°C for nine to 15 days without refeeding, up to 75 per cent of the cells became immunofluorescent positive and showed particles by electron microscopy.

Recent studies by a number of investigators have shown that both direct and indirect immunofluorescence techniques detect cells which produce herpes-type virus particles. Earlier work by Fink, Malmgren, Karon, and Orr (1965); Fink, Manaker, Dalton, and Cranford (1966); and Henle and Henle (1966) revealed a good correlation between electron microscopic and immunofluorescent determinations of virus-producing cells. This firm but independent correlation was surprising because the Fink-Malmgren direct antibody reagent was made in rabbits against centrifugal concentrates of human leukemic plasma containing type C particles while Henle and Henle used an indirect test which employed selected pools of human gamma globulin. In addition, since approximately 10^6 virus particles were necessary for an electron microscopic search to be positive, this particle visualization technique was believed to be far less sensitive in the detection of small quantities of virus than either immunofluorescent method.

The original studies of Fink et al. (1964, 1965) are important not only because they appeared to provide the first detection technique supplementary to electron microscopy, but also because the reagent and the procedure seemed to suggest the possibility that two widely different groups of viruses (type C and herpes type) might be associated with leukemia and lymphoma in man.

Using an indirect immunofluorescent method, Henle, Hummeler, and Henle (1966); and Mayyasi, Schidlovsky, Bulfone, and Buscheck (in press) then showed that human sera which were immunofluorescent positive contained antibodies directed against the virion. This was evident from electron microscopic determination of antibody coating and agglutination of virus particles extracted and concentrated from Burkitt cell lines. Additional studies by Henle and Henle (1966) revealed that pulse exposure of cells containing herpes-type virus to thymidine H^3 resulted in the labeling of both viral and cellular deoxyribonucleic acid (DNA). Later, fluorescent cells showed the label to be present in the cytoplasm whereas it remained restricted to the nucleus in nonfluorescent cells. The labeling of cellular DNA was substantially lower in cells lethally x-irradiated four to seven days prior to exposure to the isotope. This treatment, however, did not prevent the labeling of immunofluorescent cells. Unequivocal proof that immunofluorescent cells are those which contain herpes-type virus was reported by zur Hausen et al. (1967), who were able to pick immunofluorescent cells for electron microscopic examination. Their results showed clearly that immunofluorescent cells contained the virus whereas none of the immunofluorescent negative cells revealed the presence of virus particles.

Several groups of investigators have employed virus-containing Burkitt's tumor cells to detect antibodies in sera from human beings by immunofluorescence (Henle and Henle, 1966), complement-fixation (Armstrong, Henle, and Henle, 1966; Gerber and Birch, 1967), immunodiffusion (Old et al., 1966), and antibody coating (Henle, Hummeler, and Henle, 1966; Mayyasi, Schidlovsky, Bulfone, and Buscheck, in press) techniques. Using appropriate immunofluorescence tests with Burkitt's lymphoma cell lines, Henle and Henle (1966) showed that the age distribution of antibodies in noncancerous American and African children revealed a pattern similar to that for other common viruses. The incidence of positive sera was high, i.e., 70 per cent at age zero to three months; declined between four to 24 months; and then at four years rose to 50 per cent where it remained until adolescence. More than 80 per cent of sera from people at age 40 showed antibodies to herpes-type virus.

Various investigators using different serological detection techniques showed that nearly all sera from Burkitt patients contain herpes-type virus antibodies and in most instances at levels higher than in sera from nondiseased controls. There is some indication that Burkitt patients in remission generally have higher levels of antibody and that with recurrence of the tumor, their antibody levels decline. Very intriguing information was reported by Old et al. (1966) who showed an unusually high incidence and level of herpes-type virus antibodies in the sera of patients with postnasal carcinoma.

Gerber and Birch (1967)—using a sensitive complement-fixation test with partially purified herpes-type virus prepared from the Burkitt P3 line by investigators of the Pfizer Company, Maywood, New Jersey—showed that 90 per cent of sera from healthy adults and patients with malignant diseases had antibodies to herpes-type virus. They also tested five species of nonhuman primates and found that all except baboons had a high incidence of complement-fixation antibodies to the P3 antigen and that none of the sera from nine species of laboratory or domestic animals reacted with this antigen. Their finding that 10 of 10 chimpanzees had relatively high levels of herpes-type virus antibody is particularly interesting in view of the report by Landon, Ellis, Zeve, and Fabrizio (in press) who have established hematopoietic cell lines from three uninoculated chimpanzees, all of which contain a herpes-type virus. The virus in the chimpanzee cell lines is antigenically similar, if not identical, to the herpes-type virus contained in the lines derived from human beings (Landon, personal communication).

Studies by various investigators have shown clearly that herpes-type virus is not related antigenically to any of the known human or animal herpes viruses, nor is it related to other nonherpetic, human and animal viruses tested. Although additional work needs to be done, evidence suggests that the herpes-type viruses in at least some of the Burkitt's lymphoma lines from patients in Africa and the United States, as well as in cell lines started from American leukemic patients, are related (Mayyasi, Schidlovsky, Bulfone, and Buscheck, in press). It is obviously important to determine whether more than one major antigenic type of the virus exists in the more than 60 virus-containing human cell lines already established.

Herpes-type virus has been detected in the peripheral leukocytes or tissues of several leukemia patients, in peripheral leukocytes from one normal person prior to the propagation of cells in tissue culture, and in biopsy materials from patients with Burkitt's lymphoma (Griffin, Wright, Bell, and Ross, 1966). In one study, investigators of the Pfizer Company, (Jensen and Wright, personal communication) used electron microscopy to detect herpes-type virus in peripheral cells from a child with congenital leukemia. The virus persisted in the cells following propagation in tissue culture. Herpes-type virus also was detected in the peripheral blood of the mother but not the father of this child. In this regard, Moore (personal communication) and Gerber and Birch (1967) established cell lines from buffy coat cells of normal, nondiseased donors. Several of these lines were shown to contain herpes-type virus. In view of this, a reevaluation of the previous assumption that the cells of lines started from leukemia and lymphoma patients are neoplastic rather than normal or nonneoplastic may be necessary. Definitive karyotypic analyses have been done, however, with several of these lines, and the results suggest that a portion of the cells in at least some of these lines are neoplastic. As an example, the chronic myeloid leukemia patient from which the M-2 (Dalton and Manaker, 1967) line was established was shown to be positive for the Philadelphia chromosome (Lucas *et al.,* 1966). Periodic chromosome analyses on the cultured cells showed retention of the Philadelphia marker.

Perhaps related to these observations is the report by Griffin, Bell, and

Adatia, (1967 a, b) who used electron microscopy to detect the presence of virus particles, which were morphologically of the herpes type, in the pulp of a tooth removed from a Burkitt's lymphoma patient with an active maxillary tumor. Similarly, they detected herpes particles in the tooth of an apparently normal child, who five years previously had been successfully treated for a Burkitt's lymphoma of the maxilla. Unfortunately, virus isolation and identification tests were not performed, and it is not known whether these particles represented herpes simplex virus, other known herpes viruses, or the herpes-type virus. Herpes simplex virus has been isolated, in fact, from biopsy specimens of Burkitt's jaw tumors (Bell *et al.*, 1966; Simons and Ross, 1965; Woodall, Williams, Simpson, and Haddow, 1965) as well as from the throats of normal children resident in the same area of Africa (Simons and Ross, 1965).

BIOLOGIC ACTIVITY OF HERPES-TYPE VIRUS

Until very recently, neither infectivity nor any other kinds of biological activity had been shown with any of the herpes-type virus isolates. The virus appeared to replicate (persist) only in the tissue culture cells in which it was originally detected, and numerous attempts to extract herpes-type virus infective for other cell cultures and for animals were unsuccessful. More recently, however, a few investigators succeeded in showing infectivity of herpes-type virus and, in several cases, apparent disease induction in animals after their inoculation with cell and cell-free materials containing the virus. Stewart, Landon, Lovelace, and Parker (1965) showed that hamsters developed a progressive encephalitic syndrome leading to death after intracerebral inoculation with human cells or cell extracts known to contain herpes-type virus. Investigators of the Pfizer Company (Durr, personal communication) confirmed this observation and showed in addition that various strains of mice developed a similar disease following intracerebral inoculation. Grace and Mitchel (personal communication) showed that newborn kittens also developed this disease following intracerebral inoculation with herpes-type virus. In none of these studies, however, were virus particles detected by electron microscopy in thin sections of neural tissue.

Henle *et al.* (1967) have detected a reasonably frequent chromosomal aberration in tissue culture lines begun from leukemia and lymphoma patients and known to contain herpes-type virus. This modification of chromosome No. 10 and the presence of replicating virus particles also occurred in some normal human cell lines following exposure to herpes-type virus.

At this point, it appears important to reiterate that while herpes-type virus particles generally are indistinguishable in morphology and size from other known members of the herpesvirus group, there are several quantitative and qualitative differences. First, Dalton (personal communication) reported apparent morphologic differences between the unidentified herpes-type virus and known members of the herpes group. Particles associated with tissue cultures of leukemia and lymphoma cells from human beings acquired a finely granular coat which was distinct from an envelope formed from the nuclear or plasma membrane. No such coat was found to develop in relation to the known herpesviruses. Increased electron density of peripherally condensed chromatin and beading of mitochondria were also characteristic of cells of the human leukemia and lymphoma tissue cultures which contain virus particles. Such features are not seen in cells infected with known herpesviruses. These investigators cautioned, however, that the beading of mitochondria could constitute nonspecific host-cell reactions to viral infection. Second, the usual finding in attempts to replicate the more common herpesviruses, especially herpes simplex virus, is that the particles almost consistently contain nucleoids (Grace and Mitchel, personal communication). Conversely, a persistent finding in the leukemia and lymphoma cell lines from human beings is that many to most of the particles of herpes-type virus are devoid of nucleoids. Third, most attempts to show herpes-type virus infectivity have been initiated with partially purified virus after the performance of various procedures including density gradient centrifugation, sonication, freeze-thaw cycles, and chromatographic column separation. With the reasonable assumption that these factors and procedures may have been deleterious to infectivity, if not antigenicity, it does not appear unusual, in retrospect, that attempts to show infectivity have been almost invariably unsuccessful. Fourth, even when apparently intact particles were separated from cells, the amount of virus (complete and incomplete) available per unit of inoculum was low and, in fact, may have been too low to initiate infection. In this regard, it is important to recall the original observation of Bryan, Calnan, and Moloney (1955) who showed with the Rous sarcoma virus that the ability to infect, period of latency, severity of disease, and the amount of virus recoverable depended on the amount of virus contained in the infecting dose. These observations were confirmed by Groupé and Rauscher (1957) and Rauscher and Groupé (1960) and recently were shown by Pienta and Groupé (1967) to apply to at least one murine leukemia virus.

Zeve, Kondratick, and Lloyd (in press) successfully transferred herpes-type virus from a Burkitt cell line (MOB-8) to another buffy coat culture

(RPMI-2367) from a human being; the latter was negative for virus and virus antigen when examined electron microscopically and immunofluorescently, respectively. By means of a Belco dual spinner flask, the MOB-8 cells were placed on one side of a millipore filter (220 mμ) and the RPMI-2367 cells were placed on the opposite side. Following cultivation for 164 hours, the RPMI-2367 cells were shown by electron microscopy to contain particles morphologically identical to herpes-type virus. Appropriate tests to determine the integrity of the millipore filter strongly suggested cell-free infection by herpes-type virus of the recipient cell line.

Grace and Mitchel (personal communication) recently showed that an apparent virusfree line of cells, started from peripheral blood cells of a myeloid leukemia patient (6410), rapidly declined in viability and died five days later after exposure to high multiplicities of herpes-type virus (derived from the HR1-K clone of the P3J Burkitt's lymphoma cell line), of the order of 500 to 1,000 virus particles per cell. Electron microscopy and direct immunofluorescent staining indicated that almost all cells were infected and that large amounts of new virus particles were produced. In contrast, a virus carrier state of 6410 cells was observed when these cells were infected with lower doses of virus ranging from one to 250 virus particles per cell. In these experiments, therefore, a clear relationship of virus yield to infecting dose was observed. With lower multiplicities of virus input, as long as three to four weeks were required for the appearance of immunofluorescence in 30 to 50 per cent of the cells. Grace and co-workers then reasoned that since virus adsorption is the first step in infection, an assay for adsorption might aid in determining the target cell capable of supporting viral replication. Following this approach, they further confirmed the biological activity of herpes-type virus by successful infection of three additional human cell lines, all of which were negative by immunofluorescence and electron microscopy prior to infection. Their studies indicate that among the cells tested by immunofluorescence and electron microscopy, only human and monkey lymphocytes or lymphoblast-like cells have the ability to adsorb virus. All such immunofluorescent positive cells, when observed with phase-contrast microscopy, were mononucleated, uniform in size, and approximately 12 μ in diameter; the nucleus occupied 75 per cent of the cell. These and other findings seem to indicate an affinity of the virus for lymphocytic- or lymphoblastic-type cells of primate origin. These conclusions appear to be supported by the work of Gerber and Birch (1967) who used complement-fixation to detect antibodies to herpes-type virus in human beings, chimpanzees, and four species of monkeys, but not in rats, guinea pigs, cats, dogs, goats, sheep, pigs, horses, and cows.

Discussion

Since no DNA virus has been found to induce leukemia or lymphoma and since all of the known leukemia and lymphoma viruses contain ribonucleic acid (RNA), it would appear logical, from the prototype diseases in animals, to concentrate the search for a counterpart agent in human beings on viruses of the medium-sized, membrane-bound, RNA variety. However, with the present stage of knowledge and experience, it would be unwise to exclude viruses of any type as potential candidates for leukemogenesis simply because no member of the group has been discovered which induces the usual forms of leukemia or lymphoma. The facts that the medium-sized, membrane-bound, RNA viruses of avian leukemia can cause kidney carcinomas as well as leukemia and that fibrosarcomas of nearly identical gross and microscopic morphology can be induced in hamsters with both polyoma (DNA) and Rous sarcoma (RNA) viruses, further caution against stereotyping all oncogenic virus-host interactions on the basis of the usually predictable tumor responses of laboratory animals to laboratory strains of tumor viruses.

After successful propagation of a virus in sufficient quantities, the next step in the search for etiologic viruses in leukemia and lymphoma of human beings is the demonstration of the capacity to induce neoplasia in some animal or tissue culture system. Obviously, testing in man will not be done. Although the production of neoplasia in animals would not constitute proof for oncogenic potential in man, it would demonstrate that this basic property is possessed by the virus and would represent important supportive evidence for the possibility of a similar action in man (Bryan, Dalton, and Rauscher, 1966). In like manner, the induction of in vitro cytoneoplasia (Bryan, Dalton, and Rauscher, 1966) in human or other cell lines would provide valuable supportive evidence, but would not alone constitute proof for the oncogenicity of the agent in man.

The oncogenic dose of Rous sarcoma virus is several orders of magnitude higher for hosts of foreign species than for the natural host (Rabotti, Grove, Sellers, and Anderson, 1966; Rabotti, Raine, and Sellers, 1965). This type of quantitative relationship also may hold for candidate viruses found in human beings tested in other animal species.

The problems of testing for oncogenicity in animal and tissue culture systems have been described by many authors. The induction of leukemia in mice, which were inoculated when newborn with specimens from human beings with leukemia, has been reported by investigators from three different laboratories (Bergol'ts, 1957; DeLong, 1960; Schwartz, Spurrier, Yates, and Maduros, 1960), but others (Girardi, Hilleman, and Zwickey, 1962; Moore, 1960) have failed to confirm this finding. Approximately 700 primates, mostly rhesus monkeys—but including animals of nine species (cynomologous, African green monkey, baboon, pig-tail macaque, stump-tail macaque, Galago, bonnet monkey, marmosets, and chimpanzees), have been inoculated when newborn with specimens from human beings with leukemia and lymphoma by investigators at the National Cancer Institute and other institutions collaborating in the Special Virus-Leukemia Program (Rauscher and Pallotta, unpublished data). No neoplastic responses have been observed thus far. However, only about 220 of these animals are more than one year of age, and the oldest are only about four years old. If a leukemogenic agent is responsible for the age peak which occurs at three to four years in children with leukemia, and if susceptible primates approach the humans in time-to-induction of disease, the primate animals would have to be observed for several additional years before their responses could be interpreted as definitely negative.

The C type viruslike particles detected by electron microscopy in specimens from human beings with leukemia have not been successfully propagated, and sufficient amounts of the candidate agent are not yet available for satisfactory tests for oncogenicity. Nevertheless, as much as possible of the candidate agent derived from patients with the natural disease is being inoculated into nonhuman primate animals and into human cells in tissue culture, in attempts to determine whether it can be propagated and whether oncogenicity can be demonstrated. The earliest tests in primates were made with electron microscope-positive fractions derived from 10 ml of leukemic plasma. Later tests involved similar fractions derived by plasmaphoresis from five to 10 times this amount of plasma. Present efforts, under the Special Virus-Leukemia Program, are directed toward (1) increasing the amount of agent in the inocula and (2) increasing the susceptibility (decreasing immunologic reactivity) of test animals. The first objective is being pursued with the use of two procedures: (1) the pooling of electron microscope-positive plasma fractions derived in successive plasmaphoreses on the same patient; and (2) the pooling of electron microscope-positive fractions from different, but clinically similar, patients. Procedures employed in attempts to increase the susceptibility of newborn primate animals include: (1) thymectomy, (2) whole-body irradiations, and (3) administration of immunosuppressive drugs.

Since many of the studies presented in this paper utilized materials derived from patients with Burkitt's lymphoma, it is important to note that herpes simplex (Bell et al., 1966; Simons and Ross, 1965; Woodall, Williams, Simpson, and Haddow, 1965), vaccinia (Dalldorf, Linsell, Barnhart, and Martyn, 1964), Bunyamwera (Wright, Bell, and Williams, 1967), an unidentified agent (Dalldorf and Bergamini, 1964) and reoviruses (Bell et al., 1966; Wright, Bell, and Williams, 1967), in addition to herpes-type virus, have been detected in materials derived from Burkitt lymphoma patients. It is of interest and possibly of significance that only herpes-type virus has been detected or isolated from leukemia patients and from Burkitt lymphoma patients, both studied in the United States. Of the above agents and in addition to herpes-type virus, reoviruses, particularly type three, appear to be most uniformly present in Burkitt's lymphoma patients. In one study, reoviruses were isolated from biopsy material from 25 of 90 patients with Burkitt's tumor in Uganda and Tanzania whereas they were isolated from only one of 21 other patients with non-Burkitt's tumors (Bell et al., 1966). Neutralizing antibody studies, which used type three reovirus, have shown that there is a relationship between this virus and Burkitt's tumor (Bell, in press). Antibody was found in 53 of 72 cases of Burkitt's tumor, but only 12 of 65 controls which consisted of a variety of other tumors in normal children. Comparable results were obtained using hemagglutination-inhibition tests on another series of serum specimens (Levy and Henle, 1966). Stanley, Walters, Leak, and Keast (1966) reported the induction of lymphomas in mice following their inoculation with spleen cells from a mouse presenting with chronic lesions which were induced after neonatal reovirus 3 infection. The disease appeared to be a manifestation of an autoimmune disease, although some features were reported to resemble Burkitt's tumor (Papadimitriou, 1966). These preliminary results and the report by Parker, Baker, and Stanley (1965) on the isolation of reovirus 3 from mosquitoes, while suggestive of a more than casual relationship with Burkitt's tumor, must obviously await confirmation. It seems clear from the studies of Kajima and Pollard (1965) and Huebner (1967) that mice of all strains carry viruses capable of inducing leukemia and lymphoma. Since these leukemia viruses are known to be helpers (Harvey, 1964; Huebner et al., 1966) for at least one of the two known murine sarcoma viruses (Hartley and Rowe, 1966; Moloney, 1966), it would appear unwarranted to ascribe an etiological role to a human isolate of a reovirus and the induction of a lymphoma in a laboratory mouse.

The case for assigning an oncogenic role to herpes-type virus at the present time is certainly as tenuous as that for other viruses. It may be strengthened by the apparent relationship of a herpesvirus to the induction of renal carcinomas in the frog and by the recent report of Churchill and Biggs (1967) and Burmester (personal communication) that the agent of Marek's disease may be a herpesvirus. Similarly, cocarcinogenic properties have been reported for herpes simplex virus when inoculated intradermally into mice in conjunction with multiple applications of 3-methylcholanthrene (Tanaka and Southam, 1965). While these and other studies presented in this paper and at this conference certainly do not detract from the need for expanded studies, they obviously have not determined definitively whether herpes-type virus is (1) an international ubiquitous passenger virus or (2) an agent related etiologically, even indirectly, to cancer in human beings.

Summary

Selected background information is presented and discussed in the light of new facts and results from studies aimed at determining whether viruses similar to, or different from, those known to be associated with the induction of leukemia and lymphoma in laboratory and domestic animals also are involved in the etiology of leukemia and lymphoma in man. Particular emphasis is placed on studies involving the establishment and experimental use of hematopoietic cell lines and of a herpes-type virus frequently associated with the cultures.

Published information and information contributed to the Special Virus-Leukemia Program of the National Cancer Institute show that as of July 1967 scientists had established over 125 cell strains from patients with cancer or other diseases and from nondiseased controls. At least 61 of the cancer- and five of the noncancer-derived lines showed a herpes-type virus by electron microscopy. The virus(es) was detected in cultures from patients and controls in laboratories in England, the United States, Africa, Australia, New Guinea, Japan, and Sweden; in the United States, the virus also was detected in cultures from several chimpanzees and from one rhesus monkey which had myeloid leukemia.

The unknown significance of these and other findings for cancer etiology is discussed in relation to the key studies which rapidly advancing technology and production of industrial quantities of virus will make possible.

REFERENCES

Anderson, D. R.: Subcellular particles associated with human leukemias seen with the electron microscope. In Defendi, V., Ed.: *Methodological Approaches to the Study of Leukemias.* Wistar Institute Symposium Monograph No. 4. Philadelphia, Pennsylvania, Wistar Institute Press, 1965, pp. 113-146.

Anderson, D. R., and Barile, M. F.: Ultrastructure of *Mycoplasma hominis. Journal of Bacteriology,* 90:180-192, July 1965.

Armstrong, D., Henle, G., and Henle, W.: Complement-fixation tests with cell lines derived from Burkitt's lymphoma and acute leukemias. *Journal of Bacteriology,* 91:1257-1262, March 1966.

Barile, M. F., Bodey, G. P., Snyder, J., Riggs, D. B., and Grabowski, M. W.: Isolation of *Mycoplasma orale* from leukemic bone marrow and blood by direct culture. *Journal of the National Cancer Institute,* 36:155-159, January 1966.

Bell, T. M.: The chemotherapy of Burkitt's tumor. Proceedings of a Conference at Kampala, Uganda, 1966. Sponsored by the U.I.C.C. (In press.)

Bell, T. M., Massie, A., Ross, M. G. R., Simpson, D. I. H., and Griffin, E.: Further isolations of reovirus type 3 from cases of Burkitt's lymphoma. *British Medical Journal,* 1:1514-1517, June 1966.

Benyesh-Melnick, M., Fernbach, D. J., and Lewis, R. T.: Studies on human leukemia. I. Spontaneous lymphoblastoid transformation of fibroblastic bone marrow cultures derived from leukemic and nonleukemic children. *Journal of the National Cancer Institute,* 31:1311-1332, December 1963.

Benyesh-Melnick, M., and Melnick, J. L.: Personal communication.

Benyesh-Melnick, M., Smith, K. O., and Fernbach, D. J.: Studies on human leukemia. III. Electron microscopic findings in children with acute leukemia and in children with infectious mononucleosis. *Journal of the National Cancer Institute,* 33:571-579, September 1964.

Bergol'ts, V. M.: Experimental studies of the aetiology of leukaemia in man. I. The discovery of leukaemic tissues from man of a cell-free factor producing leukaemia in mice. *Problems of Hematology and Blood Transfusion,* 2:10-21, 1957.

Bernhard, W.: The detection and study of tumor viruses with the electron microscope. *Cancer Research,* 20:712-727, June 1960.

Bernhard, W., and Leplus, R.: *Fine Structure of the Normal and Malignant Human Lymph Node.* Oxford, England, Pergamon Press; Paris, France, Gauthier-Villars; New York, New York, Macmillan, 1964, 101 pp.

Bryan, W. R., Calnan, D., and Moloney, J. B.: Biological studies on the Rous sarcoma virus. III. The recovery of virus from experimental tumors in relation to initiating dose. *Journal of the National Cancer Institute,* 16:317-335, August 1955.

Bryan, W. R., Dalton, A. J., and Rauscher, F. J.: The viral approach to human leukemia and lymphoma; Its current status. *Progress in Hematology,* 5:137-179, September 1966.

Bryan, W. R., Moloney, J. B., O'Connor, T. E., Fink, M. A., and Dalton, A. J.: Viral etiology of leukemia: Combined Clinical Staff Conference at the National Institutes of Health. *Annals of Internal Medicine,* 62:376-399, February 1965.

Burger, C. L., Harris, W. W., Anderson, N. G., Bartlett, T. W., and Kniseley, R. M.: Virus-like particles in human leukemic plasma. *Proceedings of the Society for Experimental Biology and Medicine,* 115:151-156, January 1964.

Burmester, B. R.: Personal communication.

Churchill, A. E., and Biggs, P. M.: Agent of Marek's disease in tissue culture. *Nature,* 215:528-530, July 29, 1967.

Clarkson, B.: Personal communication.

Coons, A. H., and Kaplan, M. H.: Localization of antigen in tissue cells. II. Improvements in a method for the detection of antigen by means of fluorescent antibody. *Journal of Experimental Medicine,* 91:1-13, January 1, 1950.

Dabich, L., Leopold, B. A., and Zarafonetis, C. J.: Immunofluorescence in human leukemia. (Abstract).(In press.)

Dales, S., and Howatson, A. F.: Virus-like particles in association with L strain cells. *Cancer Research,* 21:193-197, February 1961.

Dalldorf, G., and Bergamini, F.: Unidentified, filtrable agents isolated from African children with malignant lymphomas. *Proceedings of the National Academy of Sciences of the U.S.A.,* 51:263-265, January 15, 1964.

Dalldorf, G., Linsell, C. A., Barnhart, F. E., and Martyn, R.: An epidemiologic approach to the lymphomas of African children and Burkitt's sarcoma of the jaws. *Perspectives in Biology and Medicine,* 7:435-449, Summer 1964.

Dalton, A. J.: Personal communication.

Dalton, A. J., Law, L. W., Moloney, J. B., and Manaker, R. A.: An electron microscopic study of a series of murine lymphoid neoplasms. *Journal of the National Cancer Institute,* 27:747-791, October 1961.

Dalton, A. J., and Manaker, R. A.: The comparison of virus particles associated with Burkitt lymphoma with other herpes-like viruses. In *Carcinogenesis: A Broad Critique* (The University of Texas M. D. Anderson Hospital and Tumor Institute at Houston, Twentieth Annual Symposium on Fundamental Cancer Research, 1966). Baltimore, Maryland, The Williams and Wilkins Company, 1967, pp. 59-90.

Dalton, A. J., and Mitchell, E. Z.: Detection of viruses with the electron microscope. In Burdette, W. J., Ed.: *Viruses Inducing Cancer—Implications for Therapy.* Salt Lake City, Utah, University of Utah Press, 1966, pp. 237-249.

Dalton, A. J., and Moloney, J. B.: Recovery of viruses from the blood of rats with induced leukemia. In Harris, R. J. C., Ed.: *The Interpretation of Ultrastructure* (Symposia of the International Society for Cell Biology). New York, New York, Academic Press, Inc., 1962, Vol. 1, pp. 385-392.

Dalton, A. J., Moloney, J. B., Porter, G. H., Frei, E., and Mitchell, E.: Studies on murine and human leukemia. *Transactions of the Association of American Physicians,* 77:52-64, 1964.

De Harven, E., and Friend, C.: Further electron microscope studies of a mouse leukemia induced by cell-free filtrates. *Journal of Biophysical and Biochemical Cytology,* 7:747-752, July 1960.

DeLong, R.: Production of leukemia in mice with cell-free filtrates from human leukemias. *Journal of Laboratory and Clinical Medicine,* 56:891-893, December 1960.

Dmochowski, L.: Electron microscope studies of leukemia in animals and men. In Hayhoe, F. G. J., Ed.: *Current Research in Leukemia.* Cambridge, England, Cambridge University Press, 1965, pp. 23-33.

———: The viral etiology of leukemia. In Berger, E., and Melnick, J. L., Eds.: *Progress in Medical Virology.* New York, New York, Hafner Publishing Company, Inc., 1961, Vol. 3, pp. 363-494.

Dmochowski, L., and Grey, C. E.: Electron microscopy of tumors of known and suspected viral etiology. *Texas Reports on Biology and Medicine,* 15:704-753, Fall 1957.

———: Studies on submicroscopic structure of leukemias of known or suspected viral origin: A review. *Blood, The Journal of Hematology,* 13:1017-1042, November 1958.

Dmochowski, L., Grey, C. E., Dreyer, D. A., Sykes, J. A., Langford, P. L., and Taylor, H. G.: Mycoplasma (pleuropneumonia-like organisms [PPLO]) and human leukemia. *Medical Record and Annals,* 57:563-568, December 1964.

Dmochowski, L., Grey, C. E., Sykes, J. A., Shullenberger, C. C., and Howe, C. D.: Studies on human leukemia. *Proceedings of the Society for Experimental Biology and Medicine,* 101: 686-690, August-September 1959.

Dmochowski, L., Padgett, F., and Gross, L.: An electron microscope study of rat leukemia induced with mouse leukemia virus (Gross). *Cancer Research,* 24:869-899, June 1964.

Dmochowski, L., Taylor, H. G., Grey, C. E., Dreyer, D. A., Sykes, J. A., Langford,

P. L., Rogers, T., Shullenberger, C. C., and Howe, C. D.: Viruses and myco-plasma (PPLO) in human leukemia. *Cancer,* 18:1345-1368, October 1965.

Durr, F.: Personal communication.

Epstein, M. A., Achong, B. G., and Barr, Y. M.: Virus particles in cultured lympho-blasts from Burkitt's lymphoma. *Lancet,* 1:702-703, March 28, 1964.

Epstein, M. A., Achong, B. G., Barr, Y. M., Zajac, B., Henle, G., and Henle, W.: Morphological and virological investigations on cultured Burkitt tumor lympho-blasts (Strain Raji). *Journal of the National Cancer Institute,* 37:547-559, October 1966.

Epstein, M. A., Achong, B. G., and Pope, J. H.: Virus in cultured lymphoblasts from a New Guinea Burkitt lymphoma. *British Medical Journal,* 2:290-291, April 29, 1967.

Epstein, M. A., Barr, Y. M., and Achong, B. G.: A second virus-carrying tissue cul-ture strain (EB2) of lymphoblasts from Burkitt's lymphoma. *Pathologie et Biolo-gie,* 12:1233-1234, December 1964.

————: The behaviour and morphology of a second tissue culture strain (EB2) of lymphoblasts from Burkitt's lymphoma. *The British Journal of Cancer,* 19:108-115, March 1965.

————: Preliminary observations on new lymphoblast strains (EB$_4$, EB$_5$) from Bur-kitt tumors in a British and a Ugandan patient. *The British Journal of Cancer,* 20: 475-479, September 1966.

Epstein, M. A., Henle, G., Achong, B. G., and Barr, Y. M.: Morphological and bio-logical studies on a virus in cultured lymphoblasts from Burkitt's lymphoma. *Journal of Experimental Medicine,* 121:761-770, May 1, 1965.

Feldman, D. G., and Gross, L.: Electron-microscopic study of the mouse leukemia virus (Gross), and of tissues from mice with virus-induced leukemia. *Cancer Re-search,* 24:1760-1784, November 1964.

Fink, M. A.: Studies of anti-"C type particle" fluorescent antibody in human leuke-mia: A status report. In *Third International Symposium for Comparative Leuke-mia Research,* July 11-13, 1967. Basel, Switzerland, Karger. (In press.)

Fink, M. A., Karon, M., Rauscher, F. J., Malmgren, R. A., and Orr, H. C.: Further observations on the immunofluorescence of cells in human leukemia. *Cancer,* 18:1317-1321, October 1965.

Fink, M. A., and Malmgren, R. A.: Fluorescent antibody studies of the viral antigen in a murine leukemia (Rauscher). *Journal of the National Cancer Institute,* 31: 1111-1122, November 1963.

Fink, M. A., Malmgren, R. A., Karon, M., and Orr, H. C.: Immunofluorescence studies in human leukemia. In Defendi, V., Ed.: *Methodological Approaches to the Study of Leukemia.* Wistar Institute Symposium Monograph No. 4. Philadel-phia, Pennsylvania, Wistar Institute Press, 1965, pp. 187-193.

Fink, M. A., Malmgren, R. A., Rauscher, F. J., Orr, H. C., and Karon, M.: Appli-cation of immunofluorescence to the study of human leukemia. *Journal of the National Cancer Institute,* 33:581-588, September 1964.

Fink, M. A., Manaker, R. A., Dalton, A. J., and Cranford, V. L.: Immunofluores-cence of tissue cultured cells derived from human lymphoid diseases. In Winqvist, G.: *Symposium on Comparative Leukaemia Research.* Oxford, England, Perga-mon Press Ltd., 1966, pp. 45-53.

Foley, G. E., Lazarus, H., Farber, S., Uzman, B. G., Boone, B. A., and McCarthy, R. E.: Continuous culture of human lymphoblasts from peripheral blood of a child with acute leukemia. *Cancer,* 18:522-529, April 1965.

Gerber, P., and Birch, S. M.: Complement-fixing antibodies in sera of human and nonhuman primates to viral antigens derived from Burkitt's lymphoma cells. *Proceedings of the National Academy of Sciences of the U.S.A.,* 58:478-484, August 1967.

Girardi, A. J., Hilleman, M. R., and Zwickey, R. E.: Search for virus in human malignancies. 2. In vivo studies. *Proceedings of the Society for Experimental Biology and Medicine,* 111:84-93, October 1962.

Grace, J., and Mitchel, E.: Personal communication.

Griffin, E. R., Bell, T. M., and Adatia, A. K.: Virus infection of teeth in Burkitt's tumour. 1. The demonstration of virus-like particles in teeth from active Burkitt's tumour. *East African Medical Journal,* 44:67-70, February 1967.

————: Virus infection of teeth in Burkitt's tumour. 2. The presence of virus-like particles in a tooth five years after clinical cure. *East African Medical Journal,* 44:71-73, February 1967.

Griffin, E. R., Wright, D. H., Bell, T. M., and Ross, M. G. R.: Demonstration of virus particles in biopsy material from cases of Burkitt's tumour. *European Journal of Cancer,* 2:353-358, December 1966.

Grist, N. R., and Fallon, R. J.: Isolation of viruses from leukaemic patients. *British Medical Journal,* 2:1263, November 14, 1964.

Groupé, V., and Rauscher, F. J.: Growth curve of Rous sarcoma virus and relationship of infecting dose to yield of virus in chick brain. *Journal of the National Cancer Institute,* 18:507-514, April 1957.

Haguenau, F., and Beard, J. W.: The avian sarcoma-leukosis complex; its biology and ultrastructure. In Dalton, A. J., and Haguenau, F., Eds.: *Tumors Induced by Viruses: Ultrastructural Studies.* New York, New York, and London, England, Academic Press, Inc., 1962, pp. 1-59.

Haguenau, F., Febvre, H., and Arnoult, J.: Mode de formation intracellulaire du virus du sarcome de Rous. Étude ultrastructurale. *Journal de Microscopie,* 1:445-454, December, 1962.

Hartley, J. W., and Rowe, W. P.: Production of altered cell foci in tissue culture by defective Moloney sarcoma virus particles. *Proceedings of the National Academy of Sciences of the U.S.A.,* 55:780-786, April 1966.

Harvey, J. J.: An unidentified virus which causes the rapid production of tumours in mice. *Nature,* 204:1104-1105, December 12, 1964.

Hayflick, L.: Mycoplasmas and human leukemia. In Defendi, V., Ed.: *Methodological Approaches to the Study of Leukemias.* Wistar Institute Symposium Monograph No. 4. Philadelphia, Pennsylvania, Wistar Institute Press, 1965, pp. 157-164.

Hayflick, L., and Koprowski, H.: Direct agar isolation of mycoplasmas from human leukaemic bone marrow. *Nature,* 205:713-714, February 13, 1965.

Heine, U., de Thé, G., Ishiguro, H., and Beard, J. W.: Morphologic aspects of Rous sarcoma virus elaboration. *Journal of the National Cancer Institute,* 29:211-223, July 1962.

Henle, G., and Henle, W.: Studies on cell lines derived from Burkitt's lymphoma. *Transactions of the New York Academy of Sciences,* 29:71-79, October 1966a.

————: Immunofluorescence in cells derived from Burkitt's lymphoma. *Journal of Bacteriology,* 91:1248-1256, March 1966b.

————: Immunofluorescence, interference and complement fixation techniques in the detection of herpes-type virus in Burkitt tumor cells. *Cancer Research.* (In press.)

Henle, W., Diehl, V., Kohn, G., zur Hausen, H., and Henle, G.: Herpes-type virus and chromosome marker in normal leukocytes after growth with irradiated Burkitt cells. *Science,* 157: 1064-1065, September 1, 1967.

Henle, W., Hummeler, K., and Henle, G.: Antibody coating and agglutination of virus particles separated from the EB_3 line of Burkitt lymphoma cells. *Journal of Bacteriology,* 92:269-271, July 1966.

Hinuma, Y., and Grace, J. T.: Cloning of immunoglobulin-producing human leukemic and lymphoma cells in long-term cultures. *Proceedings of the Society for Experimental Biology and Medicine*, 124:107-111, January 1967.

Howatson, A. F., and Almeida, J. D.: An electron microscope study of polyoma virus in hamster kidney. *Journal of Biophysical and Biochemical Cytology*, 7:753-760, July 1960.

Howatson, A. F., McCulloch, E. A., Almeida, J. D., Siminovitch, L., Axelrad, A. A., and Ham, A. W.: Studies in vitro, in vivo, and by electron microscope of a virus recovered from a C3H mouse mammary tumor: Relationship to polyoma virus. *Journal of the National Cancer Institute*, 24:1131-1151, May 1960.

Huebner, R. J.: The murine leukemia-sarcoma virus complex. *Proceedings of the National Academy of Sciences of the U.S.A.*, 58:835-842, September 1967.

Huebner, R. J., Hartley, J. W., Rowe, W. P., Lane, W. T., and Capps, W. I.: Rescue of the defective genome of Moloney sarcoma virus from a noninfectious hamster tumor and the production of pseudotype sarcoma viruses with various murine leukemia viruses. *Proceedings of the National Academy of Sciences of the U.S.A.*, 56:1164-1169, October 1966.

Hummeler, K., Tomassini, N., and Hayflick, L.: Ultrastructure of a mycoplasma (Negroni) isolated from human leukemia. *Journal of Bacteriology*, 90:517-523, August 1965.

Iwakata, S., and Grace, J. T., Jr.: Cultivation in vitro of myeloblasts from human leukemia. *New York State Journal of Medicine*, 64:2279-2282, September 15, 1964.

Jensen, E., and Wright, B.: Personal communication.

Jensen, E. M., Korol, W., Dittmar, S. L., and Medrek, T. J.: Virus containing lymphocyte cultures from cancer patients. *Journal of the National Cancer Institute*, 39:745-754, October 1967.

Kajima, M., and Pollard, M.: Detection of viruslike particles in germ-free mice. *Journal of Bacteriology*, 90:1448-1454, November 1965.

Laidlaw, P. P., and Elford, W. J.: A new group of filterable organisms. *Proceedings of the Royal Society of London*, 120:292-303, 1936.

Landon, J. C., Ellis, L. B., Zeve, V. H., and Fabrizio, D. P. A.: Herpes-type virus in cultured leukocytes from chimpanzees. *Journal of the National Cancer Institute*. (In press.)

Landon, J. L.: Personal communication.

Levine, P. H., Horoszewicz, J. S., Grace, J. T., Chai, L. S., Ellison, R. R., and Holland, J. F.: A relationship between the clinical status of leukemic patients and virus-like particles in their plasma. *Cancer*, 20:1563-1577, October 1967.

Levy, J. A., and Henle, G.: Indirect immunofluorescence tests with sera from African children and cultured Burkitt lymphoma cells. *Journal of Bacteriology*, 92:275-276, July 1966.

Lucas, L. S., Whang, J. J. K., Tjio, J. H., Manaker, R. A., and Zeve, V. H.: Continuous cell culture from a patient with chronic myelogenous leukemia. I. Propagation and presence of Philadelphia chromosome. *Journal of the National Cancer Institute*, 37:753-759, December 1966.

Mayyasi, S. A., Schidlovsky, G., Bulfone, L. M., and Buscheck, F. T.: The coating reaction of the herpes-type virus isolated from malignant tissues with an antibody present in sera. *Virology*. (In press.)

Minowada, J., Klein, G., Clifford, P., Klein, E., and Moore, G. E.: Studies of Burkitt lymphoma cells. I. Establishment of a cell line (B35M) and its characteristics. *Cancer*, 20:1430-1437, September 1967.

Moloney, J. B.: The application of studies in murine leukemia to the problems of human neoplasia. In Fiennes, R. N. T-W., Ed.: *Some Recent Developments in*

Comparative Medicine. London, England, Academic Press, Inc., 1966, pp. 251-258.

Moore, A. E.: Induction of tumors in newborn mice by inoculation of preparations of human tissues. (Abstract) *Proceedings of the American Association for Cancer Research,* 3:135, March 1960.

Moore, G. E.: Personal communication.

Moore, G. E., Gerner, R. E., and Minowada, J.: Studies of normal and neoplastic human hematopoietic cells in vitro. In *The Proliferation and Spread of Neoplastic Cells* (The University of Texas M. D. Anderson Hospital and Tumor Institute at Houston, Twenty-first Annual Symposium on Fundamental Cancer Research, 1967). Baltimore, Maryland, The Williams and Wilkins Company, 1968, pp. 41-63.

Murphy, W. H., and Furtado, D.: Isolation of viruses from children with acute leukemia. *University of Michigan Medical Bulletin,* 29:201-228, July-August 1963.

Negroni, G.: Isolation of viruses from leukaemic patients. *British Medical Journal,* 1:927-929, April 11, 1964.

O'Conor, G. T., and Rabson, A. S.: Herpes-like particles in an American lymphoma: Preliminary note. *Journal of the National Cancer Institute,* 35:899-903, November 1965.

Okano, H., Kunii, A., and Furth, J.: An electron microscopic study of leukemia induced in rats with Gross virus. *Cancer Research,* 23:1169-1175, September 1963.

Old, L. J., Boyse, E. A., Oettgen, H. F., de Harven, E., Geering, G., Williamson, B., and Clifford, P.: Precipitating antibody in human serum to an antigen present in cultured Burkitt's lymphoma cells. *Proceedings of the National Academy of Sciences of the U.S.A.,* 56:1699-1704, December 1966.

Papadimitriou, J. M.: Electron microscopic findings of a murine lymphoma associated with reovirus type 3 infection. *Proceedings of the Society for Experimental Biology and Medicine,* 121:93-96, January 1966.

Parker, L., Baker, E., and Stanley, N. F.: The isolation of reovirus type 3 from mosquitoes and a sentinel infant mouse. *Australian Journal of Experimental Biology and Medical Science,* 43:167-170, February 1965.

Pienta, R. J., and Groupé, V.: Relationship of infecting dose to recovery of Rauscher murine leukemia virus (RMLV) in random bred Swiss mice. *Cancer Research,* 27:1096-1100, June 1967.

Porter, G. H., III, Dalton, A. J., Moloney, J. B., and Mitchell, E. Z.: Association of electron-dense particles with human acute leukemia. *Journal of the National Cancer Institute,* 33:547-556, September 1964.

Prince, A. M., and Adams, W. R.: Virus-like particles in human plasma and serum from leukemic, hepatic, and control patients. (Abstract) *Federation Proceedings,* 24:175, April 1965.

Pulvertaft, R. J. V.: A study of malignant tumours in Nigeria by short-term tissue culture. *Journal of Clinical Pathology,* 18:261-273, May 1965.

Rabotti, G. F., Grove, A. S., Jr., Sellers, R. L., and Anderson, W. R.: Induction of multiple brain tumours (gliomata and leptomeningeal sarcomata) in dogs by Rous sarcoma virus. *Nature,* 209:884-886, February 26, 1966.

Rabotti, G. F., Raine, W. A., and Sellers, R. L.: Brain tumors (gliomas) induced in hamsters by Bryan's strain of Rous sarcoma virus. *Science,* 147:504-506, January 29, 1965.

Rabson, A. S., O'Conor, G. T., Baron, S., Whang, J. J., and Legallais, F. Y.: Morphologic, cytogenic and virologic studies in vitro of a malignant lymphoma from an African child. *International Journal of Cancer,* 1:89-106, January 1966.

Rauscher, F. J., and Groupé, V.: Importance of the infecting dose on growth patterns of Rous sarcoma virus (RSV) in chick brain. *Journal of the National Cancer Institute,* 25:1391-1404, December 1960.

Rauscher, F. J., and Pallotta, A. J.: Unpublished data.

Reyniers, J. A., and Sacksteder, M.: Personal communication.

Schwartz, S. O., Spurrier, W., Yates, L., and Maduros, B. P.: Studies in leukemia. XV. The induction of leukemia in Swiss mice with human leukemic brain extracts. *Blood, The Journal of Hematology,* 15:758-760, May 1960.

Simons, P. J., and Ross, M. G. R.: The isolation of herpes virus from Burkitt tumours. *European Journal of Cancer,* 1:135-136, October 1965.

Smith, K. O., Benyesh-Melnick, M., and Fernbach, D. J.: Studies on human leukemia. II. Structure and quantitation of myxovirus-like particles associated with human leukemia. *Journal of the National Cancer Institute,* 33:557-570, September 1964.

Stanley, N. F., Walters, M. N.-I., Leak, P. J., and Keast, D.: The association of murine lymphoma with reovirus type 3 infection. *Proceedings of the Society for Experimental Biology and Medicine,* 121:90-93, January 1966.

Stewart, S. E., Landon, J., Lovelace, E., and Parker, G.: Burkitt tumor: Brain lesions in hamsters induced with an extract from SL-1 cell line. In Defendi, V., Ed.: *Methodological Approaches to the Study of Leukemias.* Wistar Institute Symposium Monograph No. 4. Philadelphia, Pennsylvania, Wistar Institute Press, 1965, pp. 93-101.

Stewart, S. E., Lovelace, E., Whang, J. J., and Ngu, V. A.: Burkitt tumor: Tissue culture, cytogenetic and virus studies. *Journal of the National Cancer Institute,* 34:319-327, February 1965.

Tanaka, S., and Southam, C. M.: Joint action of herpes simplex virus and 3-methylcholanthrene in production of papillomas in mice. *Journal of the National Cancer Institute,* 34:441-451, April 1965.

Woodall, J. P., Williams, M. C., Simpson, D. I. H., and Haddow, A. J.: The isolation in mice of strains of herpes virus from Burkitt tumours. *European Journal of Cancer,* 1:137-140, October 1965.

Wright, D. H., Bell, T. M., and Williams, M. C.: Burkitt's tumour: A review of clinical features, treatment, pathology, epidemiology, entomology and virology. *East African Medical Journal,* 44:51-61, February 1967.

Yamaguchi, J., Hinuma, Y., and Grace, J. T., Jr.: Structure of virus particles extracted from a Burkitt lymphoma cell line. *Journal of Virology,* 1:640-642, June 1967.

Yohn, D. S., and Grace, J. T.: Immunofluorescent studies in human leukemia. (Abstract) *Proceedings of the American Association for Cancer Research,* 7:78, April 1966.

Zeve, V. H., Kondratick, J. N., and Lloyd, B. J.: In vitro cell free transfer of Burkitt associated virus to human leukocytes. *Science.* (In press.)

Zeve, V. H., Lucas, L. S., and Manaker, R. A.: Continuous cell cultures from a patient with chronic myelogenous leukemia. II. Detection of a herpes-like virus by electron microscopy. *Journal of the National Cancer Institute,* 37:761-773, December 1966.

Zur Hausen, H., Henle, W., Hummeler, K., Diehl, V., and Henle, G.: Comparative study of cultured Burkitt tumor cells by immunofluorescence, autoradiography, and electron microscopy. *Journal of Virology,* 1:830-837, August 1967.

Theoretical Considerations of the Effect of an Immunologic Rejection Response on the Growth of Tumor[*]

HERMAN D. SUIT, M.D., PH.D., AND
GEORGE W. BATTEN, JR., PH.D.

Department of Radiotherapy, The University of Texas M. D. Anderson Hospital and Tumor Institute at Houston, Houston, Texas; and Department of Mathematics, The University of Houston, Houston, Texas

ONE OF THE MORE PROMISING avenues of research in cancer therapy is the attempt to understand the killing of tumor cells in a growing lesion by an immunologic rejection response. At the present time, experimental data demonstrate that there is an immunologic rejection response directed against tumor cells in most of the experimental animal systems studied. However, sufficient experiments have not been performed to permit a detailed description of the quantitative aspects of such a rejection response. We are in the process of attempting some experiments in that direction and will report here the results of our preliminary and theoretical work. We have developed a tumor model and an immunologic rejection response model and have analyzed the effect of a rejection response in modifying tumor control probability following a specified radiation treatment. This report represents a continuation of earlier work (Suit and Wette, 1967; Suit and Batten, 1968).

We believe that development of these models is of value because it facilitates quantitative thinking about a particular subject and is helpful in the planning of laboratory experiments.

---

*This investigation was supported by U. S. Public Health Service Grant Nos. CA 5047, IK 3-CA-22-738, and FR 00258 from the National Cancer Institute, National Institutes of Health.

51

Models for Consideration of Interaction of Radiation Dose (D) to Tumor and an Immunologic Rejection Response (IRR)

1. The tumor is comprised of M (a finite number) viable tumor cells at the start of treatment. Nonviable tumor cells are not present at the time therapy is initiated.

2. Tumor destruction requires that all cells be killed by radiation dose or immunologic rejection response. That is, there should be no tumor cell lethal factors in the host-tumor relationship other than those pertaining directly to the IRR and there is no natural mortality of tumor cells.

3. Killing of tumor cells by irradiation may be described by one of the models which stipulates that the number of cells surviving a specified dose should follow a Poisson distribution. Simple multitarget or multihit models could be used for this purpose.

4. Proliferation of the viable tumor cells is a simple birth process, which is considered probabilistic. No allowance is made for the spontaneous or natural death of cells.

5. A constant fraction of the nonviable tumor cells undergoes lysis and is removed from the tumor site per time period. That is, the loss of cells from the tumor is a simple decay process (considered probabilistic).

6. The immunologic rejection response, or IRR, is considered to be characterized by the following properties:

    a. The magnitude of the IRR increases during the growth phase of the tumor but too slowly to cause regression of tumor. The IRR develops to a maximum level at the time of therapy. This level of IRR is sustained by the host throughout the post-treatment period.

    b. This IRR reacts against an absolute number of cells per unit of time. That is, a constant and absolute number of tumor cells is reacted against by the IRR following irradiation.

    c. The IRR reacts equally against viable cells and cells killed either by the irradiation or the IRR. That is, the sensitized lymphocytes (and any reacting humoral antibodies) cannot distinguish between viable and nonviable cells, as long as the nonviable are metabolically active and are intact. Further, an IRR reaction against a viable tumor cell is lethal to that cell.

7. Variations occur in the values assigned to the parameters. All computations assume a day-to-day variation in the various parameters of the model, as follows:

    a. α is the total number of cells reacted against by the IRR per time period.

b. β is the fraction of nonviable cells which lyse and is removed from the tumor site per time period.

c. q is the expected fractional increase in viable cells per time period. The day-to-day variation in α, β, and q is such that the number of cells affected by each process has a binomial distribution.

Further, in certain calculations, a standard error is assigned to the parameters α, β, q, and M. This refers to a variation from animal to animal and not a variation from time period to time period.

In summary, at completion of radiation treatment of the tumor model, a certain number of tumor cells remains and the IRR has developed to a maximum. Then, during each time period following irradiation, there will be three reactions:

1. A constant proportion (β) of the radiation-killed cells undergoes lysis and is removed from the tumor site.

2. A constant fraction $(q\text{-}1)$ of the viable cells divides.

3. An absolute number (α) of viable and nonviable tumor cells is reacted against by the IRR with equal probability.

Mathematical Method

Since the effect of the IRR on the viable cells depends on the total number of viable and nonviable cells, the model is nonlinear; and a convenient, closed algebraic expression for tumor control probability (TCP) in terms of the parameters M, α, β, q, and the number of cells which survived radiation treatment cannot be expected. Furthermore, because of the large numbers of cells involved, direct calculation of the various transition probabilities is not possible. For these reasons, the computations for this paper were done by the so-called "Monte Carlo" method, in which the model was simulated directly on a digital computer.

Specifically, let us assume that the state of the tumor at any time is described by two numbers: V, the number of viable cells; and K, the number of dead cells. A subscript will be used to denote time; thus, (V_i, K_i) will denote the state of the tumor at the end of the "ith"-period. In particular, since the tumor begins with M-viable and zero-dead cells, we have $V_0 = M$, $K_0 = 0$. In the first period, the tumor is irradiated; therefore, V_1 is a random variable of a Poisson distribution with a mean value equal to the expected number of cells surviving treatment; that is, the mean equals M times the survival fraction. Therefore, the number of killed cells is $K_1 = V_0 - V_1$.

After the first time period, the process is different. Consider the ith-period after irradiation. At the beginning of this period, the tumor state is (V_i, K_i). First, the dead cells are lysed and the viable cells replicate (β and q processes). Then the number V of viable cells equals V_i plus a binomially distributed random variable whose mean is the number of cells expected to divide and whose maximum is V; the number K of dead cells equals K_i minus a binomially distributed random variable with mean $\beta \cdot K_i$ and maximum β. Then the IRR occurs; and the number of viable cells killed by this process is a truncated binomially distributed random variable with mean $\alpha V/(V+K)$ and maximum is alpha; that is, if ω is a random variable with mean $\alpha V/V+K$ and maximum ω dose α, let ω' be the minimum of ω and V; then $V_i + 1 = V - \omega'$ and $K_i + 1 = K + \omega'$.

For details of the Monte Carlo method, the reader is referred to standard works (*e.g.* Hammersley and Handscomb, 1964).

Performance of the Model

As an introduction to the analysis of disappearance of radiation-killed cells and the repopulation of the tumor, inspect Figure 1 which has been

Fig. 1.—Graphic representation of the disappearance of radiation-killed cells ($\beta = 0.5$) and the repopulation of an irradiated tumor.

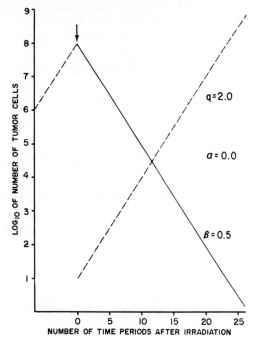

LOG$_{10}$ OF NUMBER OF TUMOR CELLS

q=2.0

a = 0.0

β = 0.5

NUMBER OF TIME PERIODS AFTER IRRADIATION

prepared for the situation where $\alpha = 0.0$. In the example shown, a tumor of 10^8 cells is irradiated and 10 cells survive. Repopulation of the tumor would occur as indicated by the solid line, assuming $q = 2.0$; similarly, removal of killed cells from the tumor site would be described by the dotted curve, assuming $\beta = 0.5$. The interest in this presentation is in the more complex situation where a significant IRR is active. Figure 2 illustrates the instance where $\alpha = 10^5$ (the IRR reacts against 10^5 tumor cells per time period) for the same tumor model shown in Figure 1, *i.e.*, $M = 10^8$, $\beta = 0.5$, and $q = 2.0$. The figure presents a family of 30 pairs of curves which demonstrates the repopulation of tumor (dotted lines) and the removal of nonviable cells (solid lines) for a series of numbers of surviving cells; the minimum number is 10 and each successive curve refers to a number of surviving cells which is larger than that for the preceding curve by a factor of 1.2. In the figure, the lowest curve for repopulation and the lowest curve for cell removal refer to a surviving number of 10 cells. For this particular set of values for the parameters, the IRR kills all surviving cells provided the number is less than approximately

Fig. 2.—Demonstration of the effect of an immunologic rejection response on repopulation of an irradiated tumor.

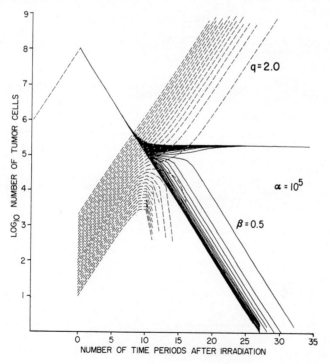

$2 \cdot 10^3$ at the end of the radiation treatment. However, for slightly greater numbers of surviving cells, the repopulation curve is only deflected by the IRR. Inspection of this graph shows that the tumor will be destroyed only if the total number of cells (nonviable and viable) decreases to a value essentially equal to α at some point during the regression of the irradiated tumor. Note that the difference between a tumor-destructive effect of the IRR and merely an effect to delay regrowth occurs over a very small range in number of cells surviving irradiation. The removal curve (solid lines) is affected by the accretion of cells to the nonviable compartment as a result of the action of the IRR; accordingly, delay in the removal curve increases as the maximum number of viable cells increases. Where the tumor recurs, the removal curve approaches an asymptote; a constant number of cells is killed by the IRR per time period and a constant fraction of those cells is removed per period.

Calculations have been made of the TCP for radiation treatments which yield a range of survival fractions of tumor cells for different values assigned to the parameters α, β, and q. Results of two sets of those cal-

Fig. 3.—Effect of the value assigned to α on position of dose-response curve along survival fraction (dose axis).

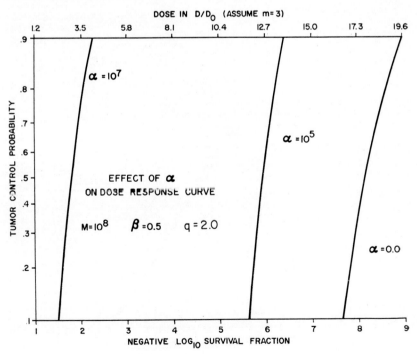

culations are presented in Figures 3 and 4 as plots of TCP against survival fraction. The abscissa at the top of the graph is scaled in terms of the corresponding radiation dose; multitarget model with $m = 3$ and radiation dose (D/D_0) given in a single fraction are used. In these computations, a standard error of 0.05 has been assigned to α and to β and a standard error of 0.10 to M. For the calculations shown in Figure 3, $M = 10^8$, $\beta = 0.5$ and $q = 2.0$. Note that α must be quite large to appreciably affect the position of the dose response curve; however, for even smaller increases in α above 10^5, the dose response curve shifts rapidly to the left. To consider the effect of a variation in β for a constant M, α, and q, examine Figure 4. The position of the curve on the dose or survival fraction axis shifts rapidly to the right with decreases in β. This is because the slower the removal of radiation-killed cells, the greater the extent of repopulation before the total number of cells decreases to a level (approximating α) where the IRR can destroy all viable cells. Simply stated, for the IRR to destroy the progeny of cells that survive irradiation, $V + K \cong \alpha$ at some time after treatment. The slopes of the dose response curves are rather similar for these various situations.

Fig. 4.—Effect of the value assigned to β on position of dose-response curve along survival fraction (dose axis).

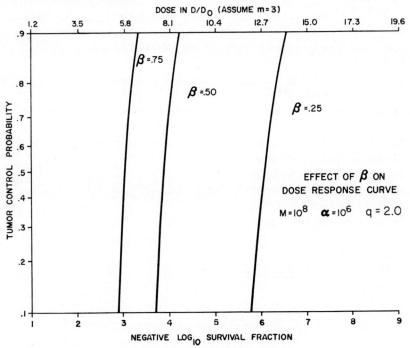

Implications of These Calculations

The effectiveness of an IRR of specified intensity in modifying TCP for a certain radiotherapy regimen would be expected to be a complex function of the following: number of tumor cells surviving treatment, number of nonviable cells in the tumor at completion of therapy, α, β, and q. For a given IRR, a maximum effectiveness would be expected, if directed against a tumor in which:

1. Cell lysis occurs during interphase and shortly after irradiation; the value of β in this situation is large. Small cells of the lymphocyte series are in this category.

2. Cell proliferation is slow, i.e., the value of q is small.

Accordingly, an IRR of specified intensity, which is directed against a given number of cells surviving irradiation, would be expected to be more effective if the tumor were a lymphoma or a seminoma than if it were a carcinoma or sarcoma; cells in carcinomas and sarcomas are more likely to pass through one or more postirradiation cell cycles before lysis. That is, β should be greater for certain of the lymphomas than for the carcinomas. The best situation for the action of an IRR might be a very slowly growing lymphoma and the worst situation a rapidly growing carcinoma or sarcoma.

There are many assumptions in the model discussed here which probably do not hold in the biological reality. First, it is not feasible that the sensitized lymphocytes or humoral antibodies have equal access to all cells within the tumor. Surviving cells are likely to be located in the hypoxic regions of a tumor where circulation is relatively inadequate, with the result that the IRR would react preferentially against the radiation-killed cells which are situated primarily in the well-vascularized portions of the lesion. There might be other bases for privileged sites within the tumor. However, as the tumor regresses and circulation improves, lymphocytes might have better access to the previously protected viable cells. Second, α is likely to be affected by the changes induced in the normal tissue surrounding the tumor. Third, the magnitude of an IRR is not likely to be constant during the period of regression: production rate of lymphocytes sensitized to a particular antigen will be affected by the lysis of radiation-killed cells. Finally, β and q almost certainly are not simple exponential processes.

Despite these legitimate reservations, the calculations presented here indicate strongly that an IRR which is effective in modifying TCP will have to be sufficient to inactivate a much larger number of viable tumor cells than simply the number which survives irradiation. This is because of the proliferation which will occur before the total number of cells has been reduced to a number approximately equal to α. In addition, any process which would increase the β/q ratio is likely to improve the effectiveness of an IRR. It may be that fractionation of radiation dose acts in that direction. During the course of irradiation, the killed cells are removed by the β process, and this process apparently would not be affected by the daily treatments. However, each treatment results in a certain delay in cell division. Hence, during therapy, cell removal would proceed at a rate near normal while proliferation of viable cells would be partially suppressed.

Many of the factors mentioned here can be subjected to quantitative evaluation in animal tumor systems.

Summary

A model tumor and a model immunologic rejection response are presented and the effect of the latter in modifying TCP following a specified radiation treatment is considered. Implications of the calculations for radiotherapy of tumors are discussed.

REFERENCES

Hammersley, J. M., and Handscomb, D. C.: *Monte Carlo Methods.* London, England, Methuen and Company, Ltd., 1964, 178 pp.

Suit, H. D., and Batten, G.: Implication of cell proliferation kinetics for radiation therapy. In *The Proliferation and Spread of Neoplastic Cells* (The University of Texas M. D. Anderson Hospital and Tumor Institute at Houston, Twenty-first Annual Symposium on Fundamental Cancer Research, 1967). Baltimore, Maryland, The Williams and Wilkins Company, 1968, pp. 423-439.

Suit, H. D., and Wette, R.: Theoretical considerations on the influence of dose fractionation on effectiveness of radiation therapy. In del Regato, J. A.: *Conference on Radiobiology and Radiotherapy* (National Cancer Institute Monograph 24). Washington, D. C., U. S. Government Printing Office, 1967, pp. 225-247.

Cellular Kinetics and Its Implication in Cancer Chemotherapy

FRANK M. SCHABEL, JR., Ph.D.

Kettering-Meyer Laboratories, Southern Research Institute,
Birmingham, Alabama

To BEGIN, I should define cellular kinetics in relation to cancer chemotherapy. Kinetics is a branch of dynamics that deals with the effects of forces on the motions of material bodies (Gove, 1961). The term is used here to describe the population kinetics of cancer cells under exposure to the cytotoxic activity of anticancer drugs. I will deal with population kinetics in describing attempts to measure the absolute numbers of cancer cells surviving drug treatment and the continuing multiplication of these cells after each dose or course of treatment. This information will be used in an attempt to establish how near we can come to the "cure" of experimental tumors with available drugs.

Theoretically, cancer arises when one normal cell changes into a malignant neoplastic cell, either by natural mutation or following chemical, viral, or radiation induction. Experimentally, my colleagues and I have repeatedly established fatal transplantable tumors of mice, rats, and hamsters—including leukemias, carcinomas, and sarcomas—by implantation of single, micromanipulator-isolated tumor cells (Schabel, 1968). Our chemotherapeutic concepts are based directly, therefore, on the probable necessity of destroying all tumor cells by drug treatment and/or immune mechanisms to achieve cure. Our work is concerned primarily with attempting to reduce the viable tumor cell population to less than one tumor cell per host animal with nonlethal doses of available drugs.

Frei and Freireich (1965) have estimated that the leukemic cell number at the time of diagnosis or relapse in many patients is about 10^{12} and that each leukemia cell weighs about 10^{-9} Gm. If one assumes that a tumor cell weighs about 10^{-9} Gm. (one billion cells per gram) on the average, then a patient with 100 Gm. of solid tumor in all sites at diagnosis

61

would have about 10^{11} tumor cells. To cure patients with tumor cell populations of this magnitude with drugs will require anticancer agents with a significant selective cytotoxicity for tumor cells as compared to vital normal cells. To reduce a population of 10^{12} tumor cells to less than one tumor cell would require a drug kill of more than 99.9999999999 per cent of the tumor cell population and a kill of not more than 99 to 99.9 per cent of vital normal cells; to kill more normal cells would be to go beyond what is probably the point of lethal toxicity for the most sensitive, vital normal cells in the bone marrow or the gut epithelium (Alexander, 1965). The few numbers cited suggest broadly the problem of successful cancer chemotherapy. Most of the anticancer agents currently available do not have selective cytotoxicity of the required order of magnitude for even the most drug-sensitive experimental tumors.

We recognize that we need better procedures for quantitating and comparing the selective cytotoxicity of known anticancer drugs and for developing improved methods for using these drugs. We have developed procedures for measuring the numbers of tumor cells surviving drug therapy in mice with leukemia L1210 (Skipper, Schabel, and Wilcox, 1964).

After parenteral implant (intraperitoneal, intravenous or intracerebral) of L1210 cells into BDF_1 mice (C57B1/6 female $\times$ DBA/2 male), life-span is related directly to the number of cells implanted, and this relationship is consistent down to one cell (Skipper, Schabel and Wilcox, 1964). Our experience in 1966 with intraperitoneally implanted cells is shown in Figure 1. There is an obvious and consistent relationship between the size of the L1210 cell implant and the median life-span of the host. The data reported here are essentially identical to those reported in 1964 (Skipper, Schabel, and Wilcox), and previous year-to-year comparisons of implant size to median life-span have been essentially identical to the 1966 experience.

The agreement between median life-span of mice implanted intraperitoneally with one micromanipulator-isolated L1210 cell and one cell isolated by dilution is very good. The mice implanted with one cell by dilution received a calculated one cell, based on log_{10} dilutions of hemacytometer-counted L1210 ascites fluid. On the basis of the Poisson distribution function, 37 per cent of mice receiving one tenth of a thoroughly mixed suspension which contained a total of 10 L1210 cells would be expected to receive no cells and not to develop leukemia. In 1966, 70 per cent of 1,675 mice implanted with one cell by dilution survived. In the absence of dilution error and 100 per cent viability of the L1210 cells, the mortality in this group—based on the Poisson distribution function— should have been 63 per cent instead of the observed 30 per cent. This

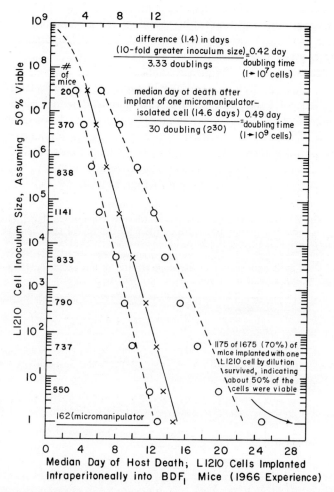

Fig. 1.—Relationship of size of inoculum to median life-span in BDF₁ mice which received intraperitoneal implants of leukemia L1210 cells. Abbreviations: ×, median; O, range.

suggests that the percentage of viable cells in the tumor cell suspensions used was about 50 per cent, on the average.

By determining the time from end of therapy to median day of death, we can estimate, from a plot such as this, the number of viable L1210 cells present at the end of therapy. We have used this procedure, along with host cure, to estimate the chemotherapeutic activity of drugs in vivo.

One of the most important observations which we have made from studies of this kind is of the first-order kinetics of drug kill of leukemia cells in vivo. By this I mean that in a random cell population, a constant percentage of the total leukemic cells, irrespective of population size, is killed by a given effective dose of a variety of different antileukemic agents. Data illustrating this principle are shown in Figure 2.

Here we have plotted the average life-span of mice implanted with $\log_{10}$ dilutions of leukemia P1534 cells and treated with a single, constant, and effective dose of vincristine. Significant and consistent percentages of kill, based on increase in life-span at each implant size, was seen. The parallel slopes of the two plots (treated and untreated) indicate constant percentage of kill by the same effective dose of vincristine over a 4 $\log_{10}$ range of implant sizes and further indicate that the doubling

Fig. 2.—Relationship between size of intraperitoneal implant and host life-span in untreated and host life-span in untreated and vincristine-treated DBA/2 mice which received implants of leukemia P1534 cells. Approximately equal per cent cell kill of all population sizes occurs, and the average doubling time of P1534 cells surviving vincristine therapy is approximately the same as that of untreated P1534 cells. Abbreviations: ●, untreated control mice; ▲, vincristine-treated mice.

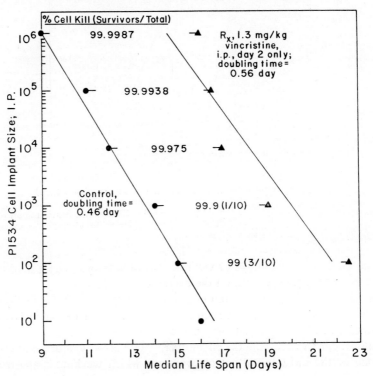

time of the leukemic cells surviving therapy was not changed by exposure to the drug. This principle of first-order cell kill kinetics by anticancer drugs is not restricted to a single tumor or a single drug; we have observed similar constant log kill of L1210 cells in vivo with representatives of the major classes of antileukemic agents, including amethopterin, 5-fluoro-uracil, cytosine arabinoside, 6-mercaptopurine, Cytoxan, and several of the active nitrosoureas (Skipper, Schabel, and Wilcox, 1964; Schabel, 1968). In addition, data based on extended observations of from six months to over a year in drug-"cured" leukemic mice indicate that treatment of mice bearing L1210 cells with representatives of the major classes of antileukemic agents did *not* result in the selection of viable leukemic cells with a long drug-induced lag phase of growth (Skipper, Schabel, and Wilcox, 1964, 1965; Schabel, 1968).

Since we do not know of any anticancer drug which will "cure" advanced experimental leukemia with a single dose lethal for 10 per cent of test subjects (LD_{10}) nor any drug with a log kill potential for any tumor cell in vivo of as much as 10^9 tumor cells, it appears that "cure" of advanced experimental tumors—and probably of tumors in man—with available drugs will require repeated dose therapy.

Using the principles of experimental plan and data analysis described, we have attempted to improve the therapeutic effectiveness of drugs in treating both experimental leukemias and experimental solid tumors.

Experimental Leukemias

1-β-D-Arabinofuranosylcytosine · HCL, otherwise known as cytosine arabinoside or arabinosylcytosine, is known to block the synthesis of deoxycytidylic acid and thus interfere with the synthesis of deoxyribonucleic acid (DNA); this action leads to the death of tumor cells in culture (see Skipper, Schabel, and Wilcox, 1967, for pertinent references to the biological activity of Ara C). 1-β-D-Arabinofuranosylcytosine (Ara C) also has consistent but not spectacular antileukemic activity against L1210 cells in mice when treatment is given once a day for 15 days or daily until death. We reasoned that multiple exposures during two average cell-doubling cycles should expose most of a metabolically random L1210 cell population to Ara C one or more times during the sensitive phase of DNA synthesis.

Results of a study to test this idea are illustrated in Figure 3. This is a graphic idealization of leukemic cell kill when Ara C is given on a daily 2- to 16-day-treatment schedule or on a multiple daily schedule every fourth day for four courses. We implanted approximately 5×10^4 viable

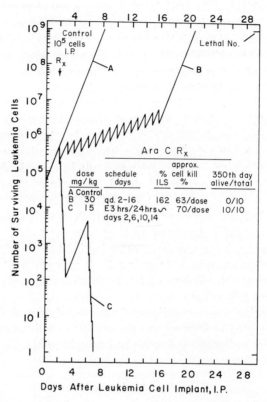

Fig. 3.—Idealization of results of a comparison of the effect of two dosage schedules on the in vivo activity of 1-β-D-Arabinofuranosylcytosine · HCL (Ara C) against L1210.

L1210 cells intraperitoneally into mice. Line A is a graphic idealization of the population kinetics of untreated mice. The median day of death in untreated control animals was day eight. Line B represents the population kinetics of mice similarly implanted and treated once a day with the LD_{10} dose of Ara C for 15 days (daily two through 16 days). Here we saw an increased life-span of 162 per cent over untreated controls, but no survivors. Assuming a constant log kill with each daily dose of drug and an unaltered doubling time in the leukemic cells surviving each dose of drug, we can calculate an approximate 63 per cent cell kill with each daily dose of Ara C. For a tumor cell with a doubling time of approximately half a day, e.g. the L1210 cell (Fig. 1), one would have to kill more than 75 per cent of the total population each day to predict ultimate cure with extended periods of daily therapy with Ara C. Since the dose used here was the LD_{10}, it is apparent that one could never predictably cure L1210 with Ara C on this dosage schedule unless the leukemic cell population at the start of therapy was very small (less than 10 viable cells). When we treat every three hours for 24 hours, every fourth day for four courses (Line C), we rarely fail to cure 100 per cent of mice. Subsequent experiments indicated that after two 24-hour courses at four-day intervals with Ara C and at the dose indicated, some animals survived. This indicates that at the end of the second course on this dose and treatment schedule, the number of surviving L1210 cells was reduced to approximately one cell per mouse. Since the dose of Ara C used (15 mg./kg./dose) on this multiple treatment schedule is the LD_{10} for this schedule, it is apparent that we are reducing the viable tumor cell population into the range of cures with approximately one-half the cumulative LD_{10} of Ara C on this schedule (Skipper, Schabel, and Wilcox, 1967; Schabel, 1968).

Hydroxyurea, another known inhibitor of DNA synthesis, shows an improvement in therapeutic activity against L1210 on multiple daily dose-multiple course therapy similar to that seen with Ara C (Schabel, 1968).

Evans, Bostwick, and Mengel (1964) reported therapeutic potentiation of Ara C by porfiromycin against two mouse leukemias, L1210 and P1534. We readily confirmed their observations. Since we had nitrosoureas significantly superior to porfiromycin when used alone, we tried using Ara C plus 1-(2-chloroethyl)-3-cyclohexyl-1-nitrosourea (CCNU) against *intravenously* implanted L1210. Intraperitoneal therapy was begun either 24 or 48 hours prior to the median day of death in untreated control mice. Twenty-four hours prior to the median day of death in untreated control mice that were intravenously implanted with L1210 cells, we can measure more than 10^8 viable L1210 cells in each mouse by sensitive bioassay (Skipper *et al.*, 1965), and the disease can be diagnosed clinically on the basis of elevated white blood cell counts (Schabel, 1968).

Figure 4 is a similar graphic illustration of the therapeutic activity of Ara C alone, CCNU alone, and Ara C plus CCNU on optimum therapy schedules for Ara C; therapy was begun 24 or 48 hours prior to median day of death in untreated control mice. At the LD_{10} of Ara C alone, lifespan was increased; but there were no survivors. CCNU alone at its optimum schedule—that is, single dose LD_{10}—reduced the viable L1210 cell population to about one cell per mouse when therapy was begun 48 hours before median day of death; but when therapy was begun 24 hours before median day of death, only very slight therapeutic activity was seen. However, when the two drugs were given in combination every three hours

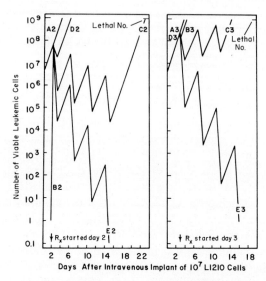

Agent	Dose, I.P. mg/kg	Schedule	% ILS	Approx. Cell kill (%)	200th Day Alive/Total
A2 Control					
B2 CCNU	40	Day 2 only	250	99.999997	4/10
C2 Ara C	15	E3 hrs/24hrs,	475	99.4/course	0/9
D2 CCNU	2.5	days 2,6,10,14	50	72/course	0/10
E2 AraC+CCNU	10+2.5		925	99.985/course	9/10
A3 Control					
B3 CCNU	50	Day 3 only	12	61	0/10
C3 Ara C	10	E3hrs/24hrs,	262	98/course	0/10
D3 CCNU	2.5	days 3,7,11,15	0	0/course	0/10
E3 Ara C+CCNU	10+2.5		400	99.982/course	4/10

Fig. 4.—Approximation of leukemia L1210 cell kill by optimal dose therapy at the LD$_{10}$ or less with 1-β-D-Arabinofuranosylcytosine · HCL (Ara C), 1-(2-chloroethyl)-3-cyclohexyl-1-nitrosourea (CCNU), or Ara C plus CCNU, beginning 48 or 24 hours prior to median day of death in untreated control mice. Abbreviation: ILS, increase in life-span.

for 24 hours, every fourth day beginning 48 hours after implant (48 hours before median day of death), 90 per cent of the treated animals survived. If combination therapy was delayed until 24 hours before median day of death, at a time when each mouse was bearing in excess of 10^8 viable leukemic cells and when the disease was clinically diagnosable on the basis of peripheral white counts, the LD$_{10}$ combination therapy (Line E3) reduced the viable leukemic cells per mouse to approximately one cell per mouse, and 40 per cent of such treated animals survived indefinitely.

This degree of therapeutic activity was seen with no more than a 99.9 per cent kill of the vital normal cells, a figure generally considered to describe lethal toxicity. These observations have been confirmed repeatedly.

I do not support the position that the combination of Ara C plus CCNU is the panacea that we all seek for human leukemia. Available clinical data indicate that Ara C is much less effective in man than in mice, probably as a result, at least in part, of the fact that (1) man deaminates Ara C to inactive arabinosyluracil very rapidly (Camiener and Smith, 1965; Creasey *et al.*, 1966), and because (2) most human tumors probably have a lower percentage of the total, viable, tumor cell population in the sensitive phase of DNA synthesis at any given time than does rapidly fulminating leukemia L1210. Similarly, the effectiveness of CCNU is still unproved in man. The only point I would make from these observations is that, at least with some experimental systems, marked therapeutic improvement of anticancer drugs can be obtained with rationally directed modifications of treatment schedules and favorable drug combinations.

Population Kinetics of Experimental Solid Tumors under Drug Therapy

We have attempted to carry over the experimental principles and concepts developed with murine leukemias to studies on the population kinetics of solid tumor cells under drug treatment in vivo. Wilcox *et al.* (1965) developed the concept that regression and regrowth of a solid tumor after temporarily affective single dose therapy with an active anticancer drug could be considered a constantly varying summation of two factors: (1) resorption of drug-killed tumor cells added to (2) continuing multiplication of tumor cells surviving the therapy.

This concept is illustrated in Figure 5. The solid line in this figure was drawn from actual data derived from an experiment in which a transplantable plasmacytoma of hamsters (Fortner, Mahy, and Cotran, 1961) was treated with a single nonlethal and noncurative dose of Cytoxan. Assuming that the tumor cells surviving therapy continue to grow at the same rate after treatment as they did before and that the drug-killed cells will be resorbed at some approximately constant rate after drug kill, one can conceive that the viable cells surviving therapy in a drug-sensitive solid tumor could be much fewer than would be estimated from observations on tumor mass after drug therapy.

Since we have a sensitive bioassay procedure for viable plasmacytoma cells in hamsters, we put this concept to direct experimental test. The results of a representative experiment of this kind are shown in Figure 6 (Skipper, 1968).

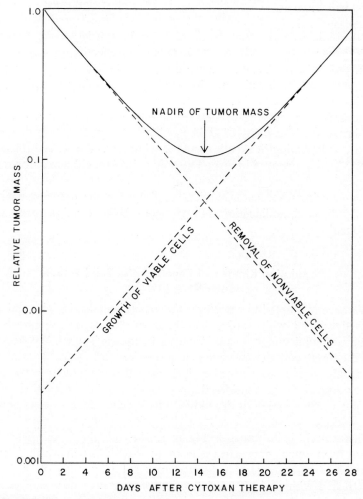

Fig. 5.—Plasmacytoma No. 1 (a hamster tumor). Regression and recurrence after administration of a single, nonlethal, and noncurative dose of Cytoxan. Initial "killing" of 99.7 per cent of the cells is shown. Solid curve shows calculated net mass of the tumor.

Hamsters received subcutaneous trocar implants of plasmacytoma No. 1. About four to five days postimplant, the tumor was large enough to be palpable (about 60 mg.). In untreated controls, it continued to grow at an approximately exponential rate for about eight to 10 additional days, at which time the increase in tumor mass became asymptotic (Line A).

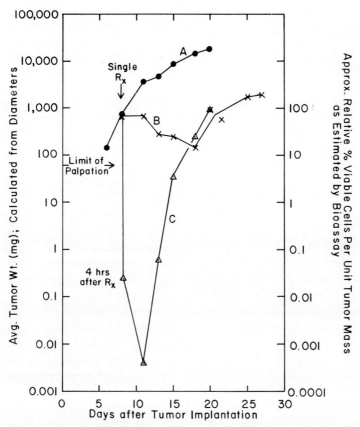

Fig. 6.—Relationships between behavior of solid tumor mass and tumor cell viability after a single dose of Cytoxan. Line **A** shows the weights of untreated control tumors. Line **B** shows the weights of treated tumors after a single dose of Cytoxan (25 mg./kg.) on day eight only; the nadir is on day 18, 10 days after treatment; about 80 per cent regression of tumor mass occurs. Line **C** shows the approximate relative per cent of viable tumor cells per unit of tumor mass as determined by in vivo bioassay; about 99.999 per cent tumor cell kill is achieved by a single dose of Cytoxan; the nadir occurs shortly after treatment. NOTE: For this study, hamsters received subcutaneous implants of plasmacytoma No. 1, a tumor which is unusually sensitive to alkylating agents, but not to other classes of antitumor agents.

After single dose treatment of animals bearing 700- to 800-mg. tumors with a nontoxic, noncurative, but effective dose of Cytoxan (Line B), the tumor mass remained essentially static for a few days and then regressed modestly, reaching a nadir in five to seven days. The tumor then resumed growth at a rate approximating its exponential rate of increase prior to drug treatment. Bioassay of the viable tumor cells before drug treatment and during the period of regression and regrowth (Line C) indicated that the viable tumor cells per unit mass of the tumor decreased four to five logs between four and 24 hours post-therapy, and that the surviving tumor cells then repopulated the tumor at a growth rate approximating that of the previously untreated tumor. Similar observations of tumor mass and bioassay of viable tumor cells after single drug treatment of mice with sarcoma 180 and mice with adenocarcinoma 755 yielded essentially the same results as those presented here for hamsters with plasmacytoma.

Two very important concepts are derived from these common observations: (1) tumor cell kill by effective drugs may be underestimated significantly from tumor mass observations following effective drug treatment, and (2) the optimum time for following sequential therapy is probably as soon after the first dose as recovery of vital normal cells will allow and not at the nadir or during obvious regrowth of the solid tumor. In attempting to test some of these principles with solid tumors in experimental animals, we have carried out some interesting experiments with adenocarcinoma 755 in mice.

The results of a typical experiment are shown in Figure 7. In this experiment, we implanted BDF_1 mice subcutaneously with adenocarcinoma 755 and allowed the tumors to grow until day seven, at which time they weighed an average of 500 mg. We then treated groups of 10 animals with one to four courses of Cytoxan followed by 6-mercaptopurine in sequence. Figure 7 is a cumulative mortality plot of these drug-treated, tumor-bearing animals. There was 100 per cent mortality in the untreated control mice; the median day of death was about 24 and the extreme length of life was about 46 days. The single dose of Cytoxan or a single course of 6-mercaptopurine failed to cure any of the treated animals, but did increase the median day of death from about 25 to about 45 days. Following a single course of the two drugs in sequence, another increase in life-span to median day of death was obtained, and in 40 per cent of the treated animals the tumors regressed completely. These animals are alive and grossly tumor-free more than 230 days postimplant. Of these 30 animals receiving two, three, or four courses of Cytoxan followed by 6-mercaptopurine, total and permanent tumor regression occurred in 28 and these animals are alive and grossly tumor-free more than 230 days postimplant. The one tumor that failed to completely regress and the one that reappeared in the two uncured animals have been passed to recipient mice and have been shown to be resistant to treatment with 6-mercaptopurine. In other experiments, we have failed to cure any mice bearing

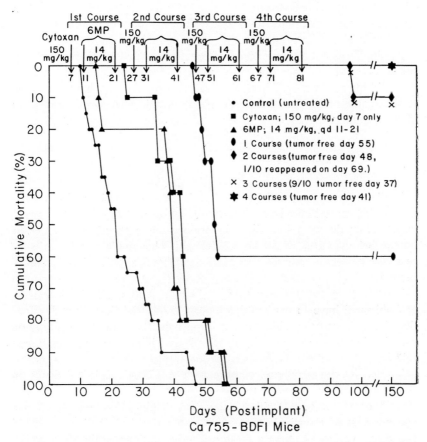

Fig. 7.—Cumulative mortality in mice with advanced adenocarcinoma 755 (mean tumor weight, 500 mg. plus or minus 100 mg.) which were given one or more non-lethal courses of sequential therapy with Cytoxan followed by 6-mercaptopurine.

500-mg. tumors with sequential Cytoxan or 6-mercaptopurine alone at up to frankly toxic doses.

Cured mice similar to those described above have been reimplanted (along with control mice of the same age which were not previously exposed to adenocarcinoma 755) with adenocarcinoma 755. All animals developed lethal tumors, and the median life-spans in previously cured and control mice were not significantly different. These observations in cured animals subsequently challenged with adenocarcinoma 755 indicate that the cured were indistinguishable from those not previously exposed to the tumor; further, they support the conclusion that multiple course therapy with Cytoxan followed by 6-mercaptopurine cured (reduced the viable cell population to less than the number of cells required to re-establish the detectable tumor) these animals.

Again, I do not support the position that sequential therapy of Cytoxan followed by 6-mercaptopurine is the panacea that we seek for treating solid tumors in man. These observations do point out, however, some of the requirements for "cure" of solid tumors in animals and probably also in man, and they suggest some of the likely requirements for the curative drug treatment of human beings with tumors.

Discussion

While my associates and I treat experimental tumors in laboratory rodents with some limited success, we recognize that this is not our real target. How do we relate these laboratory observations to diseases in human beings? Little of the knowledge which has made our limited success with tumors in animals possible is available for application to tumors in man.

To "cure" a tumor—any tumor—in man with available drugs, we probably will have to use multiple course sequential therapy with effective single drugs or combinations of drugs, since we know of no drug or combination of drugs capable of selectively killing 10^9 or more tumor cells in man or animals at single LD_{10} doses or less.

To predict the likelihood of cure with any known selected drugs or course of therapy, we need to know a great deal about the population kinetics of the tumor cell with which we are dealing. For example, if only one per cent of the viable tumor cell population is in active cell cycle (synthesizing DNA), then a totally effective antimetabolite drug active only against cells synthesizing DNA would result in a maximum tumor cell destruction of only one per cent. It seems apparent that the antimetabolites may have maximum application against tumors with a relatively high percentage of the viable tumor cells in an active DNA synthesis cycle. This renews the desirability of the often discussed but yet-to-be-demonstrated stimulator to tumor cell growth. If we knew of a compound that would stimulate metabolically inactive but viable tumor cells to enter into active DNA synthesis, we should be able to increase greatly the log kill of that tumor cell population by antimetabolites, such as amethopterin, Ara C, hydroxyurea, or the purine analogues.

The cytotoxic activity of the alkylating agents against tumor cells, irrespective of the metabolic state of the cells, makes them very attractive anticancer agents, but generally vital normal cell recovery from alkylating agent toxicity takes a long time. Drugs with significant cytotoxicity for vital normal cells cannot be given repeatedly at a time interval shorter than that required for total vital normal cell recovery from the previous dose. If the tumor cells surviving the first course of sequential therapy replace the number killed by drug faster than normal vital cells can recover, extension of life will result, but cure (reduction to less than the

Fig. 8.—Matching cancer cell population size, per cent cell kill per dose or course, rate of cancer cell recovery, and rate of host recovery from sublethal drug toxicity. A, approximate size of cancer cell population at beginning of treatment (e.g. at diagnosis of leukemia or perhaps after surgical therapy in the instance of solid tumors). B, approximate size of surviving (viable) cancer cell population after a *single* dose or course of treatment; approximately the same per cent of the proliferating cells is killed, regardless of number, by a given dose (in vivo exposure) of a specific drug or radiation. This per cent kill by a given dose is related to the sensitivity of the type of cancer. C1, rate of recovery of the cancer cell population resulting from proliferation of cells that survive treatment; this rate is usually comparable to the doubling time of the untreated tumor cell population (C2). D, host recovery time (time at which a second dose or course may be administered without significant or unacceptable cumulative host toxicity). D1, hypothetical illustration in which host recovery time is shorter than recovery time of the cancer cell population. D2, hypothetical illustration in which the recovery time for the cancer cell population is shorter than the host recovery time. NOTE: A continued, constant per cent tumor cell kill might be expected until drug resistance intervened or unless or until tumor cells metastasized to anatomic sites where exposure to drug was relatively poor, e.g. the central nervous system. If, with the use of any tolerated dosage level or any spacing in the administration of a given agent, it is impossible to destroy neoplastic cells (with or without host-immune assistance) faster than they are replaced by the proliferation of surviving cells, tumor cell eradication will be impossible.

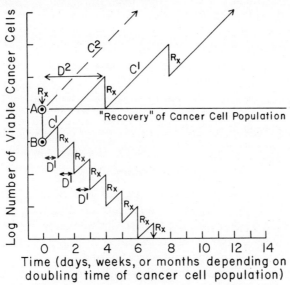

minimum number of tumor cells necessary to allow regrowth of the tumor after therapy is terminated) by sequential treatment with such agents is theoretically impossible. Figure 8 graphically illustrates the simplest tumor cell kinetic circumstances under which success or failure to cure tumors with sequential drug therapy may be visualized (Skipper, 1967).

The most promising areas of future research in the chemotherapeutic control of cancer are:

(1) Searching for new agents with an even greater selective cytotoxicity for tumor cells than those now known,

(2) Searching for highly active compounds, such as the alkylating agents and nitrosoureas, with a shorter vital normal cell recovery time than those now known, and

(3) Extending the very promising work which is being conducted by both clinical and experimental cancer chemotherapists in the demonstration and development of drug combinations with greater therapeutic activity than the component agents alone and with additive, or less than additive, combination toxicity for vital normal cells.

My associates and I think that we are beginning to understand many of the dynamic factors involved in the population kinetics of tumor cells in some experimental tumors. That some of these principles can be applied effectively to clinical cancer chemotherapy in man is evidenced by the success of Hertz and his associates in treating women with choriocarcinoma or related trophoblastic diseases with methotrexate alone or methotrexate plus actinomycin D (Ross *et al.*, 1965); the experience of Burkitt, Clifford, and others in treating Burkitt's lymphoma with alkylating agents, methotrexate, or vincristine (Burchenal and Burkitt, 1967); Farber's success in treating Wilms' tumor with surgical therapy plus dactinomycin (actinomycin D) and/or local irradiation (Farber, 1966); and the success of several active groups, including Drs. Frei and Freireich at The University of Texas M. D. Anderson Hospital and Tumor Institute at Houston, in managing acute lymphatic leukemia with several different sequential multiple drug-treatment programs (Frei and Freireich, 1965).

Acknowledgments

The work reported in this paper that was conducted in the Kettering-Meyer Laboratories of the Southern Research Institute was supported by Contract PH43-65-594 with the Cancer Chemotherapy National Service Center, National Cancer Institute, National Institutes of Health, and by Grant T-111 from the American Cancer Society.

In presenting this report, the author wishes to point out that the concepts, experimental designs, and data analyses presented were a result of the joint efforts of H. E. Skipper, the late W. S. Wilcox, W. R. Laster, Jr., D. P. Griswold, Jr., J. G. Mayo, and M. W. Trader. Excellent technical support was provided by M. H. Witt, J. A. Bowers, C. M. Andrews, A. Brazier, L. Mattil, and their laboratory associates.

REFERENCES

Alexander, P.: *Atomic Radiation and Life*. 2d edition. Baltimore, Maryland, Penguin Books, 1965, 296 pp.

Burchenal, J. H., and Burkitt, D. P., Editors: *Treatment of Burkitt's Tumour* (UICC Monograph Series, Vol. 8). Berlin and Heidelberg, Germany, and New York, New York, Springer-Verlag, 1967, 268 pp.

Camiener, G. W., and Smith, C. G.: Studies of the enzymatic deamination of cytosine arabinoside. I. Enzyme distribution and species specificity. *Biochemical Pharmacology*, 14:1405-1416, October 1965.

Creasey, W. A., Papac, R. J., Markiw, M. E., Calabresi, P., and Welch, A. D.: Biochemical and pharmacological studies with 1-β-D-arabinofuranosylcytosine in man. *Biochemical Pharmacology*, 15:1417-1428, October 1966.

Evans, J. S., Bostwick, L., and Mengel, G. D.: Synergism of the antineoplastic activity of cytosine arabinoside by porfiromycin. *Biochemical Pharmacology*, 13:983-988, July 1964.

Farber, S.: Chemotherapy in the treatment of leukemia and Wilms' tumor. *Journal of the American Medical Association*, 198:826-836, November 21, 1966.

Fortner, J. G., Mahy, A. G., and Cotran, R. S.: Transplantable tumors of the Syrian (golden) hamster. II. Tumors of the hematopoietic tissues, genitourinary organs, mammary glands, and sarcomas. *Cancer Research*, 21:199-234, July 1961.

Frei, E., III, and Freireich, E. J.: Progress and perspectives in the chemotherapy of acute leukemia. In Goldin, A., Hawking, F., and Schnitzer, R. J., Eds.: *Advances in Chemotherapy*. New York, New York, Academic Press, Inc., 1965, Vol. 2, pp. 269-298.

Gove, P. B., Editor: *Webster's Third New International Dictionary of the English Language* (unabridged). Springfield, Massachusetts, G. and C. Merriam Company, 1961, 2,662 pp.

Ross, G. T., Goldstein, D. P., Hertz, R., Lipsett, M. B., and Odell, W. D.: Sequential use of Methotrexate and actinomycin D in the treatment of metastatic choriocarcinoma and related trophoblastic diseases in women. *American Journal of Obstetrics and Gynecology*, 93:223-229, September 15, 1965.

Schabel, F. M., Jr.: In vivo leukemic cell kill kinetics and "curability" in experimental systems. In *The Proliferation and Spread of Neoplastic Cells* (The University of Texas M. D. Anderson Hospital and Tumor Institute at Houston, Twenty-first Annual Symposium on Fundamental Cancer Research, 1967). Baltimore, Maryland, The Williams and Wilkins Company, 1968, pp. 379-408.

Skipper, H. E.: Kinetic considerations associated with therapy of solid tumors. In *The Proliferation and Spread of Neoplastic Cells* (The University of Texas M. D. Anderson Hospital and Tumor Institute at Houston, Twenty-first Annual Symposium on Fundamental Cancer Research, 1967). Baltimore, Maryland, The Williams and Wilkins Company, 1968, pp. 213-233.

————: Some types of quantitative and kinetic information worth seeking and considering in the design of therapeutic trials. In Burchenal, J. H., and Burkitt, D. P., Eds.: *Treatment of Burkitt's Tumour* (UICC Monograph Series, Vol. 8). Berlin and Heidelberg, Germany, and New York, New York, Springer-Verlag, 1967, pp. 122-125.

Skipper, H. E., Schabel, F. M., Jr., and Wilcox, W. S.: Experimental evaluation of potential anticancer agents. XIII. On the criteria and kinetics associated with "curability" of experimental leukemias. *Cancer Chemotherapy Reports,* 35:1-111, February 1964.

————: Experimental evaluation of potential anticancer agents. XIV. Further study of certain basic concepts underlying chemotherapy of leukemia. *Cancer Chemotherapy Reports,* 45:5-28, April 1965.

————: Experimental evaluation of potential anticancer agents. XXI. Scheduling of arabinosylcytosine to take advantage of its S-phase specificity against leukemia cells. *Cancer Chemotherapy Reports,* 51:125-165, June 1967.

Skipper, H. E., Schabel, F. M., Jr., Wilcox, W. S., Laster, W. R., Jr., Trader, M. W., and Thompson, S. A.: Experimental evaluation of potential anticancer agents. XVIII. Effects of therapy on viability and rate of proliferation of leukemic cells in various anatomic sites. *Cancer Chemotherapy Reports,* 47:41-64, August 1965.

Wilcox, W. S., Griswold, D. P., Laster, W. R., Jr., Schabel, F. M. Jr., and Skipper, H. E.: Experimental evaluation of potential anticancer agents. XVII. Kinetics of growth and regression after treatment of certain solid tumors. *Cancer Chemotherapy Reports,* 47:27-39, August 1965.

Angiography in Childhood Neoplasia

SIDNEY WALLACE, M.D.

Department of Diagnostic Radiology,
The University of Texas M. D. Anderson Hospital and
Tumor Institute at Houston, Houston, Texas

ANGIOGRAPHY, *e.g.,* arteriography, venography, and lymphangiography, is of considerable value in the diagnosis and treatment of pediatric patients with neoplasia. These techniques also foster a greater understanding of the morphologic and physiologic changes involved in cancer.

Arteriography

TECHNIQUE

The techniques currently utilized, *i.e.,* direct arterial puncture and arterial catheterization, have been described in the medical literature in detail. Arterial catheterization (Seldinger, 1953) is employed most frequently via the femoral artery. At present, selective arteriography performed with a preformed catheter is the preferred method. Needles, wire guides, and catheters suitable for use in the pediatric age group are available (Desilets, Ruttenberg, and Hoffman, 1966).

SUBTRACTION.—The subtraction technique (Ziedses des Plantes, 1934) by which extraneous shadows are neutralized is a procedure complementary to angiography and may be done photographically or electronically. Our modification of the photographic method was devised by Seymour Sterling, Albert Einstein Medical Center, Philadelphia, Pennsylvania (Fig. 1).

The equipment required includes:

1. Light source. The Blu-Ray copier ordinarily is used for film duplication.

2. Radiographic film.

3. Commercial film. Single emulsion film is used in the first step to make the "negative."

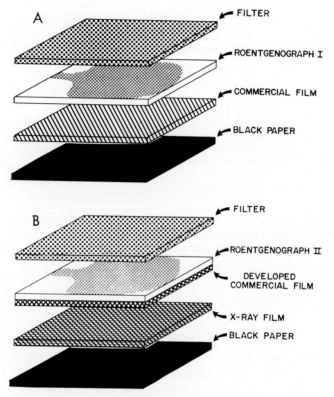

Fig. 1.—Subtraction technique (Seymour Sterling, Albert Einstein Medical Center, Philadelphia, Pennsylvania). **A**, in the initial step, the above sandwich is passed through the Blu-Ray copier. The commercial film is processed in the usual manner. **B**, the final step consists of the passage of the second sandwich through the Blu-Ray copier. The permanent record is on x-ray film which is processed in the usual manner.

4. Processing unit. This can be any method employed for routine radiographic processing.

5. Filters. These are made by exposing radiographic film to the Blu-Ray copier at different light settings. The filter regulates the amount of light striking the film "sandwich." The specific filter used depends on the density of the radiograph to be subtracted.

6. Black paper. This absorbs the transmitted light, lessening the effect of any reflected light.

The results obtained with this procedure are illustrated in Figure 2, which shows the carotid arteriogram of an eight-year-old female with a recurrent ependymoma. The opacification of the tentorial artery—a cavernous branch of the internal carotid artery—with a subsequent tumor

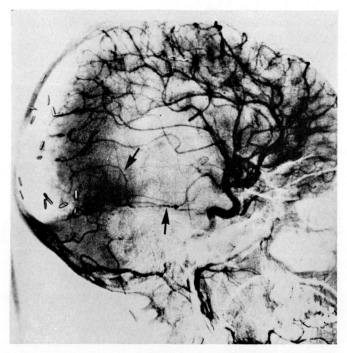

Fig. 2.—A recurrent ependymoma invading the tentorium is being supplied by the tentorial artery, a branch of the cavernous portion of the internal carotid artery.

stain, provides the additional information that the ependymoma invaded the tentorium (Wallace, Goldberg, Leeds, and Mishkin, 1967). The subtraction technique makes information, which by necessity must be present, more obvious.

CRITERIA

Absolute arteriographic criteria for malignant disease are few. There are two fairly dependable findings which are seen primarily with malignant disease.

1. Abrupt and irregular changes in caliber of vessels are manifestations of invasion of the vessels by malignant disease.

2. Perivascular laking of contrast material outside the vessels probably is representative of the new vascularity of the tumor.

Secondary findings include:

1. Distortion, displacement, and occlusion of normal vessels.

2. Hypervascularity. The number of vessels opacified increases.

3. Tumor stain. A capillary blush is seen in the tumor area.

4. Arteriovenous shunting. The filling of veins during the arterial phase represents rapid circulation.

These secondary findings are not specific for malignant disease; they also may be found in patients with occlusive vascular disease, inflammation, necrosis, and benign neoplasms.

APPLICATIONS

Arteriography has been of assistance in: (1) localizing the lesion, (2) establishing the specific diagnosis, (3) delineating the blood supply of the lesion, and (4) determining residual disease and thereby aiding in the evaluation of the effect of therapy.

Cerebral arteriography is performed most frequently by direct puncture of the carotid or vertebral vessels. In children, the technique may be done easily via retrograde femoral artery catheterization. Multiple vessels may be studied arteriographically after one arterial puncture.

JUVENILE ANGIOFIBROMA OF NASOPHARYNX.—In addition to intracranial disease, arteriography can be used in the diagnosis and management of nasopharyngeal lesions, such as juvenile angiofibromas. Opacification of the vessels nourishing this richly vascular neoplasm permits confirmation of the diagnosis since biopsy is a dangerous procedure in this instance. The surgical treatment frequently is complicated by exsanguination. Knowledge of the vascular supply is, therefore, of the utmost importance in planning the therapeutic approach. In the child shown in Figure 3, the external carotid artery supplies the lesion; whereas in the child shown in Figure 4, the external carotid artery and the inferior cavernous sinus branch of the cavernous portion of the internal carotid artery are the major sources of tumor nourishment (Wallace, Goldberg, Leeds, and Mishkin, 1967).

ABDOMINAL ARTERIOGRAPHY.—The differential diagnosis of abdominal lesions is improved by arteriography (Baum, Kuroda, and Roy, 1965; Hope and Dorus, 1965). This is especially true in the evaluation of retroperitoneal masses. Retrograde femoral artery catheterization with selective injection of the specific visceral vessel is the preferred approach. However, in the examination of smaller children and in the search for unknown sites of primary lesions, a midline aortagram may be safer and may yield more information.

PHEOCHROMOCYTOMA.—The importance of the localization of a lesion is illustrated by the child shown in Figure 5, who was evaluated for hypertension by Singleton at Texas Children's Hospital, Houston, Texas. The

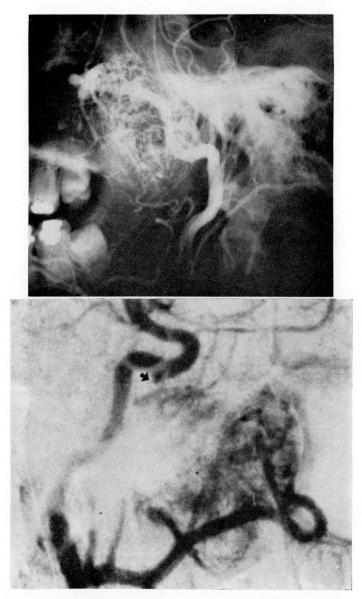

Fig. 3 (above).—Angiofibroma of the nasopharynx supplied by the external carotid artery.

Fig. 4 (below).—Angiofibroma of the nasopharynx supplied by both the external carotid artery and the inferior cavernous sinus branch (arrow) of the cavernous portion of the internal carotid artery.

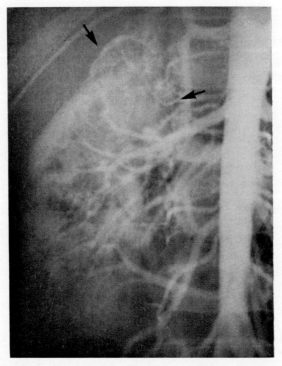

Fig. 5.—Pheochromocytoma. This very vascular adrenal neoplasm was opacified in an aortogram. (Courtesy of E. Singleton, Texas Children's Hospital, Houston, Texas.)

aortogram opacified a very vascular adrenal neoplasm, a pheochromocytoma. When combined with the clinical and laboratory findings, the angiographic pattern, although not pathognomonic, established the diagnosis and site of involvement (Boijsen, Williams, and Judkins, 1966; Kahn and Nickrosz, 1967). Pheochromocytomas are usually richly vascular lesions; however, at times they can show relatively few abnormal vessels (Weber, Janower, and Griscom, 1967). Adrenal venography has been used to great advantage in demonstrating pheochromocytomas (Reuter, Blair, Schteingart, and Bookstein, 1967). Care must be taken to prepare for any crisis which might be precipitated by the intravascular injection.

NEUROBLASTOMA.—Neuroblastoma, a frequent neoplasm of childhood, can be opacified (Fig. 6). In the child shown in Figure 6, the inferior adrenal artery originated from the renal artery, outlining a richly vascular lesion. Another child, a five-year-old female, was examined to

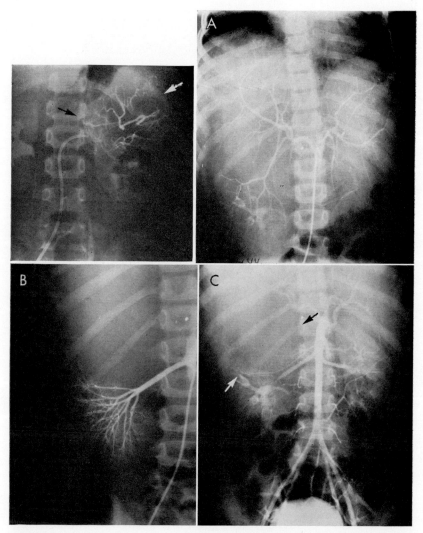

Fig. 6 (above left).—Neuroblastoma. The inferior adrenal artery originated from the renal artery and outlined a richly vascular lesion. (From U. S. Naval Hospital, San Diego, California.)

Fig. 7 (above right and below).—Neuroblastoma. **A,** selective hepatic arteriography demonstrates displacement and distortion of the intrahepatic branches. This probably is caused by extensive metastasis. **B,** selective renal arteriography demonstrates the distorted and depressed right kidney. **C,** the aortogram demonstrates the adrenal vessels originating from the right renal artery and the abdominal aorta. The pelvocaliceal system of the right kidney is displaced. The kidney is not invaded. The suprarenal lesion is a neuroblastoma.

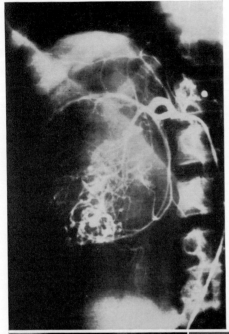

Fig. 8 (above).—Wilms' tumor. Renal angiography demonstrates the abnormal vessels in the Wilms' tumor. (Courtesy of E. Boijsen, University of Lund, Sweden).

Fig. 9 (below).—Wilms' tumor. Selective renal angiography demonstrates the abnormal vessels more clearly, especially when only a few can be opacified. A, early arterial phase; B, late arterial and capillary opacification.

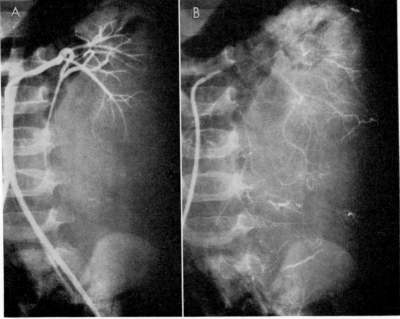

delineate more specifically the etiology of a right upper quadrant mass. Selective hepatic arteriography revealed marked distortion of the intra-hepatic branches which probably was caused by extensive infiltrative metastases. A distorted and depressed right kidney with a normal, al-though displaced, vascular pattern was seen after right renal artery injec-tion. A midline aortagram verified the existence of a right adrenal mass, a neuroblastoma (Fig. 7).

WILMS' TUMOR.—A frequent differential diagnostic problem is the evaluation of the enlarged kidney with distortion of the pelvo-caliceal system (Boijsen, 1959; Greenberg, Altman, and Litt, 1967; Puyau, 1965). A variety of conditions could be indicated, among them—Wilms' tumors, cystic kidneys, or hydronephrosis. In most Wilms' tumors, pathologic ves-sels can be seen by careful scrutiny of the vascular pattern. The more selective approach allows better filling of these abnormal vessels (Figs. 8 and 9). Occasionally, especially when studied by a midline aortogram,

Fig. 10.—Bilateral Wilms' tumor. The midline aortogram opacifies the vessels to each kidney. There are only a few abnormal vessels in the left Wilms' tumor (arrow). The majority of the lesion was necrotic. No obvious tumor vessels are seen in the right Wilms' tumor. The renal vessels merely are displaced.

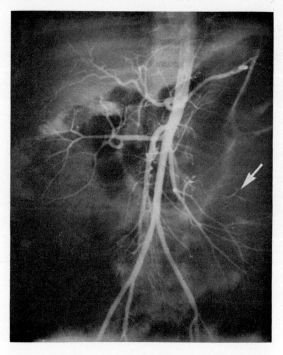

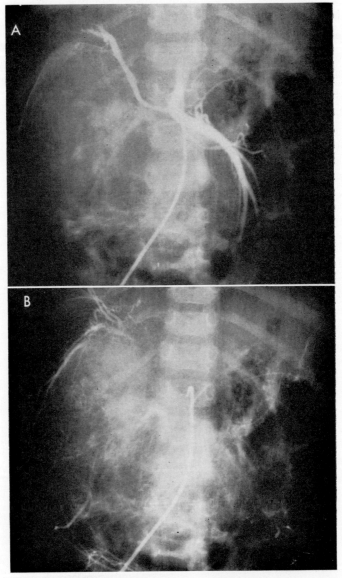

Fig. 11.—Leiomyoma. The selective celiac arteriogram demonstrates a large lesion attached to the capsule of the liver and fed by the celiac vessels. A, early arterial phase; B, late arterial and capillary phases. (Courtesy of S. Baum, Graduate Hospital, University of Pennsylvania, Philadelphia, Pennsylvania.)

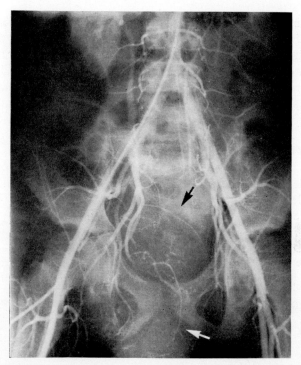

Fig. 12.—Undifferentiated sarcoma of the pelvis. The lesion is supplied primarily by the right internal iliac artery. The limits of the lesion are delineated by the vascular supply. There is also opacification of the metastases in the body of the fifth lumbar and in the right ischium.

the Wilms' tumor may appear relatively avascular. Figure 10 is the aortogram of a seven-month-old child with a bilateral Wilms' tumor. Only a few abnormal vessels are seen in the huge left lesion. The majority of the mass was necrotic tumor. The tumor on the right was avascular, producing the effect of a mass in the renal hilum. In patients under one year of age, an aortogram is performed rapidly with fewer complications. Pathologic vessels in the Wilms' tumor are distinctly different from the vascular changes seen with polycystic disease, multiple cysts, and hydronephrosis.

Other abdominal and retroperitoneal neoplasms can be demonstrated to some advantage. A leiomyoma adherent to the liver is seen in the selective celiac arteriogram shown in Figure 11. Knowledge of the vascular supply facilitated the use of a surgical approach. A pelvic sarcoma (Fig. 12) is supplied primarily by the right internal iliac artery which directed selective intra-arterial chemotherapy. Tumor vascularity may be of significance in predicting the effect of radiotherapy and chemotherapy. The angiographic criterion of vascular invasion by the tumor and the vascularity of the metastases to the bony pelvis are noted in Figure 12 (arrows).

BONE AND SOFT TISSUE TUMORS OF EXTREMITIES.—Evaluation of bone tumors and soft tissue tumors of the extremities can be assisted by arteriography (Halpern and Freiberger, 1965). Determining the extent and character of the neoplasm is extremely helpful in planning the therapeutic approach. Figure 13 demonstrates a very vascular giant cell tumor of bone. There seems to be some correlation between the degree of vascularity and the degree of malignancy. Conversely, in an osteoid osteoma— a benign lesion—a specific diagnosis can be established when the vascular nidus is demonstrated. This nidus must be removed for cure (Lindbom, Lindvall, Söderberg, and Spjut, 1960).

Fig. 13.—Giant cell tumor of the tibia. A, arterial phase reveals an increased vascularity in the lesion of the proximal tibia. The vessels are tortuous and irregular. B, in the venous phase, there is early shunting to the veins with excellent opacification of the popliteal vein.

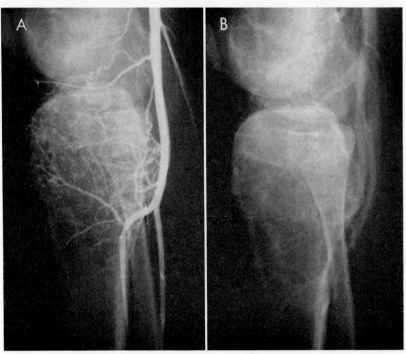

Venography

Venography, in particular vena cavography, has considerable application in the child with neoplasia (Hellman and Tristan, 1963; Tucker, 1965). Inferior vena cavography can be accomplished as an adjunct to the intravenous pyelogram (Allen, Morse, Frye, and Clatworthy, 1964; Ducharme and Ellis, 1964; Greenberg, Altman, and Litt, 1967). Injection into the saphenous vein in the foot will allow the performance of this study as the initial phase of an intravenous pyelogram. Tourniquets applied to each lower extremity limit the admixing of blood and allow better opacification. When two thirds of the predicted amount of contrast material has been injected, the ipsilateral tourniquet is released, allowing a

Fig. 14.—Minimal distortion of the inferior vena cava was caused by a Wilms' tumor of the right kidney.

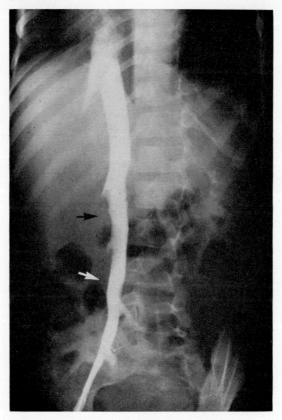

larger bolus of the radiopaque substance to fill the inferior vena cava. Two separate injections will allow anterior-posterior and lateral projections to be made. Collateral circulation may be present in both the abnormal and normal cases. Under normal circumstances with a crying child or during the Valsalva maneuver, collateral circulation to the vertebral plexus may be visualized. Changes in the inferior vena cava itself are more specific. Retroperitoneal masses must be large enough to distort or obstruct the inferior vena cava; lymph nodes and lesions such as Wilms' tumor, neuroblastoma, and hepatoblastoma fit this size criterion. Two patients with Wilms' tumor illustrate these findings. Figure 14 demon-

Fig. 15.—Both iliac veins are obstructed by metastases from a Wilms' tumor. Collateral circulation is seen via the vertebral and paravertebral plexuses. (Courtesy of E. Singleton, Texas Children's Hospital, Houston, Texas.)

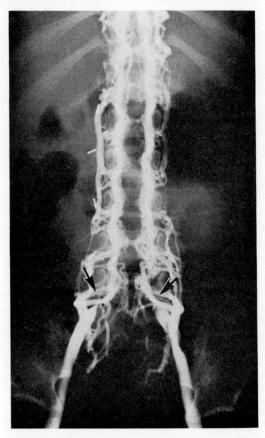

strates distortion of the inferior vena cava. Metastases from a Wilms' tumor obstructed the inferior vena cava in Figure 15. Knowledge of the projection of a Wilms' tumor into the renal vein and inferior vena cava is valuable in planning surgical procedures. For the most part, vena cavography provides information of a secondary nature about lesions which are adjacent to the inferior vena cava on the right side of the retroperitoneal space and which are large enough and in positions strategic enough to produce changes.

Lymphangiography

Lymphangiography, the radiographic demonstration of the lymphatic system by the intralymphatic injection of radiopaque contrast material, is the most direct method now available for the evaluation of the lymphatics and nodes.

TECHNIQUE

The technical aspects of this procedure have been described by Wallace *et al.* (1961). There are a few modifications of this technique for application to the pediatric age group. The child must be premedicated adequately and his feet must be secured to prevent undue motion. The intradermal injection of 0.25 cc. of 5% Patent Blue V (alphazurine 2G) into the first interdigital web space is, in essence, an intralymphatic injection. Following a small longitudinal incision, a lymphatic is isolated, dissected and cannulated with a 27- or 30-gauge needle-catheter assembly. The amount of Ethiodol, an ethyl ester of poppyseed oil, injected depends on the height of the child and the nodal configuration. The patient must be monitored carefully by image intensification or radiographic control to minimize the amount injected. A one-year-old child usually requires approximately 2 cc. injected into each lower extremity. Multiple radiographic projections are taken at the completion of the injection and again in 24 hours so that the lymphatic and nodal phases may be seen in their entirety; this facilitates a more accurate diagnosis.

The most difficult aspect of lymphangiography is its interpretation (Wallace, Jackson, Dodd and Greening, 1965). A thorough knowledge of the normal lymphatic drainage is essential. Both lymphatic and nodal phases should be evaluated. A "normal" study means little, since microscopic changes are beyond the competence of the examination.

NORMAL

Normal nodes vary in size and number, and an inverse relationship exists between the two factors. The afferent lymphatics enter the marginal sinus while the efferent vessels exit through the hilum. The internal architecture has a homogeneous or reticular pattern (Fig. 16).

Fig. 16.—Normal lymphangiogram. A, lymphatic phase; B, nodal phase.

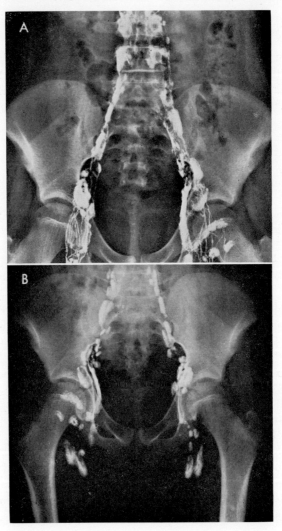

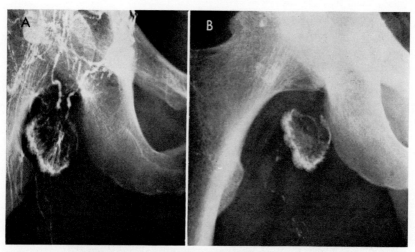

Fig. 17.—Lymphangiogram. A, the lymphatic phase reveals multiple vessels pass-ing through a defect in a node. This is the site of the hilum and an area of fatty re-placement. The defect is a normal one. B, the nodal phase reveals the site of the hilum. Any defect permeated by the lymphatics without displacement or distortion of the lymphatics is probably of no significance.

FALSE-POSITIVES

False-positive interpretation of nodal disease has provoked consider-able criticism of lymphangiography. A proper evaluation must have a multidimensional approach, including tomography. A high percentage of false-positives may be caused by fatty replacement and fibrosis of nodal parenchyma. In general, these spurious defects usually will be traversed by lymphatic channels traced in the lymphatic phase (Fig. 17).

CARCINOMA

Carcinomatous changes in the lymphatic system are usually at the local site of drainage from a known primary lesion. Tumor emboli enter the node via the afferent lymphatics and frequently obstruct the marginal sinus; the result is a moth-eaten appearance. The elongated shape is transformed to a more rounded contour or to a crescent shape (Fig. 18). In contrast to the false-positive defects, lymphatic channels do not tra-verse the area replaced by carcinoma but are distorted and circumvent the carcinomatous focus. When the lymphatic pathways become ob-structed by the proliferating tumor, the collateral circulation may be the only residual evidence of massive replacement of nodal tissue.

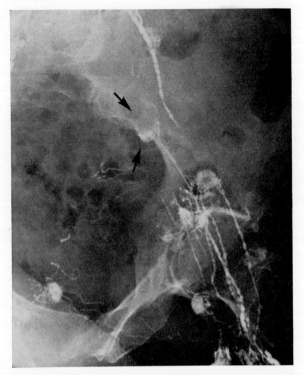

Fig. 18.—Metastatic carcinoma of the iliac node has resulted in the crescent-shaped deformity of the node. The lymphatic channels do not permeate the defect within the node. Multiple lymphatics are obstructed and collateral circulation is opacified.

The modes of metastasis are determined by the normal anatomical distribution of lymph drainage, the variations of normal, and the collateral pathways available in the event of interference with normal flow.

LYMPHOMA

Lymphomatous disease produces an early change in the intrinsic nodal architecture. The margin of the node is intact, for the most part, until the late stages of the disease. Distortion or obstruction of the lymphatics also occurs as a late phenomenon. Differentiation of certain types of lymphoma can be made by careful scrutiny of these patterns (Fig. 19). Nodal involvement is usually more generalized by the time it is seen, in contrast to metastatic carcinoma, which is locally distributed. The nodes involved by lymphoma frequently are enlarged, and there may be an over-all increase in the number of nodes opacified.

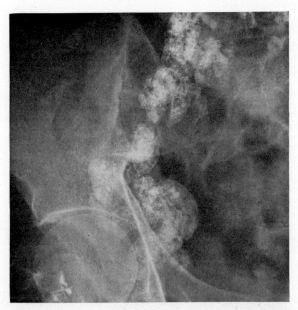

Fig. 19.—Lymphoma. The primary change is in the internal nodal architecture. The margin of the node remains intact until late in the course of the disease. This patient had lymphosarcoma.

MELANOMA

When melanomas and sarcomas metastasize, they may produce similar lymphangiographic changes. The lymphatics do not penetrate these usually well-outlined tumor deposits (Fig. 20).

APPLICATIONS

Lymphangiography can be used in children with neoplasia to: (1) determine the gross extent and nature of the disease, (2) guide surgical treatment (node dissection), (3) assist in more exact portal placement in radiotherapy, and (4) assess the effect of radiotherapy and chemotherapy.

Determining the gross extent and nature of the neoplastic disease is the primary diagnostic function of lymphangiography. It has been used to great advantage to assist in staging and following lymphomatous disease. Figure 21 shows an eight-year-old male with lymphosarcoma whose urinary tract was obstructed partially by involved para-aortic nodes.

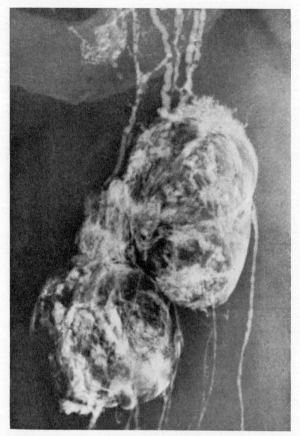

Fig. 20.—Melanoma. This pattern frequently is seen with metastatic melanoma.

Another patient, a 12-year-old male with reticulum cell sarcoma, was examined because of abdominal pain and vomiting (Fig. 22). His complaints proved to be caused by nodal invasion of the duodenum. Radiation therapy to this area produced a rapid remission. In children with neuroblastoma, opacification of the para-aortic nodes leads to a more exact evaluation of the extent of disease (Fig. 23).

The radiopaque material remains within the nodes for varying lengths of time (as long as five years in our series), which allows repeated follow-up evaluations. Hence, a child with a normal examination may be watched for subsequent macroscopic evidence of disease. Exacerbations may be recognized earlier. The effect of therapy may be judged more accurately.

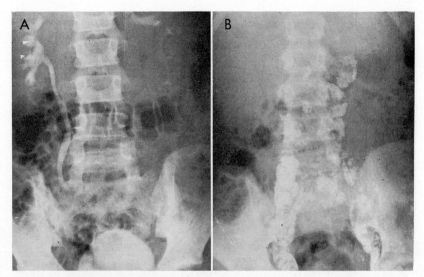

Fig. 21.—Lymphosarcoma of the para-aortic and pelvic nodes with partial obstruction of the urinary tract. A, the intravenous pyelogram demonstrates partial obstruction and distortion of the right ureter; B, the lymphangiogram reveals the changes in the urinary tract to be caused by enlarged involved nodes.

Retroperitoneal node dissections are at best very difficult. Opacification of these nodes offers considerable assistance toward a complete dissection. This is demonstrated by the one-year-old child shown in Figure 24, who was treated for a teratocarcinoma of the testicle by a para-aortic node dissection. Immediately prior to the end of the surgical procedure, a radiograph of the abdomen taken in the operating room revealed many residual nodes. These nodes were dissected and the procedure was completed.

A few months after the removal of a right Wilms' tumor along with the adjacent para-aortic nodes, the child shown in Figure 25 was found to have a mass in the right lower abdomen. Demonstration of a lymphocele, a localized collection of lymph secondary to transection of lymphatics, solved the problem and assisted in the further treatment of the patient.

Lymphography represents the only nonexcisional approach to the differential diagnosis of diseases involving the lymphatic system. As a macroscopic procedure which documents patterns of growth of the disease processes, its results must be correlated with all other information available.

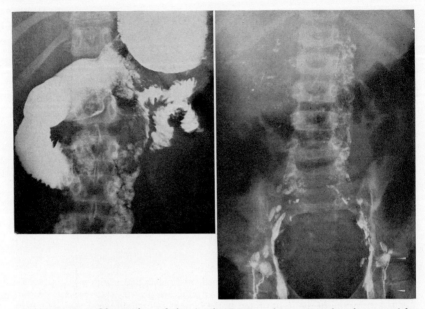

Fig. 22 (left).—Obstruction of the duodenum was demonstrated to be caused by enlarged nodes involved by reticulum cell sarcoma.

Fig. 23 (right).—Neuroblastoma. The abnormal para-aortic nodes are partially replaced by neuroblastoma. The primary lesion of the right adrenal also is partially opacified.

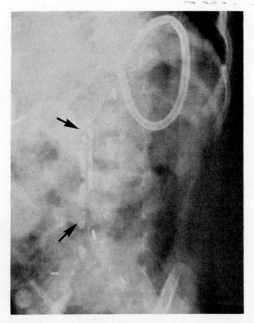

Fig. 24.—Teratocarcinoma of the testicle. A para-aortic node dissection was assisted by this examination. A radiograph made during the operative procedure revealed residual nodes along the inferior vena cava. With this information, the dissection was completed more adequately.

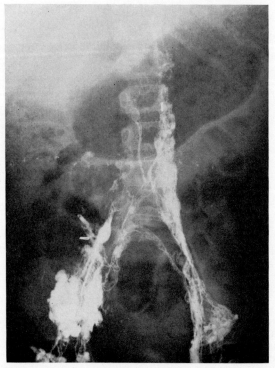

Fig. 25.—Lymphocele formation following the removal of the right kidney and adjacent para-aortic nodes. A mass was palpated in the right abdomen. Lymphangiogram demonstrated the mass to be caused by a lymphocele.

Complications

Complications of all these procedures may be caused by hypersensitivity to the agents employed. The oil-based contrast media, Ethiodol, used in lymphangiography has additional risks. All patients examined by means of lymphangiography will experience a temporary pulmonary diffusion block. For this reason, close monitoring is essential to limit the amount of contrast material which gains access to the lungs. In the presence of pre-existing pulmonary disease, lymphangiography is contraindicated. The procedure also is contraindicated in children with cardiac shunts.

The problems encountered during arteriography include hemorrhage and thrombosis. Careful application of the technique, a minimum of vascular trauma, and close postarteriographic observation help to minimize complications.

The complications resulting from the use of these procedures in children are comparable to those seen in adults. To justify the examinations, the procedural risks must be few in comparison to the benefits which result from the information acquired.

REFERENCES

Allen, J. E., Morse, T. S., Frye, T. R., and Clatworthy, H. W.: Vena cavagrams in infants and children. *Annals of Surgery,* 160:568-574, October 1964.

Alpert, S., Metcalf, W., Vreede, A. A., and Meng, C. H.: Right hepatectomy for hamartoma in an eleven-month-old infant: A case report. *Annals of Surgery,* 165: 286-292, February 1967.

Arvay, N., and Picard, J. D.: *La lymphographie; Étude radiologique et clinique des voies lymphatiques normales et pathologiques.* Paris, France, Masson and Company, 1963, 305 pp.

Baum, S., Kuroda, K., and Roy, R. H.: The value of special angiographic techniques in the management of patients with abdominal neoplasms. *The Radiologic Clinics of North America,* 3:583-599, December 1965.

Berdon, W. E., Baker, D. H., and Santulli, T. V.: Factors producing spurious obstruction of the inferior vena cava in infants and children with abdominal tumors. *Radiology,* 88:111-116, January 1967.

Boijsen, E.: Angiographic studies of the anatomy of single and multiple renal arteries. *Acta radiologica,* Suppl. 183:1-135, 1959.

Boijsen, E., Williams, C. M., and Judkins, M. P.: Angiography of pheochromocytoma. *The American Journal of Roentgenology, Radium Therapy and Nuclear Medicine,* 98:225-232, September 1966.

Desilets, D. T., Ruttenberg, H. D., and Hoffman, R. B.: Percutaneous catheterization in children. *Radiology,* 87:119-122, July 1966.

Ducharme, J., and Ellis, F.: Inferior vena cavagram: An aid in the diagnosis of abdominal tumors in children. *The Journal of the Canadian Association of Radiologists,* 15:38-41, March 1964.

Greenberg, L. A., Altman, D. H., and Litt, R. E.: Cystic enlargement of the kidney in infancy. *Radiology,* 89:850-856, November 1967.

Halpern, M., and Freiberger, R. H.: Arteriography in orthopedics. *The American Journal of Roentgenology, Radium Therapy and Nuclear Medicine*, 94:194-206, May 1965.

Hellman, D. C., and Tristan, R. A.: Inferior vena cavography in the detection of abdominal extension of pelvic cancer. *Radiology*, 81:416-427, September 1963 .

Hope, J. W., and Borns, P. F.: Radiologic diagnosis of primary and metastatic carcinoma in infants and children. *The Radiologic Clinics of North America*, 3:353-374, December 1965.

Kahn, P. C., and Nickrosz, L. V.: Selective angiography of the adrenal glands. *The American Journal of Roentgenology, Radium Therapy and Nuclear Medicine*, 101:739-749, November 1967.

Lindbom, A., Lindvall, N., Söderberg, G., and Spjut, H.: Angiography in osteoid osteoma. *Acta radiologica*, 54:327-333, November 1960.

Puyau, F. A.: Renal arteriography in infancy. *Pediatrics*, 36:789-790, November 1965.

Reuter, S. R., Blair, A. J., Schteingart, D. E., and Bookstein, J. J.: Adrenal venography. *Radiology*, 89:805-814, November 1967.

Rusznyak, I., Foldi, M., and Szabo, G.: *Lymphatics and Lymph Circulation*. Oxford, England, Pergamon Press, 1960, 853 pp.

Seldinger, S. I.: Catheter replacement of needle in percutaneous arteriography: A new technique. *Acta radiologica*, 39:368-376, May 1953.

Tucker, A. S.: The roentgen diagnosis of abdominal masses in children. Intravenous urography vs. inferior venacavography. *The American Journal of Roentgenology, Radium Therapy and Nuclear Medicine*, 95:76-90, September 1965.

Wallace, S., Goldberg, H., Leeds, N., and Mishkin, M.: The cavernous branches of the internal carotid artery. *The American Journal of Roentgenology, Radium Therapy and Nuclear Medicine*, 101:34-46, September 1967.

Wallace, S., Jackson, L., Dodd, G. D., and Greening, R. R.: Lymphangiographic interpretation. *The Radiologic Clinics of North America*, 3:467-485, December 1965.

Wallace, S., Jackson, L., Schaffer, B., Gould, J., Greening, R. R., Weiss, A., and Kramer, S.: Lymphangiograms: Their diagnostic and therapeutic potential. *Radiology*, 76:179-199, February 1961.

Weber, A. L., Janower, M. L., and Griscom, N. T.: Radiologic and clinical evaluation of pheochromocytoma in children: Report of 6 cases. *Radiology*, 88:117-123, January 1967.

Ziedses des Plantes, B. G.: *Planigraphie en subtractie*. Utrecht, The Netherlands, Kemik en Zoon, N. V., 1934, 112 pp.

Evaluation of Neoplasia in Childhood with Techniques in Nuclear Medicine*

MERLE K. LOKEN, M.D., PH.D.

Department of Radiology, University of Minnesota Hospitals,
University of Minnesota, Minneapolis, Minnesota

NUCLEAR MEDICINE involves the development, evaluation, and propagation of various uses of radioactive materials in the diagnosis and management of disease. To this end, consideration must be given to the physical and chemical properties of radioisotopes, to the availability and performance of devices for measurement of radioactivity, and to the radiation hazards to patients and clinic personnel.

The field of nuclear medicine had its beginning shortly after the discovery of radioactivity by Antoine Henri Becquerel in 1896. However, in the 50 years that followed, few radioactive materials other than radium and its related products were used to any great extent by practicing physicians. Since the end of World War II, there has been a steady increase in the availability of reactor-produced radioactive materials, so that today there are several hundred radiopharmaceuticals available for use in medicine and medical research.

The growth in availability of radioisotopes has been paralleled by rapid advances in nuclear instrumentation. Such factors as cost, versatility, sensitivity, and speed and reliability of obtaining data have been major considerations in this development. Most of the instruments employ a scintillation crystal detector coupled with a spectrometer for analysis of gamma ray energies. Beyond that, the instruments differ according to their particular application. For assay of radioactivity, a scaler may be used. If information is desired on the rate of radioisotope uptake and clearance from an organ, *e.g.,* in a study of the function of a renal trans-

*This work was sponsored in part by grants from the U.S. Public Health Service (No. 1T01CA05190-01 and No. HE NB 11237-01), the American Cancer Society (institutional grant), and the Graduate School, University of Minnesota.

plant, then ratemeters and strip chart recorders usually are employed (Loken, Staab, Vernier, and Kelly, 1964). Scintiphotograms of body organs containing radioactivity are obtained with a rectilinear scanner or scintillation camera (Loken, 1965; Loken, Telander, and Laxdal, 1966; Loken, Telander, and Salmon, 1965; Loken, Wigdahl, Gilson, and Staab, 1966). The camera is an instrument of relatively recent design and is used primarily for studies in which dynamic function data are desired in addition to scintiphotograms. Scintiphotography with xenon[133] (Xe^{133}) gas is used routinely in our clinic for evaluation of cerebral blood flow and pulmonary function (Loken and Westgate [1967]; Pierce, Loken, and Resch [1967]). With the aid of computer analyses, specific information on regional cerebral blood flow and regional pulmonary function are obtained.

Scope of Nuclear Medicine

A summary of our clinical uses of radioactive pharmaceuticals is given in Table 1. These uses may be divided into five general areas, each of

TABLE 1.—SUMMARY OF CLINICAL USES OF RADIOACTIVE
PHARMACEUTICALS IN THE NUCLEAR MEDICINE CLINIC,
UNIVERSITY OF MINNESOTA HOSPITALS

A. LABORATORY TECHNIQUES	B. DYNAMIC FUNCTION
1. Blood volume	1. Thyroid
2. Red cell mass	2. Kidney
3. Red cell survival	3. Liver
4. Fat absorption	4. Lung
5. Vitamin B_{12} absorption	5. Pancreas
6. Radiopharmaceutical preparation	6. Bone
	7. Heart

C. ORGAN VISUALIZATION		D. REGIONAL BLOOD FLOW
1. Brain	7. Spleen	1. Brain
2. Thyroid	8. Kidney	2. Heart
3. Lung	9. Bone	3. Lung
4. Heart	10. Pancreas	4. Extremities
5. Stomach	11. Subarachnoid space	5. Liver
6. Liver	12. Placenta	

E. THERAPY
1. Hyperthyroidism
2. Thyroid carcinoma
3. Polycythemia vera
4. Leukemia
5. Effusions
6. Subarachnoid tumors
7. Carcinoma of cervix
8. Carcinoma of head and neck

which includes several specific procedures. Certain aspects of each of these procedures relate directly to the diagnosis and management of neoplasia in childhood. All of the laboratory techniques listed may be used in certain situations for either diagnosis or management purposes. Organ scintiphotography is important for the demonstration of tumors and other disease conditions. Function and blood flow measurements of the organs listed are performed routinely in our clinic as are measurements of blood flow to the heart and extremities. These studies may also relate to the evaluation of children with tumors.

Radioisotopes began to be used in therapy shortly after they became available in reasonable quantities following World War II. The initial enthusiasm expressed for therapeutic applications of internal emitters has waned somewhat in recent years because of the lack of specificity of radioisotopes for tissues to be irradiated. Iodine[131] (I^{131}) and phosphorus[32] (P^{32}) were among the first radioisotopes to be used for therapeutic purposes. I^{131} was and still is used in the management of hyperthyroidism and thyroid carcinomas which take up a significant amount of radioactive iodine. P^{32} has been used successfully in the control of polycythemia vera and some leukemias. It occasionally has been used effectively for palliation of pain in patients with metastatic disease to bone. Recently, studies initiated at our institution have utilized colloidal gold for the management of subarachnoid tumors in children. Results of these studies have been encouraging, particularly in controlling spread of medulloblastoma along the cerebrospinal axis (Kieffer, D'Angio, and Nowak, 1966).

Organ Scintiphotography

A detailed discussion of all procedures in nuclear medicine mentioned in previous paragraphs is beyond the scope of a single report. This presentation therefore will be restricted to developments in organ visualization which relate to the diagnosis and/or follow-up care of children with neoplastic disease.

The thyroid was among the first organs to be scanned successfully. It continues to be one of the organs most frequently studied by scintiphotography despite some controversy concerning the necessity of the procedure; many thyroid abnormalities, including thyroid nodules, are detectable by simple palpation. The thyroid scan with I^{131} or technetium[99m] (Tc^{99m}) is nonetheless helpful in determining whether a palpable nodule is nonfunctioning "cold," in which case the probability of malignancy is considerably greater (approximately 20 per cent). If a palpable thyroid nodule is "hot" to either iodine or technetium, a diagnosis of functioning adenoma can be made since the probability of malignancy in this situation is essentially nonexistent.

Among the many organs which can be visualized by scintiphotography, the brain occupies an important place. "Positive" brain scintiphotograms typically are obtained in patients with an alteration of the permeability of the blood-brain barrier. This breakdown of the barrier will be localized to the immediate area of the lesion so that the radioactive material used for the study will be concentrated selectively. A large variety of isotopes has been used in brain scintiphotography; the emphasis today is on the use of mercury[197] chlormerodrin and Tc[99m] (Loken, Telander, and Salmon, 1965; Quinn, Ciric, and Hauser, 1965). More recently, indium[113m] (In[113m]) chelates also have been shown to be acceptable agents for these studies (Wagner, Stern, and Goodwin, 1967). Scintiphotography of the brain can be performed in an accurate and atraumatic manner and thus can serve as an excellent screening procedure. This technique can be used to diagnose primary or metastatic tumors as well as to demonstrate the presence of an abscess, subdural hematoma, or cerebral vascular accident. In practice, any patient suspected of having a tumor of the brain or meninges should be studied by this technique, whose over-all accuracy in the detection of brain disease is about 90 per cent.

We have performed more than 3,000 brain scintiphotograms during the past four years and have published a number of summaries of this work (Loken, Hewel, and French, 1967; Loken, Telander, and Laxdal, 1966; Loken, Telander, and Salmon, 1965; Loken, Wigdahl, Gilson, and Staab, 1966). The brain scintiphotogram is of value in the detection of the initial lesion and in the follow-up of these patients. This follow-up may include surgical therapy, radiation therapy, or the use of chemotherapeutic agents. Certain problems do occur in the management of brain lesions after scintiphotography, such as increased uptake of the radioisotope in the area of the bone flap during the immediate postoperative period. Problems also are encountered in the evaluation of posterior fossa lesions, the posterior fossa is a common site for brain tumors in children. We have found that a high percentage of tumors localized in the posterior fossa (approximately 70 per cent) may be demonstrated by the use of careful technique.

The liver may be visualized scintiphotographically with a wide variety of radiopharmaceuticals. Colloidal gold[198], I[131] attached to Rose Bengal, Cholografin and colloidal albumin, and Tc[99m] complexed with colloidal albumin or colloidal sulfur have been used (Loken, Staab, and Shea, 1966). At present, most of our liver scans are performed with technetium[99m] sulfur colloid, which is made daily in our laboratories. This material provides excellent visualization of the liver and also is taken up by the reticuloendothelial cells of the spleen. We currently are determining whether useful information on liver function also might be obtained with the sulfur colloid.

We are using sequential liver scanning in pediatric patients who are receiving radiation therapy to the abdomen for various malignant diseases. This technique permits an evaluation of liver damage secondary to radiation as well as liver regeneration after completion of radiation therapy (Fig. 1). These scans, together with tests of function, are also of importance in the evaluation of patients treated with chemotherapeutic agents.

Pulmonary scintiphotography is rapidly increasing in popularity. The agent routinely used in our clinic for these studies is macroaggregated albumin labeled with Tc[99m] (Bugby and Loken, 1966b). This material must be made up daily in our laboratories because of the very short half-life (six hours) of technetium. Macroaggregated albumin labeled with I[131] is available commercially and also may be used, but is less desirable because of the greater radiation exposure to the patient in addition to the lesser resolution obtained because of the higher energy gamma rays from I[131]. The use of a radioactive gas, such as Xe[133], is a more physiological approach to the evaluation of pulmonary perfusion and ventilation and is used with increasing frequency in our clinic for this purpose. To study effectively the passage of Xe[133] through the lungs, it is necessary to use a camera device which can view both lungs simultaneously and can register the very rapid change in radioactivity that occurs as the gas diffuses from the alveoli to the blood capillaries or vice versa (Bugby and Loken, 1966b; Loken and Westgate, 1967).

Chlormerodrin labeled with either mercury[203] (Hg[203]) or mercury[197] (Hg[197]) is used effectively for scanning of the kidneys. Despite the selective localization of these radioisotopes in the kidneys, this technique has not been accepted widely as a means of evaluating renal disease. The basic problem is that it is difficult, if not impossible, to distinguish between a malignant tumor and other defects of the kidney, such as cysts. Nonetheless, useful information is obtained from scintiphotograms concerning location, size, and function of the kidneys. Kidney scans are used routinely at our institution to aid in the placement of lead shielding over the kidneys during radiation therapy to the abdomen. In this instance, both anterior and posterior kidney scintiphotograms are obtained. An iron complex with Tc[99m] for scintiphotography of kidneys currently is being evaluated in our laboratories.

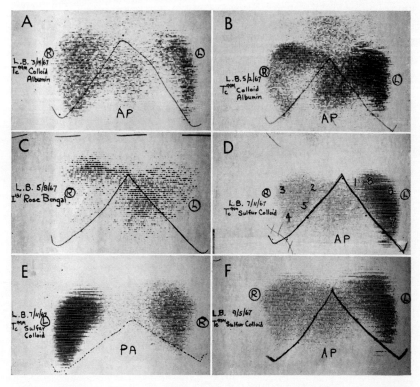

Fig. 1.—A series of liver and spleen scans on a five-year-old patient is shown. This patient had a right nephrectomy for Wilms' tumor in February, 1967. Radiation therapy was started on March 7, 1967. **A**, scan A was performed with technetium[99m] colloidal albumin on March 14, 1967, and shows the liver to be approximately normal in size, but with some irregularity in the uptake of radioactive material. The spleen appears slightly enlarged. **B**, scan B was obtained on May 2, 1967, with technetium[99m] colloidal albumin. This scan shows relatively more uptake in the spleen than in the liver, thus indicating some depression of liver function. A large filling defect, which was thought to be secondary to radiation therapy, is present in the liver. **C**, for verification, scan C was performed with Rose Bengal on May 8, 1967. It shows a defect which fits very well with the radiation fields used in the treatment of the patient. **D**, scan D was performed on July 11, 1967, with still another agent, technetium[99m] sulfur colloid. This study shows the spleen to be larger and more sharply visualized than on earlier studies, thus indicating further depression of liver function. There does appear to be some return to a more uniform distribution of uptake in the liver, which suggests liver regeneration after completion of therapy. The numbers on this scan were the sites of sequential spot counts taken on successive studies with technetium[99m] sulfur colloid; radiologists determined regional liver function, in a semiquantitative fashion, by comparing the counts obtained over the liver with those obtained over the spleen. **E**, scan E was performed as part of the same study and shows the liver and spleen from the posterior projection. **F**, scan F was performed on August 5, 1967, with technetium[99m] sulfur colloid and shows further improvement in function of the liver as indicated by a more uniform scan pattern. The spleen appears to be about the same size as on the previous study.

Several radiopharmaceuticals are used for scintiphotography of the spleen. The agent of current interest is mercury hydroxypropane labeled with Hg^{197} (Bugby and Loken, 1966a; Wagner, Weiner, McAfee, and Martinez, 1964). This agent is quite specific for localization of the spleen because of its attachment to red cells which then are sequestered selectively by this organ. In addition to its utilization for evaluation of spleen size and location, this technique permits useful data to be obtained on function.

Scintiphotography provides the only way of visualizing the pancreas without surgical exploration. The material used, selenomethionine labeled with selenium^{75} (Se^{75}) is incorporated into proteins synthesized by the pancreas. Selenomethionine also is taken up by other organs involved with protein synthesis so that the liver is seen on scintiphotograms, frequently to the detriment of pancreatic visualization. A single scan of the pancreas is of limited value because frequently it is not obtained at a time when the concentration of radioactivity in the organ is the highest. In addition, the pancreas is quite variable in its anatomic configuration so that difficulty is encountered in evaluating the scintiphotogram without prior knowledge of the organ's normal anatomy. Recent studies with the scintillation camera, which permits frequent time-lapse scintiphotograms to be obtained after the administration of selenomethionine, have shown the greatest promise to date for obtaining clinically useful scintiphotograms of the pancreas.

The skeleton may be examined effectively with one of several radioactive materials; emphasis currently is placed on the use of strontium^{87m} (Sr^{87m}) or fluorine^{18} (F^{18}). Use of the fluorine isotope requires the laboratory to be in close proximity to a linear accelerator or cyclotron; F^{18} is a short-lived radionuclide which must be produced, transferred, and utilized quickly. Sr^{87m} is obtained, as are Tc^{99m}, In^{113m}, and certain other radionuclides, from a generator. Consequently, Sr^{87m} can be used effectively despite its very short physical half-life of 2.8 hours.

Bone scans performed in our clinic with either Sr^{87m} or strontium^{85} (Sr^{85}) have detected bone lesions well before they can be detected by ordinary roentgenography (Loken and MacGibbon, 1967). Either of these gamma-emitting isotopes of strontium will localize selectively in areas of increased osteoblastic activity. This permits both primary and metastatic cancers to be detected. However, the appearance of radioactive strontium in these lesions cannot always be distinguished from its appearance in benign processes such as Paget's disease, osteomyelitis, and, to some degree, osteoarthritis.

Scintiphotography of the heart is used primarily for the evaluation of pericardial effusions which may be the result of either an inflammatory or a malignant condition. With the use of albumin labeled with Tc^{99m}, excellent scintiphotograms of the heart are obtained by scanning. These scans then are correlated with chest x-ray films obtained at a relatively long focal skin distance with the patient in a position similar to the one used for the scan.

Scintiphotography of the gastrointestinal tract is just beginning to develop. Excellent representations of the esophagus, stomach, and bowel have been obtained with one of several radioisotopes. Tc^{99m} administered orally is used most commonly for these studies. Whether this technique will yield fruitful results in the detection of tumors or other lesions of the gastrointestinal system remains to be seen.

Technetium-labeled albumin and Xe^{133} dissolved in saline are used effectively to study the subarachnoid space. The Xe^{133} distributes itself throughout the cerebrospinal fluid more rapidly than the technetium-labeled albumin, but also diffuses out of the subarachnoid space more rapidly. A scintiphotographic device such as the scintillation camera thus is necessary for the study. We are using technetium-labeled albumin routinely to visualize abnormalities in the subarachnoid space as well as in the ventricular system of the brain (Hodak, Chou, and Loken, 1966). The advantage of this approach over conventional myelography or cisternography is that both of the radioisotopic agents are administered in physiological solutions and do not have to be removed as do the usual x-ray contrast media.

Summary

All but a few of the procedures listed in Table 1 have been developed within the past five years. The same is true for the scintiphotographic techniques discussed above, indicating the rapid growth of nuclear medicine. At the present time, about 10 per cent of all diagnostic procedures employing radiation involve radioisotopic techniques. It seems reasonable to expect that this percentage may triple or even quadruple within the next decade so that nuclear medicine may well achieve a status comparable to that of diagnostic radiology in terms of the number of procedures performed in the evaluation of patients. To achieve this goal, continuous attention must be given to the reliability of all procedures in nuclear medicine, particularly those which are relatively new. Procedural simplicity consistent with reliability also should be emphasized. In addition, the aim of nuclear medicine should be to maintain rigid control of radiation exposure. This is particularly important in procedures performed on children, regardless of whether the diagnosis of neoplasia is entertained.

REFERENCES

Bugby, R. D., and Loken, M. K.: Spleen studies with mercurihydroxypropane-197. (Abstract) *Journal of Nuclear Medicine,* 7:350, May 1966a.

Bugby, R. D., and Loken, M. K.: Visualization of the lung by methods of scintiphotography. *The American Journal of Roentgenology, Radium Therapy and Nuclear Medicine,* 97:850-859, August 1966b.

Hodak, J., Chou, S., and Loken, M. K.: Scintiphotography of the subarachnoid space. (Abstract) *Journal of Nuclear Medicine,* 7:344, May 1966.

Keiffer, S. A., D'Angio, G. J., and Nowak, T. J.: Laboratory studies of intrathecal radiogold with a new rationale for its use. *Radiology,* 87:1120-1121, December 1966.

Loken, M. K.: Radioactive isotope. *Minnesota Medicine,* 48:1138-1143, September 1965.

Loken, M. K., Hewel, C., and French, L. A.: Comparison of scintiscanning with 203-chlormerodrin and special radiographic procedures in the evaluation of brain pathology. *Archives of Neurology,* 17:437-440, October 1967.

Loken, M. K., and MacGibbon, J. D.: The use of strontium-87m for bone scanning. (Abstract) *Journal of Nuclear Medicine,* 8:273, April 1967.

Loken, M. K., Staab, E. V., and Shea, A. S.: [131]I colloidal albumin as an agent for scanning liver and spleen. *Investigative Radiology,* 1:295-300, July-August 1966.

Loken, M. K., Staab, E. V., Vernier, R. L., and Kelly, W. D.: Radioisotope renograms in kidney transplants. *Journal of Nuclear Medicine,* 5:807-810, October 1964.

Loken, M. K., Telander, G., and Laxdal, S.: Conventional scanning vs. scintillation camera. A comparison for evaluation of brain pathology. *Minnesota Medicine,* 49:237-241, February 1966.

Loken, M. K., Telander, G. T., and Salmon, R. J.: Technetium[99m] compounds for visualization of body organs. *Journal of the American Medical Association,* 194: 152-156, October 11, 1965.

Loken, M. K., and Westgate, H. D.: Evaluation of pulmonary function using [133]xenon and the scintillation camera. *The American Journal of Roentgenology, Radium Therapy and Nuclear Medicine,* 100:835-843, August 1967.

Loken, M. K., Wigdahl, L. O., Gilson, J. M., and Staab, E. V.: [197]Hg and [203]Hg chlormerodrin for evaluation of brain lesions using a rectilinear scanner and scintillation camera. *Journal of Nuclear Medicine,* 7:209-218, March 1966.

Pierce, R., Loken, M. K., and Resch, J.: Cerebral blood flow measurements following the inhalation of [133]xenon. *Geriatrics,* 22:115-121, August 1967.

Quinn, J. L., Ciric, I., and Hauser, W. N.: Analysis of 96 abnormal brain scans using technetium[99m] (pertechnetate form). *Journal of the American Medical Association,* 194:157-160, October 11, 1965.

Wagner, H. N., Jr., Stern, H. S., and Goodwin, H. S.: Comparison of indium-113m chelates and technetium-99m pertechnetate as brain scanning agents. (Abstract) *Journal of Nuclear Medicine,* 8:261, April 1967.

Wagner, H. N., Jr., Weiner, I. M., McAfee, J. G., and Martinez, J.: 1-Mercuri-2-hydroxypropane (MHP). A new radiopharmaceutical for visualization of the spleen by radioisotope scanning. *Archives of Internal Medicine,* 113:696-701, May 1964.

Wilms' Tumor: A Current Plan of Treatment and Review of 50 Patients

CEDRIC J. PRIEBE, JR., M.D.,*

WILLIAM A. NEWTON, M.D., AND

H. WILLIAM CLATWORTHY, JR., M.D.

Departments of Surgery, Pathology, and Pediatrics, Ohio State University College of Medicine; and Division of Pediatric Surgery and Department of Pathology and Hematology, Division of Department of Pediatrics, Children's Hospital, Columbus, Ohio

RECENT ENTHUSIASTIC REPORTS (Farber, 1966; Howard, 1965; Johnson, Maceira, and Koop, 1967) which show improved survival rates in patients with Wilms' tumor (nephroblastoma) since the advent of dactinomycin therapy spurred us to review our experience at the Columbus Children's Hospital. In so doing, we reassessed the "risk period," the diagnostic value of infusion pyelography and vena cavography, and the place of primary and secondary surgical therapy, irradiation, and chemotherapy.

Wilms' tumor continues to rank as the second most common extracranial solid malignant tumor encountered in childhood, exceeded only by neuroblastoma. Fifty patients with this disease were seen at this institution during the 15-year-period from 1952 to 1966.

Clinical Management

During this time interval, a standard program for the management of abdominal solid tumors in children was in effect. Patients referred to this institution with abdominal mass lesions which did not transilluminate were admitted promptly, evaluated rapidly, and operated on—usually within 24 hours. Preoperative appraisal included a complete history and

---

*Dr. Priebe is now attending surgeon (pediatric) at Roosevelt Hospital, New York, New York.

physical examination, routine blood and urine studies, a high-infusion intravenous pyelogram, an inferior vena cavagram, a chest x-ray film and bone survey for metastases, a bone marrow examination, and more recently vanilmandelic acid determinations on the urine.

In the children with Wilms' tumors, intravenous pyelograms showed distortion of the collecting system and displacement of the involved kidney. However, in five no function was seen in the involved kidney. For this reason, when a diagnosis of tumor was considered, we turned to the high-infusion pyelogram technique to obtain better nephrograms and better outlines of the collecting systems. Our procedure for this study, which utilizes the rapid injection of a double dose of Hypaque, has been described elsewhere (Rowe, Morse, and Frye, 1967).

The inferior vena cavagram was of primary value in detecting tumor extension into the lumen of the inferior vena cava. Total obstruction of the vena cava was frequently merely the result of the pressure effect of a large tumor and did not mitigate against successful surgical excision. These findings are in contrast to those observed in patients with neuroblastoma in whom caval obstruction usually was associated with a tumor which could not be completely resected surgically.

After their rapid evaluation, patients usually were explored through a long transverse supraumbilical incision, dividing both rectus sheaths and extending deep into the flank involved. After a preliminary evaluation, including a careful visualization and palpation of the opposite kidney for evidence of bilateral disease, the involved kidney and the adjacent adrenal gland were removed. This was accomplished by first dividing the renal vessels centrally. Great care was taken to avoid undue manipulation of the tumor and accidental rupture of its capsule. Regional lymph nodes, particularly along the periaortic chain, were resected with the specimen if possible, or if not, after the removal of the major mass. Silver clips were positioned to outline the tumor bed which was not reperitonealized and the abdomen which was closed in layers.

Postoperative irradiation was administered to the site of the tumor in all patients. Those under two years of age received 2,000 r; those over two years up to 3,000 r. Since 1958 most patients also were treated with at least one course of dactinomycin, consisting of 15 mg./kg./day for five days, the first dose being given on the day of operation. More recently, some patients also received planned repeated courses of this drug.

Postoperative follow-up management was directed jointly by the surgeon and the chemotherapist. Under ideal conditions, evaluations, including chest x-ray films, were done at two-month intervals for a year and then every three months for about three years. Inferior vena cavagrams and high-infusion pyelograms were repeated after about six months and then done as indicated to search for recurrent tumors and contralateral kidney disease. With frequent examinations, metastases and recurrent tumor can be identified earlier and additional irradiation, chemotherapy, or surgical therapy can be suggested. All surviving patients then were examined annually to evaluate the long-range effect of the combined treatment program.

Period of Risk

In earlier evaluations, we considered Collins' risk period (Collins, 1958) as the best guide for a survival time that could be equated with an expected cure in patients with Wilms' tumor. This period is equal to the age of the child at the time of diagnosis plus the gestational period of nine months and represents the length of time that an embryonic tumor could have been present. It is based on the theory that once treated, any residual or metastatic tumor should regrow at the original rate and thus be recognized within the risk period. Collins found that only two of 340 patients developed a tumor recurrence after the risk period and subsequently died. In our series, all patients who died had evidence of recurrent tumor before the end of this risk period. Thus, Collins' risk period proved to be of excellent prognostic value; however, it is cumbersome and requires long-risk periods in older children.

Other investigators (Sukarochana and Kiesewetter, 1966; Johnson, Maceira, and Koop, 1967; Farber, 1966) found a two-year period of freedom from disease to be a practical guide to prognosis. Platt and Linden (1964), in a study of the criteria for survival in 89 children from the California Tumor Registry, found that Collins' risk period and a fixed two-year risk period were of identical prognostic value. Each method had three probable exceptions. In contrast, four of our 50 patients who were free of tumor two years after diagnosis subsequently died. These same patients had demonstrable tumors within three years. Thus, the two-year risk period appears too short for equation with a probable cure in patients with Wilms' tumor; however, it does give a useful guide for comparing various series and treatment programs. We therefore conformed to this method of evaluating our series.

Two-Year Survival Rate

Twenty-one of our 28 surviving patients have been tumor free for more than two years. Twenty-two patients already have died. Thus, our over-all two-year, tumor-free survival rate has been 21/43 or 49 per cent.

One of the 21 tumor-free patients, who was referred to our hospital following surgical procedures complicated by operative rupture of the tumor, developed an abdominal recurrence two years and 10 months later and is still living with tumor. To obtain more useful statistics, we classified this patient as living with tumor; he has not been included in the two-year survival group in the analyses which follow.

Six of our patients are still within the two-year risk period. Two of these have persistent tumor. One additional patient, who is just beyond the risk period, has pulmonary metastases.

Factors Affecting Survival

We have found the survival rate in our series to be related closely to the patient's age and extent of disease at the time of diagnosis, as well as to the development of pulmonary metastases.

AGE

The importance of age in relation to prognosis has been stressed by Gross (1953), Lattimer, Melicow, and Uson (1958), and Snyder, Hastings, and Pollack (1962). Six of seven infants, or 85 per cent, under one year of age have remained tumor free for two years (Fig. 1). In this young age group, a two-year survival probably can be equated with cure. In the group over one year of age, our two-year survival rate fell to 40 per cent.

Fig. 1.—Those patients who have survived tumor free for two years (white), those who are living with tumor or who are still within the risk period (stippled), and those who have died (black) are shown in relation to their age at the time of the diagnosis.

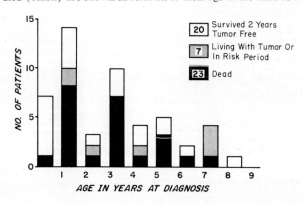

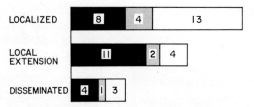

Fig. 2.—Survival in all 50 patients is related to the extent of disease at the time of diagnosis (see Figure 1 for explanation of white, stippled, and black bars).

EXTENT OF DISEASE

We classified Wilms' tumors as (1) localized, (2) locally extended, or (3) disseminated. Localized tumors have been contained entirely within the capsule of the kidney. Those locally extended have penetrated through the capsule or involved regional lymph nodes or the inferior vena cava. Disseminated tumors have metastasized to the lungs or more rarely, to the liver, bones, or brain.

As expected, our best results were among patients with localized tumors (Fig. 2). Sixty-two per cent survived the two-year risk period. Six of the seven children under one year of age had such localization of their tumors.

In all patients in whom local extension was present, the survival rate decreased to 29 per cent.

Eight patients had disseminated disease at the time of diagnosis, yet, three of these are tumor free 3, 7, and 9 years after diagnosis.

Results of Treatment

We, like others (Farber, 1966; Howard, 1965; Johnson, Maceira, and Koop, 1967), found recent results of treatment of patients with Wilms' tumor encouraging (Fig. 3). Prior to the discovery of dactinomycin, when treatment consisted of surgical excision and irradiation of the primary tumor, only four of 16, or 25 per cent, of our patients survived the two-year risk period. In contrast, since the routine addition of initial dactinomycin therapy, 14 of 24 patients, or 58 per cent, successfully survived this period. Eight additional children are still living, but four of these have demonstrable tumor. Two other patients were treated in a somewhat different manner. One, a six-year-old girl who initially had pulmonary metastases and whose care was begun elsewhere, was treated with nitrogen mustard and dactinomycin, total excision of the tumor, and

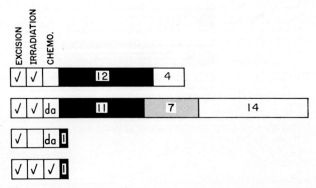

Fig. 3.—The results of initial therapy with excisional surgical procedures, irradiation, and chemotherapy, usually with dactinomycin, are presented graphically (see Figure 1 for explanation of white, stippled, and black bars).

irradiation of the lung metastases, but no abdominal irradiation. Her metastases were resolved and she is now living seven years after treatment. The remaining patient, a four-year-old girl who also had initial pulmonary metastases, received nitrogen mustard in addition to surgical excision and irradiation of the tumor. She is now free of tumor nine years later.

Dactinomycin Therapy

Because of the great improvement in survival rates among our patients after the addition of dactinomycin therapy, we believe that this drug should be used routinely. Fortunately, there are only a few undesirable side effects associated with its administration and they are controllable. Although it appears that more children have experienced transient leukopenia, severe anorexia, or malaise during postoperative irradiation since the addition of initial dactinomycin therapy, no patient has died as a result of such treatment. When these symptoms become severe, a temporary cessation of irradiation for several days usually has enabled the patient to recover sufficiently to allow the therapy to continue.

A study of those patients with localized tumor (Fig. 4) suggested an effect of the drug against metastatic tumor cells which are not yet detectable clinically. Ten of 13, or 77 per cent, of those initially treated with dactinomycin in this group have survived the two-year risk period, as opposed to three of eight, or 38 per cent, of those who did not receive it.

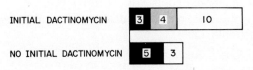

Fig. 4.—The results of therapy both with and without initial dactinomycin are compared in 25 patients with only localized tumor at the time of diagnosis (see Figure 1 for explanation of white, stippled, and black bars).

At the present time we are cooperating with the Children's Cancer Study Group A in a controlled study of patients without disseminated disease to learn more about the value of repeated courses of dactinomycin given six weeks postoperatively and then every three months for one to two years.

An early summation of our results in such a group of 42 patients is presented in Figure 5. As stated previously, only four of 16, or 25 per cent, of patients who did not receive initial dactinomycin therapy successfully survived the two-year risk period. With the addition of only a planned initial course of dactinomycin, four of nine patients, or 44 per cent, survived the risk period, and four others are still living, two with probable persistent tumor. Thirteen patients, however, received both initial and planned repeated courses of dactinomycin. Nine of these survived the two-year risk period; two additional patients are tumor free, but still within the risk period. Only one patient has died and one other is living with tumor. Our present two-year survival rate is thus 9/10, or 90 per cent, in those patients without initial metastases who received both initial and planned repeated courses of dactinomycin. This promising rate has encouraged us to suggest that all patients should receive such therapy, because the advantageous effects of the drug are much reduced once a metastatic tumor has become clinically apparent. Of 11 patients who were

Fig. 5.—The results of treatment in 42 patients who had either localized or locally extended tumor are related to therapy without initial dactinomycin, with only a planned initial course of dactinomycin, and with both initial and planned repeated courses of the drug (see Figure 1 for explanation of white, stippled, and black bars).

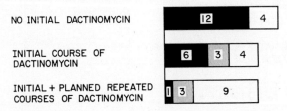

given initial or additional courses of dactinomycin only after the later appearance of metastases, nine have died and the remaining two are living with demonstrable tumor.

Lung Metastases

Anyone studying survival in patients with Wilms' tumor must analyze carefully the appearance of lung metastases, which are the usual cause of death among those with this disease. Twenty-four patients in this series were known to develop such metastases. In seven, the metastases were present at the time the diagnosis was established. Three of these patients survived the two-year risk period successfully. Each was given 1,500 to 2,500 r of pulmonary irradiation; in addition, one received initial nitrogen mustard therapy, the second had repeated courses of dactinomycin, and the third had a combination of these drugs. All four patients who died received initial and subsequent courses of dactinomycin.

Seventeen patients developed pulmonary metastases later in the course of their disease. Eleven of these were treated with pulmonary irradiation and subsequent courses of dactinomycin. Eight of those who were so treated have died, and the other three are living with tumor. Because of this poor experience with the management of late pulmonary metastases, we studied the development of this problem in the 42 patients who initially did not have disseminated disease. In this group (Fig. 6), lung metastases occurred in eight (50 per cent) of 16 patients who did not receive initial dactinomycin, in seven (54 per cent) of 13 who had only a planned initial course of dactinomycin, but in only two (15 per cent) of 13 who

Fig. 6.—The development of lung metastases in those patients initially with no disseminated tumor is related to their treatment without dactinomycin, with only a planned initial course of dactinomycin, and with both initial and planned repeated courses of the drug. The striped bars signify patients who developed lung metastases and the clear bars indicate those who did not.

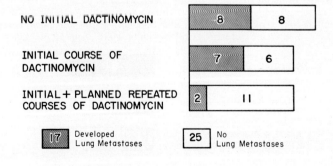

had both initial and planned repeated courses of dactinomycin. These findings correlate well with our previously noted survival statistics and lend further support to the use of planned repeated courses of dactinomycin in all patients to help prevent the development of clinical lung metastases.

Surgical excision of controlled pulmonary metastases also was done in selected cases. Three children underwent six thoracotomies for excision of residual, isolated pulmonary metastases after initial response to irradiation and chemotherapy. Although all eventually died, one lived four and one-half years and another nine years after operation. We plan to continue this aggressive treatment program.

Other Metastases

Of the entire group of 50 patients, only four children were known to develop liver metastases. Bony metastases occurred in two patients and intraspinal and brain metastases each appeared only once. We have not been able to produce survival with our present modes of therapy once these metastatic lesions have appeared.

Secondary Abdominal Operation

Repeated abdominal operations to remove locally recurrent disease were attempted in five patients. All subsequently died. In an attempt to control such recurrent or persistent local disease in its early stages, the concept of the "second look" abdominal operation was applied in five patients about 10 years ago. In all five, no intra-abdominal tumor was found. In spite of this, one patient subsequently died of lung metastases. This reemphasizes the fact that the cause of death in patients with Wilms' tumor is usually not locally recurrent disease, but systemic disseminated tumor with lung metastases.

Conclusions

From this analysis of 50 patients with Wilms' tumor, it is apparent that the addition of dactinomycin chemotherapy to standard management with surgical excision and irradiation of the primary tumor increased the two-year tumor-free survival rate substantially. Dactinomycin was most effective in preventing clinical lung metastases when given both initially at the time of surgical therapy and in planned repeated courses in six weeks and then every three months for one to two years. Although our patients must be followed for a longer period of time before statistically significant survival rates can be obtained, evidence that one should use both initial and planned repeated courses of dactinomycin in all patients with Wilms' tumor is accumulating rapidly.

Secondary operations for locally recurrent tumor as well as second look procedures were not worthwhile.

Summary

A standard management program for patients with Wilms' tumor was presented. Fifty patients, most of whom were treated in this manner either with or without the addition of dactinomycin chemotherapy, were studied retrospectively.

Survival for two years without evidence of tumor was found to be a practical risk period, but it could not be equated with eventual cure. Our two-year survival rate was closely related to the patient's age and the extent of the tumor at the time of diagnosis, as well as to the development of lung metastases. Concentration on the prevention of lung metastases encouraged the use of both initial and planned repeated courses of dactinomycin, with strikingly good results on early evaluation.

REFERENCES

Collins, V. P.: The treatment of Wilms's tumor. *Cancer*, 11:89-94, January-February 1958.

Farber, S.: Chemotherapy in the treatment of leukemia and Wilms' tumor. *Journal of the American Medical Association*, 198:826-836, November 21, 1966.

Gross, R. E.: Embryoma of the kidney (Wilms' tumor). In *The Surgery of Infancy and Childhood*. Philadelphia, Pennsylvania, W. B. Saunders Company, 1953, pp. 588-605.

Howard, R.: Actinomycin D in Wilms' tumour: Treatment of lung metastases. *Archives of Disease in Childhood*, 40:200-202, April 1965.

Johnson, D. G., Maceira, F., and Koop, C. E.: Wilms' tumor treated with actinomycin D: The relationship of age and extent of disease to survival. *Journal of Pediatric Surgery*, 2:13-21, February 1967.

Lattimer, J. K., Melicow, M. M., and Uson, A. C.: Wilms' tumor: A report of 71 cases. *Journal of Urology*, 80:401-416, December 1958.

Platt, B. B., and Linden, G.: Wilms's tumor—A comparison of 2 criteria for survival. *Cancer*, 17:1573-1578, December 1964.

Rowe, M. I., Morse, T. S., and Frye, T. R.: Infusion pyelography in infancy and childhood. *Journal of Pediatric Surgery*, 2:215-220, June 1967.

Snyder, W. H., Jr., Hastings, T. N., and Pollack, W.: Wilms' tumor: Embryoma of the kidney. In Benson, C. D., Mustard, W. T., Ravitch, M. M., Snyder, W. H., Jr., and Welch, K. J., Eds.: *Pediatric Surgery*. Chicago, Illinois, Year Book Medical Publishers, Inc., 1962, Vol. 2, pp. 860-899.

Sukarochana, K., and Kiesewetter, W. B.: Wilms' tumor: Factors influencing long-term survival. *Journal of Pediatrics*, 69:747-752, November 1966.

Platelet Replacement*

EMIL J FREIREICH, M.D.,

JOHN A. SHIVELY, M.D., AND

DAVID S. DE JONGH, M.D.

*Departments of Developmental Therapeutics and Pathology,
The University of Texas M. D. Anderson Hospital and
Tumor Institute at Houston, Houston, Texas*

FOR THE OPTIMAL MANAGEMENT of neoplastic diseases in childhood, the replacement of platelets in the patient's circulation provides an important mode of supportive therapy (Djerassi, Farber, and Evans, 1963; Freireich, 1966; Zucker and Lundberg, 1966). It is particularly crucial in the treatment of patients with leukemia in whom thrombocytopenia sufficient to result in hemorrhage is regularly present and in whom effective chemotherapy is assisted greatly by a decrease in the risk of hemorrhage. Much of the pioneer work in establishing platelet replacement therapy as a practical and useful method of treatment was accomplished in children with neoplastic disease, particularly leukemia (Farber and Klein, 1957; Freireich *et al.,* 1963). Because platelets have a life-span of 10 days or less in normal individuals and even shorter in patients with leukemia and other malignant diseases, a major obstacle for adequate replacement therapy is the large quantity of material required (Aas and Gardner, 1958). Studies in children allow the collection resources from adult donors to be combined with the smaller blood volume of pediatric recipients. This combination is probably a major reason for the success of many of the early studies in the pediatric age group.

Background

Virtually all of the essential facts relating to platelet replacement were described by Duke in 1910. He recognized the clinical syndrome associ-

*The work on this project was supported in part by U. S. Public Health Service Grant No. CA 08859.

ated with thrombocytopenia and described three patients who had a hemorrhagic disease characterized by petechiae. He introduced the bleeding time test bearing his name, which consists of puncturing the ear lobe and observing the time required for hemorrhage to stop. He also examined the blood and observed that the concentration of the small bodies, known as blood platelets, was decreased greatly. Duke even used a method for the direct enumeration of the number of platelets in the blood. He then described the direct transfusion of blood from volunteer donors into the three patients mentioned above and observed that the bleeding stopped, the number of platelets in the blood increased significantly, and the results of the bleeding time test turned toward normal. Shortly thereafter, citrate was introduced as an effective anticoagulant which permitted whole blood to be stored at refrigerator temperatures, thus permitting creation of blood banks. We now realize that storage at refrigerator temperatures results in a rapid loss of the ability of platelets to circulate in the recipient (Levin and Freireich, 1964). Because blood bank procedures were so effective for red cell transfusion, direct transfusion of fresh blood rarely was attempted.

With the introduction of nonwettable silicone and plastic surfaces in the handling of blood, interest in the transfusion of platelets revived (Gardner, Howell, and Hirsch, 1954). The pioneering work of Farber and his group indicated the potential usefulness of platelet transfusion in the supportive therapy for children with malignant diseases (Farber and Klein, 1957). What remained to be developed were the techniques for efficient collection and transfusion of platelets. Klein developed a closed system for the separation of platelets from whole blood (Klein, Arnold, Earl, and Wake, 1956); and Kliman described the repeated plasmapheresis of blood donors as a technique for increasing greatly the availability of platelets for transfusion (Kliman, Gaydos, Schroeder, and Freireich, 1961).

Indications for Platelet Replacement

A quantitative estimation of the degree of platelet depression in the patient is essential for platelet replacement. Adequate assessment of the concentration of platelets requires an accurate, direct, platelet counting method. The method introduced by Brecher and co-workers, which utilizes a direct chamber count with a phase contrast microscope, provides a reproducible, effective method for measuring accurately the concentration of platelets in whole blood (Brecher, Schneiderman, and Cronkite, 1953).

Platelets also can be counted by electronic blood cell counting instruments, but the estimations then must be made on platelet-rich plasma freed of red cells (Bull, Schneiderman, and Brecher, 1965).

The intensity of the hemorrhagic diathesis in the patient is related directly to the degree of thrombocytopenia: the more severe the depression of platelet count the greater the likelihood that the patient will demonstrate the hemorrhagic diathesis (Gaydos, Freireich, and Mantel, 1962). The most common hemorrhagic manifestations are petechiae of the skin and mucous membranes; gross hemorrhage, such as bleeding from mucous membranes, hematuria, and intracranial hemorrhage occur less frequently. For platelet counts in excess of 100,000/cu. mm., the risk of hemorrhage does not differ significantly from the risk in individuals with normal platelet counts (*i.e.,* 250,000/cu. mm.). While mild hemorrhagic manifestations are observed when platelet counts are between 20,000 and 100,000, gross major bleeding is observed rarely (less than one per cent of days at these levels). In contrast, when platelet counts are below 1,000/cu. mm., patients will have gross, major bleeding on 30 per cent of the days that the platelet count is depressed so severely. It must be emphasized that other disturbances of the blood coagulation system will aggravate the hemorrhagic diathesis resulting from thrombocytopenia alone. Thus, patients who have hemorrhage should be examined carefully for other abnormalities which must be adequately managed if platelet replacement is to be effective.

Patients with platelet counts lower than 50,000/cu. mm. who have a hemorrhagic diathesis indicated by petechiae or gross bleeding have an indication for platelet replacement transfusion. In the absence of a hemorrhagic diathesis, moderately severe thrombocytopenia (*i.e.,* platelet count between 10,000 and 50,000/cu. mm.) carries only a moderate risk of bleeding and often can be managed without platelet transfusion. However, patients who have severe thrombocytopenia (*i.e.,* platelet counts below 10,000/cu. mm.) and particularly patients with platelet counts below 1,000/cu. mm. have such a high risk of developing hemorrhage that platelet transfusion is indicated even in the absence of clinical bleeding.

Patients undergoing therapy for malignant diseases will show rapid changes in platelet counts. Myelosuppressive therapy combined with a shortened platelet life-span in the sick patient can cause a rapid fall in the platelet count (Freireich *et al.,* 1963). Frequent platelet counts, at least two every week are essential for the recognition and management of thrombocytopenia.

Technique of Platelet Transfusion

The most effective platelet transfusion product is freshly collected platelets, transfused immediately to the recipient. The interval between the start of the phlebotomy in the donor and the completion of the transfusion in the recipient should be kept below six hours, if possible. Platelets lose viability quickly in vitro (Levin and Freireich, 1964). After 24 hours of storage in anticoagulant acid citrate dextrose (ACD) solution at refrigerator temperature, the number of transfused platelets remaining in the circulation of the recipient one hour after transfusion is only half the number observed with fresh platelets. After 48 hours of storage in vitro, there are essentially no viable platelets remaining. Moreover, the life-span of those platelets which do circulate is greatly shortened, so that virtually all are removed from the circulation within one day after transfusion. Thus, fresh platelets are the optimal product.

The platelets may be transfused as whole blood, platelet-rich plasma, or platelet concentrates. When the patient is bleeding actively and requires replacement of red cells, plasma, and platelets, the ideal replacement product is fresh whole blood. If the patient does not need replacement of red cells, then platelet-rich plasma is the simplest and most effective platelet transfusion product. More than 90 per cent of the platelets in whole blood should be present in the platelet-rich plasma. However, the ideal platelet transfusion product is platelet concentrates. In the preparation of platelet concentrates, good technique is essential, since 50 per cent or more of the platelets in the platelet-rich plasma can be lost if the concentrates are not prepared properly (Levin, Pert, and Freireich, 1965). There are several effective techniques for the preparation of platelet concentrates (Aster and Jandl, 1964; Flatow and Freireich, 1966; Shively, Sullivan, and Chiu, 1966; Chappell, 1966). The simplest and most effective is acidification of the platelet-rich plasma with additional ACD solution, prior to centrifugation (Shively, Sullivan, and Chiu, 1966). In the acidified plasma, platelet aggregation and clumping are inhibited greatly; and smooth, effective concentrates can be regularly prepared. The use of platelet concentrates permits salvaging of red cells and plasma for conventional blood bank purposes and provides the smallest volume for injection to the recipients, many of whom are quite ill and unable to tolerate the large plasma and blood volume which otherwise would be required for adequate platelet replacement.

Dosage and Frequency of Treatment

One unit of platelets is considered to be the number of platelets derived from one unit of whole blood which contains 1–1.5×10^{11} platelets. If platelet-rich plasma or platelet concentrates are prepared, between 0.7–1.25×10^{11} platelets will be derived from each unit of whole blood. These quantities frequently are referred to as one unit of platelet-rich plasma or platelet concentrate. The average increase in the concentration of platelets in peripheral blood observed depends on both the number of platelets injected and the size of the recipient (Freireich *et al.*, 1963). For a child with one square meter of body surface area (a body weight of approximately 30 kg.), transfusion of 10^{11} platelets (one unit of platelets) will result in an average increase in circulating platelet count of 12,000/cu. mm. For very small children with 0.5 square meter body surface area (a body weight of 10 kg.), transfusion of one unit of platelets will give an increment of approximately 25,000/cu. mm.; whereas in an adult with two square meters (body weight of approximately 70 kg.), four units of platelets would be needed to produce an average increase of 25,000/cu. mm.

Transfused platelets in a normal individual have a life-span of up to 10 days. However, in children with neoplastic disease, particularly patients with acute leukemia, the survival period is appreciably shorter; the median half-life (50 per cent survival) is between 36 and 48 hours. Factors known to be associated with shortened platelet life-span include fever and infection, gross bleeding, and massive splenomegaly. Patients with these complications have an even shorter platelet life-span and will require larger doses of platelets at more frequent intervals. Patients who are in better condition will require less frequent treatment. In the average patient, treatment at two- to four-day intervals is usually adequate, if the appropriate increments are accomplished with each transfusion. As an example, for a child with one square meter of body surface area, who has a platelet count of 10,000/cu. mm., transfusion of four units of platelets would give an expected average increment of 50,000/cu. mm., and four days later the platelet count would have fallen from 60,000 to 30,000. Treatment with two to four units of platelets two to three times a week thereafter would maintain the platelet count in excess of 20,000 for most of the time. This would be quite effective replacement therapy for such an individual.

Evaluation of Response to Therapy

The objective of therapy with platelet transfusion is the control and prevention of bleeding. For patients who have thrombocytopenia with hemorrhage, adequate quantities of platelets must be transfused to produce cessation of hemorrhage. Clearly, an adequate dosage in this instance is the amount required to control the bleeding. If the platelet count is elevated by transfusion to levels in excess of 20,000 and hemorrhage persists, then careful evaluation of the patient must be undertaken to identify other contributing causes of bleeding, such as local lesions or disturbances of the coagulation mechanism.

Once bleeding is controlled, sufficient platelet transfusion should be given to prevent recurrence of hemorrhage. The most reliable guide to platelet replacement therapy is the concentration of platelets in the peripheral blood. Clinical hemorrhage can be controlled with small quantities of platelets, which produce only minor increases in the concentration of circulating blood platelets (Freireich, Schmidt, Schneiderman and Frei, 1959). However these increases are short-lived, and hemorrhage is likely to recur. If the platelet count is elevated well out of the range where hemorrhage is likely, that is, if the platelet count is maintained between 20,000 and 50,000/cu. mm., the likelihood of recurrent bleeding is diminished greatly (Han, Stutzman, Cohen and Kem, 1966; Hersh, Bodey, Nies, and Freireich, 1965). If the patient's bone marrow recovers adequately to maintain his platelet count, then therapy is discontinued.

Complications of Platelet Transfusion

As with the transfusion of any blood product in man, one of the greatest risks is transfusion hepatitis. The careful screening of donors may be of value in reducing the frequency of this complication. Keeping the number of donors used in a platelet transfusion program to a minimum also is helpful. The number of donors needed can be reduced by using platelets collected by plasmapheresis and by developing donor populations that donate frequently and at regular intervals.

The other side effect which occurs regularly after platelet transfusion is a febrile reaction. This reaction is always self-limited. It occurs during transfusion or up to 12 hours after its completion. It usually is of short duration and lasts less than 24 hours. The febrile reaction can be associated with chills, hives, or flushing of the skin. No dangerous side effects have been observed. There is an isoantigen system in platelets which differs from that associated with red cell transfusion (Shulman, Marder,

Hiller, and Collier, 1964). Even in the presence of very high concentrations of platelet antibodies, the transfusion of large quantities of platelets will be associated with febrile reactions, but not with more serious or more threatening complications. The procedures for detecting platelet isoantibodies and isoantigens are complex, and the routine grouping and typing of platelets are difficult and elaborate processes. Because isoimmunization to platelets seldom occurs particularly in patients who are receiving immunosuppressive chemotherapy, it is possible to transfuse platelets over a long period of time with infrequent occurrence of resistance to platelet transfusion (Flatow and Freireich, 1966). If platelet isoimmunization does develop, then appropriate screening procedures can help to select compatible platelets, and platelet transfusion therapy can continue (Aster, Levin, Cooper, and Freireich, 1964).

Selection of Donors

Use of plasmapheresis can increase greatly the available supply of platelets for transfusion. In children with malignant diseases, the use of parents and relatives frequently has proved effective. An adult donor can give two units of platelets twice a week for extended periods of time with no depletion (Kliman, Carbone, Gaydos, and Freireich, 1964). As a result, one or two donors are adequate for good replacement therapy in a patient. Many patients with acute leukemia are treated for periods up to three months with twice weekly transfusions from one donor. Limiting the number of donors minimizes the risk of isoimmunization and of transfusion hepatitis. The selection of parents as donors further minimizes the risk of isoimmunization because of shared antigens with the patient. Thus, plasmapheresis procedures have proved invaluable in effective platelet replacement programs. The collection of platelets as a by-product of whole blood is also very useful and will supplement the available supply of platelets for replacement.

Summary

The replacement of platelets is a relatively simple, practical, and useful form of supportive therapy. The intelligent application of platelet replacement therapy can greatly assist physicians in the treatment of children with neoplastic diseases, particularly those with leukemia. With adequate platelet replacement therapy, the risk of morbidity and mortality from hemorrhage can be virtually eliminated. Control of hemorrhage can increase the effectiveness of the treatment regimen and produce better control of the malignant disease. In addition, parents appreciate the opportunity to participate in the treatment of their children by serving as platelet donors; they especially desire to participate during periods when their children must be hospitalized. The equipment is now sufficiently simple and inexpensive, so that platelet replacement can and should be practiced widely in the supportive therapy of children with neoplastic diseases.

REFERENCES

Aas, K., and Gardner, F. H.: Survival of blood platelets labeled with chromium. *Journal of Clinical Investigation,* 37:1257-1268, July 1958.

Aster, R. H., and Jandl, J. H.: Platelet sequestration in man. *Journal of Clinical Investigation,* 43:843-869, May 1964.

Aster, R. H., Levin, R. H., Cooper, H., and Freireich, E. J.: Complement fixing platelet iso-antibodies in serum of transfused persons. Correlation of antibodies with platelet survival in thrombocytopenic patients. *Transfusion,* 4:428-440, November-December 1964.

Brecher, G., Schneiderman, M., and Cronkite, E. P.: Reproducibility and constancy of the platelet count. *American Journal of Clinical Pathology,* 23:15-26, January 1953.

Bull, B. S., Schneiderman, M. A., and Brecher, G.: Platelet counts with the Coulter counter. *American Journal of Clinical Pathology,* 44:678-688, December 1965.

Chappell, W. S.: Platelet concentrates from acidified plasma: A method of preparation without the use of additives. *Transfusion,* 6:308-309, July-August 1966.

Djerassi, I., Farber, S., and Evans, A. E.: Transfusions of fresh platelet concentrates to patients with secondary thrombocytopenia. *New England Journal of Medicine,* 268:221-226, January 31, 1963.

Duke, W. W.: The relation of blood platelets to hemorrhagic disease: Description of a method for determining the bleeding time and coagulation time and report of three cases of hemorrhagic disease relieved by transfusion. *Journal of the American Medical Association,* 55:1185-1192, 1910.

Farber, S., and Klein, E.: The nature and control of bleeding in acute leukemia and other thrombocytopenic states: A review of a ten year program of research. *Annals of Paediatric Fenniae,* 3:348-362, 1957.

Flatow, F. A., and Freireich, E. J: Effect of splenectomy on the response to platelet transfusion in three patients with aplastic anemia. *New England Journal of Medicine,* 274:242-248, February 3, 1966.

———: The increased effectiveness of platelet concentrates prepared in acidified plasma. *Blood, The Journal of Hematology,* 27:449-459, April 1966.

Freireich, E. J: Effectiveness of platelet transfusion in leukemia and aplastic anemia. *Transfusion,* 6:50-54, January-February 1966.

Freireich, E. J, Kliman, A., Gaydos, L. A., Mantel, N., and Frei, E., III: Response to repeated platelet transfusion from the same donor. *Annals of Internal Medicine,* 59:277-288, September 1963.

Freireich, E. J, Schmidt, P. J., Schneiderman, M. A., and Frei, E., III: A comparative study of the effect of transfusion of fresh and preserved whole blood on bleeding in patients with acute leukemia. *New England Journal of Medicine,* 260:6-11, January 1, 1959.

Gardner, F. H., Howell, D., and Hirsch, E. O.: Platelet transfusions utilizing plastic equipment. *Journal of Laboratory and Clinical Medicine,* 43:196-207, February 1954.

Gaydos, L. A., Freireich, E. J, and Mantel, N.: The quantitative relation between platelet count and hemorrhage in patients with acute leukemia. *New England Journal of Medicine,* 266:905-909, May 3, 1962.

Han, T., Stutzman, L., Cohen, E., and Kem, U.: Effect of platelet transfusion on hemorrhage in patients with acute leukemia. *Cancer,* 19:1937-1942, December 1966.

Heish, E. M., Bodey, G. P., Nies, B. A., and Freireich, E. J: Causes of death in acute leukemia. A ten-year study of 414 patients from 1954-1963. *Journal of the American Medical Association,* 193:105-109, July 12, 1965.

Jandl, J. H., and Aster, R. H.: Increased splenic pooling and the pathogenesis of hypersplenism. *The American Journal of the Medical Sciences,* 253:383-398, April 1967.

Klein, E., Arnold, P., Earl, R. T., and Wake, E.: A practical method for the aseptic preparation of human platelet concentrates without loss of other blood elements. *New England Journal of Medicine,* 254:1132-1133, June 14, 1956.

Kliman, A., Carbone, P. P., Gaydos, L. A., and Freireich, E. J: Effects of intensive plasmapheresis on normal blood donors. *Blood, The Journal of Hematology,* 23: 647-656, May 1964.

Kliman, A., Gaydos, L. A., Schroeder, L. R., and Freireich, E. J: Repeated plasmapheresis of blood donors as a source of platelets. *Blood, The Journal of Hematology,* 18:303-309, September 1961.

Levin, R. H., and Freireich, E. J: Effect of storage up to 48 hours on response to transfusions of platelet rich plasma. *Transfusion,* 4:251-256, July-August 1964.

Levin, R. H., Pert, J. H., and Freireich, E. J: Response to transfusion of platelets pooled from multiple donors and the effects of various technics of concentrating platelets. *Transfusion,* 5:54-63, January-February 1965.

Shively, J. A., Sullivan, M. P., and Chiu, J. S.: Transfusion of platelet concentrates prepared from acidified platelet-rich plasma. *Transfusion,* 16:302-307, July-August 1966.

Shulman, N. R., Marder, B. J., Hiller, M. D., and Collier, E. M.: Platelet and leukocyte iso-antigens and their antibodies: Serologic physiologic and clinical studies. In Moore, C. V., and Brown, E. B., Eds.: *Progress in Hematology.* New York, New York, Grune and Stratton, Inc., 1964, Vol. 4, pp. 222-304.

Zucker, M. B., and Lundberg, A.: Platelet transfusions. *Anesthesiology,* 27:385-398, July-August 1966.

The Problem of Infection in Children with Malignant Disease*

GERALD P. BODEY, M.D., AND

EVAN M. HERSH, M.D.

*Department of Developmental Therapeutics, The University of Texas
M. D. Anderson Hospital and Tumor Institute at Houston,
Houston, Texas*

WITH THE AVAILABILITY of effective cancer chemotherapy there has been an increasing awareness of infection as a major cause of morbidity and mortality in children with neoplastic diseases. In most cases, chemotherapeutic agents must be administered for four to eight weeks before maximum antitumor effect is achieved. It is during this period of time that the patient is most susceptible to infectious complications. Hence, prompt diagnosis and effective management of infection have become integral parts of the successful treatment of patients with malignant diseases.

Figure 1 illustrates graphically that infection is the major cause of death in children 10 years old or younger who have acute leukemia. The data were obtained from a study of patients with acute leukemia who underwent autopsy at the National Institutes of Health in the period from 1955 to June 1963 (Hersh, Bodey, Nies, and Freireich, 1965). The figure shows that the incidence of hemorrhage as a cause of death in children was reduced by 50 per cent after platelet transfusion became available as a therapeutic measure. However, infection continued to be the major cause of mortality during the entire period, accounting for 70 per cent of deaths.

*This investigation was supported in part by grant No. CA 10042-02 from the U. S. Public Health Service.

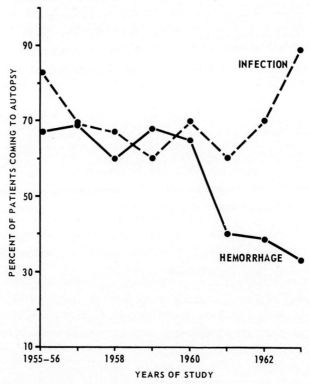

Fig. 1.—The incidence of fatal hemorrhage in children with acute leukemia was reduced significantly after platelet transfusions became available. Infection continues to be the major cause of death in these children.

The Incidence and Types of Infection in Malignant Diseases

The incidence of infection was determined in children with cancer at The University of Texas M. D. Anderson Hospital and Tumor Institute at Houston. Charts of all patients 10 years old and younger who underwent autopsy from January 1, 1962 to June 30, 1967 were reviewed. Infection was not considered to be present if organisms were isolated from heart blood cultures only, unless other evidence of infection was found. Some of these patients were highly febrile prior to death, and the heart blood culture may have been an accurate indication of septicemia.

Table 1 indicates the incidence of infection in children with each of the three major types of malignant diseases. Of the 98 subjects who underwent autopsy, 69 per cent had infections. The incidence of infection

TABLE 1.—INFECTIONS IN PEDIATRIC CANCER PATIENTS AT AUTOPSY
JANUARY 1, 1962 TO JUNE 30, 1967

	SOLID TUMORS		LYMPHOMA		ACUTE LEUKEMIA		TOTAL	
	No.	Per Cent	No.	Per Cent	No.	Per Cent	No.	Per Cent
Total autopsies	44	—	11	—	43	—	98	—
Subjects with infection	20	45	9	82	39	91	68	69
Deaths resulting from infection	6	13	5	45	34	79	45	46

was about twice as high in subjects with acute leukemia as in those with
solid tumors. Infection was responsible for death in the majority of subjects with acute leukemia, accounted for death in nearly half of subjects
with lymphoma, but seldom caused death in subjects with solid tumors.
Of all subjects dying of infection, 79 per cent had acute leukemia and
only 13 per cent had solid tumors.

Table 2 lists the various types of infection found in this series of autopsy subjects. Pneumonia was the most common type and occurred with
equal frequency in subjects with hematologic and nonhematologic cancers. Septicemia occurred in 44 per cent of those studied. It was 12 times
more frequent in patients with acute leukemia than in those with solid
tumors and twice as frequent in subjects with acute leukemia as in those

TABLE 2.—TYPES OF INFECTIONS IN PEDIATRIC CANCER PATIENTS AT AUTOPSY
JANUARY 1, 1962 TO JUNE 30, 1967

TYPE OF INFECTION	SOLID TUMORS		LYMPHOMA		ACUTE LEUKEMIA		TOTAL	
	No. of Infec- tions	% of Sub- jects	No. of Infec- tions	% of Sub- jects	No. of Infec- tions	% of Sub- jects	No. of Infec- tions	% of Sub- jects
Septicemia	1	5	3	33	26	67	30	44
Pneumonia	13	65	5	56	22	56	40	59
Pyelonephritis	5	25	0	0	2	5	7	10
Enterocolitis	1	5	3	33	9	23	13	19
Mouth infection and pharyngitis	3	15	1	11	6	15	10	15
Cellulitis	1	5	1	11	6	15	8	12
Peritonitis	1	5	0	0	4	10	5	7
Meningitis	1	5	0	0	4	10	5	7
Disseminated cytomegalic inclusion disease	0	0	0	0	3	8	3	4
Disseminated candidiasis	0	0	0	0	1	3	1	1
Miscellaneous	1	5	2	22	8	21	11	16
Total infections	27	—	15	—	91	—	133	—
Subjects with infection	20	—	9	—	39	—	68	—
Subjects with multiple infections	4	20	4	44	29	74	37	54

with lymphoma. Eighty-seven per cent of all cases of septicemia occurred in patients with acute leukemia. Pyelonephritis occurred with frequency only in subjects with solid tumors, whereas enterocolitis occurred more often in subjects with hematologic cancers. Multiple infections were found in 54 per cent of the patients. They occurred in only 20 per cent of subjects with solid tumors compared to 44 per cent of those with lymphoma and 74 per cent of those with acute leukemia.

Organisms Responsible for Infection

The organisms isolated from patients dying of septicemia in the present series are listed in Table 3; 37 organisms were isolated from 30 patients. Multiple organisms were isolated from the blood of five patients. *Pseudomonas* sp. was isolated most frequently; it was found in 47 per cent of patients with fatal septicemia. *Escherichia coli* also was isolated frequently, occurring in 33 per cent of the 30 patients. Only 11 per cent of the organisms were gram-positive cocci. It is noteworthy that there was only one case of fatal *Staphylococcus aureus* septicemia in this series.

These results are similar to those found by Hersh, Bodey, Nies, and Freireich (1965) in a study of patients with acute leukemia who underwent autopsy at the National Institutes of Health. In the group with fatal septicemia, 34 per cent of the deaths were caused by *Pseudomonas* sp., 13 per cent by *E. coli,* 12 per cent by *Klebsiella* sp., 5 per cent by *Staph. aureus,* and 23 per cent by fungi. Figure 2, taken from that study, illustrates the changing incidence of these organisms in the pediatric population from 1955 to June 1963. During the early years, *Staph. aureus* was a frequent cause of fatal septicemia; but when the semisynthetic penicillins became available, no fatal cases of staphylococcal septicemia were

TABLE 3.—ORGANISMS ISOLATED FROM
PATIENTS WITH FATAL SEPTICEMIA

ORGANISM	NUMBER OF SUBJECTS
Pseudomonas sp.	14
Escherichia coli	10
Enterobacter sp.	3
β Streptococcus	3
Proteus mirabilis	2
Proteus vulgaris	2
Klebsiella sp.	1
Clostridium sp.	1
Staphylococcus aureus	1
TOTAL	37

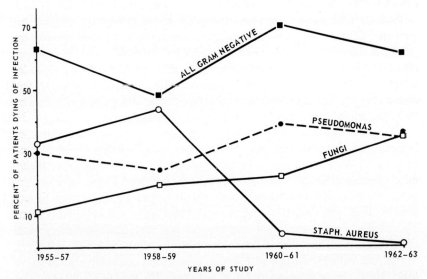

Fig. 2.—The incidence of *Pseudomonas* sp. and fungi causing fatal septicemia in children with acute leukemia increased from 1955 to 1963. However, *Staph. aureus* septicemia which often caused death from 1955 to 1959 was seldom fatal thereafter.

observed. *Pseudomonas* sp. septicemia occurred frequently and increased during the later years of the study. Fungi also occurred more frequently in the later years. The incidence of gram-negative organisms as the cause of fatal septicemia did not change appreciably during the years of the study.

Thirty-seven sites of infection were associated with the 30 cases of fatal septicemia in this series. Septicemia occurred without any demonstrable focus of infection in only two cases. Thirteen cases were associated with respiratory infections, 12 with infection of the gastrointestinal tract, seven with cellulitis, four with meningitis, and one with pyelonephritis.

Infections with gram-negative bacilli are a serious problem in patients with cancer, especially in those with hematologic malignant diseases. Many of these organisms are normal inhabitants of the gastrointestinal tract and probably enter the bloodstream through the ulcerations which frequently result from cancer chemotherapy. Unfortunately, these organisms are ubiquitous and cannot be eliminated readily from the environment of the susceptible patient. The explanation for the peculiar sensitivity of patients with acute leukemia to infection with *Pseudomonas* sp. remains a mystery. The fatality rate for patients with infections caused by this organism approaches 100 per cent, and survival from onset of septicemia is often only 24 hours (Forkner, Frei, Edgecomb, and Utz, 1958).

Patients with cancer are also susceptible to infection with unusual organisms. Septicemias caused by *Serratia marcescens, Listeria monocytogenes, Bordetella bronchiseptica, Bacteroides distasonis,* and several species of *Clostridium* have been observed in these patients. Many episodes of systemic salmonellosis occur in patients with cancer (Han, Sokal, and Neter, 1967). These organisms may infect tumor masses or cause meningitis, pneumonia, peritonitis, or urinary tract infections.

Bloodstream invasion by multiple organisms is a frequent occurrence in patients with acute leukemia. Bodey, Nies, and Freireich (1965) found that such infections occurred in 12 per cent of patients with acute leukemia. Combinations of *Pseudomonas* sp., *E. coli,* and *Staph. aureus* were most common. Gram-positive cocci usually appeared first in the bloodstream, and gram-negative bacilli and fungi were secondary invaders. The fatality rate in these patients was 92 per cent, and median survival after recovery of the second organism from the blood was only two days.

Patients with Hodgkin's disease are considered susceptible to tuberculosis. However, in a study of 1,100 patients with Hodgkin's disease, less than 2 per cent developed active tuberculosis (Silver, 1963). In several studies of patients with acute leukemia, the incidence of tuberculosis was no higher than in the general population (Abbatt and Lea, 1957; Lowther, 1959). Although the incidence is not unusually high with most malignant diseases, patients with prolonged fever of unknown etiology should be investigated for the presence of tuberculosis. Too often this infection is first diagnosed at autopsy.

Fungal infections, once considered a medical curiosity, are now a frequent complication of hematologic cancers (Hutter and Collins, 1962; Schumacher, Ginns, and Warren, 1964). Although uncommon in the pediatric population at Anderson Hospital, fungal infections have been observed with increasing frequency elsewhere and are as common in children as in adults. In an autopsy study of 51 subjects with Hodgkin's disease, Casazza, Duvall, and Carbone (1966) found 10 with fungal infections. Four of the patients died from these infections. The fungi causing infection were *Cryptococcus neoformans, Histoplasma capsulatum, Nocardia* sp., and *Candida* sp. Bodey (1966a) studied the incidence of fungal infections in 454 patients with acute leukemia. A total of 161 patients had fungal infection, excluding thrush, and in 61 per cent this infection was responsible for death. Fourteen per cent of the 454 patients died of fungal infections. Disseminated candidiasis and pulmonary aspergillosis were the most common types of infection, but occasionally cryptococcosis, histoplasmosis, and mucormycosis were seen. These infections were seldom diagnosed before death since the organisms were rarely isolated from culture specimens. For example, *Candida* spp. were isolated from the blood cultures of only 25 per cent of patients with disseminated candidiasis.

Several viral infections have been reported as the cause of serious and, at times, fatal complications in patients with cancer. Giant cell pneumonia caused by the measles virus has been observed in the absence of a rash. The virus may persist for long periods of time in the respiratory tract of leukemic patients, whereas it is not recoverable from normal patients 48 hours after the rash has disappeared (Mitus, Enders, Craig, and Holloway, 1959). Varicella is the exanthem seen most frequently in children with cancer. Like adults who contract chickenpox, these patients tend to develop severe pneumonia which may be fatal (Pinkel, 1961). Liver necrosis also may occur with this infection. Herpes zoster infection is common in patients with lymphomas and may become generalized. Occasionally patients die because of this infection. A few patients with acute leukemia and lymphoma have died from overwhelming herpes simplex infection. Patients may have disseminated infection without any visible herpetic lesions.

Cytomegalic inclusion disease has been observed with increasing frequency in children with malignant diseases (Bodey, Wertlake, Douglas, and Levin, 1965). Although infected patients usually die because of bacterial or fungal infections, the cytomegalovirus is capable of causing fatal pneumonitis and myocarditis. Some patients have died of hemorrhage or protracted diarrhea which led to electrolyte imbalance and occurred secondary to infected gastrointestinal ulcers. Cytological examination or viral cultures of urinary sediment and sputum or gastric washings may be used to establish the diagnosis.

Infection caused by *Pneumocystis carinii,* a protozoan, has been seen increasingly, especially in children with hematologic malignant diseases (Hendry and Patrick, 1962). Clinically, the disease is characterized by progressive dyspnea and cyanosis with few physical findings in the chest. The chest x-ray film usually reveals hazy perihilar infiltrates with sparing of the peripheral lung fields. Although the organisms have been observed in bronchial secretions, the diagnosis usually is established from lung biopsy. Evidence suggests that patients with hematologic cancers also are susceptible to infection with *Toxoplasma gondii*. Infection occurring in patients with hematologic cancers may represent initial exposure or recrudescence of chronic quiescent disease. Infection may be manifested as lymphadenitis, pneumonitis, myocarditis, or encephalitis, or as a maculopapular rash. One patient with acute leukemia died of cardiac arrhythmias secondary to *Toxoplasma gondii* myocarditis (Wertlake and Winters, 1965).

Factors Responsible for Infection

Many factors have been recognized as partially responsible for the high incidence of infection in patients with cancer. Table 4 lists those factors which could be determined in the group of autopsy cases at this institution. Since gamma globulin determinations and studies of immune competence were not performed routinely, an assessment of the role of immunologic deficiencies in these patients was not possible. The majority of patients with all types of malignant diseases received cancer chemotherapy during the month prior to death.

Local factors, such as tumor metastases and operative procedures, played an important role in the infection occurring in subjects with nonhematologic cancers. Of the cases of pneumonia, 80 per cent were associated with pulmonary metastases, aspiration, or tracheostomy. Three of five subjects with pyelonephritis had neurogenic bladder problems because of metastatic disease in the spinal cord. The single cases of meningitis, peritonitis, and enterocolitis occurring in patients with solid tumors were associated with tumor involvement and operative procedures in the area of infection. Similar local factors were seldom apparent in the infections occurring in subjects with hematologic malignant diseases.

Most of the infections in patients with acute leukemia or lymphoma were associated with granulocyte levels less than 1,000/cu. mm. blood on the day prior to death. Granulocytopenia was not present regularly in subjects with nonhematologic cancers. Granulocyte levels less than 100/cu. mm. were found in 51 per cent of the infected subjects with acute leukemia. Of the 133 infections observed in this study, 61 per cent occurred in subjects with acute leukemia who had granulocytopenia.

The relationship between granulocytopenia and severity of infection is shown in Table 5. Only 30 per cent of the 26 cases of pneumonia alone were associated with granulocytopenia, compared to 97 per cent of the 30 cases of septicemia. Granulocyte levels less than 100/cu. mm. were

TABLE 4.—FACTORS ASSOCIATED WITH INFECTION

INFECTION ASSOCIATED WITH	SOLID TUMORS No.	Per Cent	LYMPHOMA No.	Per Cent	ACUTE LEUKEMIA No.	Per Cent
Local factors	18	67	3	20	2	2
Granulocytopenia ($<$ 1,000 granulocytes/cu. mm.) blood	6	22	9	60	81	89
Chemotherapy	19	70	12	80	83	91
TOTAL	27	—	15	—	91	—

TABLE 5.—THE ROLE OF GRANULOCYTOPENIA IN
PNEUMONIA AND SEPTICEMIA

	PER CENT OF SUBJECTS WITH GRANULOCYTE LEVELS			TOTAL NUMBER
	> 1,000	< 1,000	< 100	
Pneumonia	70	30	8	26
Pneumonia with septicemia	0	100	57	14
All septicemia	3	97	60	30

found seven and a half times more often in the subjects with septicemia alone than in those with pneumonia alone. Thirty-five per cent of cases of pneumonia were associated with septicemia. Pneumonia resulted in septicemia only in patients with granulocytopenia. Bodey, Buckley, Sathe, and Freireich (1966) found a relationship between circulating leukocytes and infection in patients with acute leukemia. Fifty-two patients, most of whom were children, were followed from diagnosis to death, a total of 17,743 days of observation. The total number of days spent at various granulocyte levels was determined for the entire group. For more than 30 per cent of the total time, the granulocyte levels were less than 1,000 granulocytes/cu. mm. blood.

The frequency of severe infections, such as pneumonia and septicemia, was related to the level of circulating granulocytes. There were 40 episodes of infection per 1,000 days with granulocyte levels less than 100/cu. mm. compared to only six infectious episodes per 1,000 days with granulocyte levels greater than 1,000/cu. mm. The incidence of infection at any granulocyte level was always greater during relapse than during remission. Similar relationships existed for lymphocytes, but the granulocyte was more important. More severe infections were observed to be associated with more severe granulocytopenia. Any episode of granulocytopenia, regardless of duration, carried a 39 per cent chance of resulting in infection. The risk of infection increased with the duration of granulocytopenia. Infection occurred in 100 per cent of patients who had less than 100 circulating granulocytes/cu. mm. for more than three weeks.

There was also a relationship between episodes of falling granulocyte levels and infection. There were 331 occasions when granulocyte levels fell during one-week periods, and 12 per cent of these resulted in severe infections. The risk of infection correlated more closely with the final level of circulating granulocytes than with the magnitude of the fall. Hence, regardless of the initial level, a fall to 2,000 granulocytes/cu. mm. resulted in only a 2 per cent incidence of severe infections whereas a fall to less than 100 granulocytes/cu. mm. resulted in a 28 per cent incidence of severe infection. The fatality rate was related to the ability of the patient to respond to infection with a granulocytosis. Considering only those patients with granulocyte levels less than 1,000/cu. mm. at the onset of severe infection, the fatality rate was 59 per cent if the granulocyte level did not rise at all during the first week of infection and a fatality rate of 27 per cent if it rose to greater than 1,000/cu. mm.

Patients with granulocytopenia have an inadequate inflammatory response to infection. They may have urinary tract infection without pyuria or pneumonia without characteristic physical signs or evidence of pulmonary infiltrates on the chest x-ray films. Recently we observed a patient with clostridial meningitis who had no leukocytosis in the cerebrospinal fluid and no inflammatory response in the meninges despite the presence of massive numbers of bacteria. Jaffé (1932) concluded from an autopsy study of leukemic subjects that in the absence of marrow granulopoiesis, no inflammatory response occurred at sites of infection. If some functioning myeloid elements were present in the marrow, these subjects had a normal inflammatory response to infection.

Most malignant diseases also are associated with other types of abnormalities in host-defense mechanisms (Hersh and Freireich, 1968). These deficiencies are listed in Table 6. Quantitative and qualitative abnormalities of lymphocyte function are characteristic of advanced solid tumors and lymphoma, especially Hodgkin's disease (Aisenberg, 1966). Lymphocyte function is assessed by skin tests for delayed hypersensitivity, by immunization and subsequent skin tests with dinitrochlorobenzene, by the in vivo lymphocyte transfer test, and by measurement of lympho-

TABLE 6.—HOST DEFENSE IN PATIENTS WITH MALIGNANT DISORDERS

IMMUNOLOGIC FUNCTION	ACUTE LEUKEMIA Relapse	ACUTE LEUKEMIA Remission	SOLID TUMOR Early	SOLID TUMOR Advanced	HODGKIN'S DISEASE Local	HODGKIN'S DISEASE Disseminated
Lymphocyte level	D	N	N	D	N	D
Delayed allergy	N	N	N	D	N or D	D
Lymphocyte transfer	?	?	N	D	D	D
Lymphocyte blastogenesis in vitro	*	N	N	?	N or D	D
Inflammatory response	D	N	N	D	N or D	D
Homograft rejection	N	N	N	N or D	N or D	D
Immunoglobulin levels	N	N	N	N	N	N or D
Antibody response	N	N	N	N or D	N	N or D
Granulocyte level	D	N	N	N	N	N or I
Phagocytosis	D	N	N	N	D	D
Reticuloendothelial system particle clearance	N or D	N or D	N	N or D	I	I

Abbreviations: D, Decreased; I, Increased; N, Normal; *, cannot be evaluated.

blastoid transformation of lymphocytes cultured in vitro with antigens or phytohemagglutinin. Characteristically, patients with disseminated Hodgkin's disease have diminished or absent delayed hypersensitivity, impaired homograft rejection, decreased inflammatory response, and poor in vitro lymphoblastogenesis in response to phytohemagglutinin (Hersh and Oppenheim, 1965). They become progressively lymphopenic with advancing disease. Similar deficiencies in host defense mechanisms are found in patients with disseminated cancers, but they are less severe and appear only in very advanced disease.

In some leukemic patients, the phagocytic capacity of granulocytes is diminished (Hirschberg, 1939). Recently reticuloendothelial function was studied by measuring the clearance rate of aggregated albumin from the blood. The rate of clearance was reduced in some patients with solid tumors and acute leukemia, although the changes were of questionable significance (Groch, Perillie, and Finch, 1965; Donovan, 1967).

Many studies of the effects of antitumor agents on human host defense mechanisms have been conducted. Levin, Landy, and Frei (1964) found that a one-month course of daily, oral 6-mercaptopurine completely inhibited the primary antibody response and the induction of delayed hypersensitivity to tularemia vaccine and the Vi antigen of *E. coli*. Figure 3 summarizes the observations of Hersh, Carbone, and Freireich (1966) and Hersh, Carbone, Wong, and Freireich (1965) concerning five-day courses of 6-mercaptopurine and methotrexate. There was no antibody response to a primary antigen given 24 hours after onset of treatment. Recovery was rapid, and the response to an antigen given 24 hours after the end of treatment was normal.

Several other aspects of host defense in man have been observed to be inhibited by chemotherapy. In the skin window technique, the initial granulocytic phase is followed by the exudation of mononuclear phagocytes (monocytes and macrophages). This phase is profoundly suppressed or completely abolished by antitumor agents (Hersh, Wong, and Freireich, 1966). Recovery is rapid after cessation of therapy.

The effects of cancer chemotherapy on the function of lymphocytes also have been investigated. The in vitro blastogenic response (per cent lymphoblasts generated among lymphocytes cultured with phytohemagglutinin) is inhibited promptly during intensive chemotherapy, but recovers rapidly on cessation of treatment (Hersh and Oppenheim, 1967).

The majority of patients with hematologic malignant diseases receive adrenal corticosteroids as either specific or supportive therapy. Many studies have implicated these agents as a factor predisposing to a variety of bacterial, viral, and fungal infections (Silver, 1963; Bodey, 1966a;

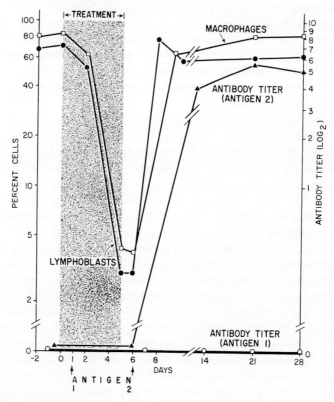

Fig. 3.—A five-day course of cancer chemotherapy inhibits antibody formation, lymphoblastoid transformation of lymphocytes cultured in vitro with antigens of phytohemagglutinin, and the exudation of mononuclear phagocytes (monocytes and macrophages) as measured by the skin window technique.

Pinkel, 1961; Bodey, Wertlake, Douglas, and Levin, 1965; Baker, 1962). The fatality rate from experimental acute and chronic bacterial infections, viral infections, and fungal infections is higher in animals receiving adrenal corticosteroids than in animals not receiving them (Robinson, 1960). Organisms are more numerous in the tissues of treated animals. Furthermore, recrudescence of infection occurs in animals with asymptomatic persistence of pathogenic organisms when they are treated with these agents.

Management of Fever and Infection

Infection should be suspected whenever fever occurs in patients with cancer. Cultures of all orifices and blood specimens should be obtained routinely whenever fever occurs. Chest x-ray films and urinalysis and any other special procedures indicated by the patient's signs and symptoms should be performed. In patients with granulocytopenia or hypogamma-globulinemia, the presence of fever almost always indicates infection. Under these circumstances, antibiotic therapy must be started immediately after initial cultures are obtained. Many of the infections occurring in this group of patients will cause death within 24 hours if not adequately managed.

Since most infections in these patients are caused by gram-negative bacilli and especially *Pseudomonas* sp., broad spectrum antibiotic coverage is necessary. Table 7 shows the activity of some of the currently available antibiotics. Therapy should be initiated with either one of the semisynthetic penicillins or cephalothin plus polymyxin B or colistin. These combinations give maximum coverage against those organisms most likely to cause infection in this group of patients. Modifications then can be made on the basis of culture data. It should be emphasized that although ampicillin is effective against many gram-negative bacilli, it is destroyed by penicillinase and consequently is ineffective against penicillin G-resistant *Staph. aureus*. Where possible, bactericidal antibiotics should be used in preference to bacteriostatic antibiotics, since the latter are more dependent on normal host defenses for eradication of infection. Parenteral antibiotics are preferable during the acute phase of an infection since some oral antibiotics have variable absorption from the gastrointestinal tract and often are tolerated poorly by these patients.

Patients with solid tumors or lymphoma who have prolonged fever of unknown origin should have repeated cultures and should be investigated for the presence of tuberculosis or fungal infection. A trial of antibiotic therapy probably is indicated since fever as a result of cancer seldom

TABLE 7.—SPECTRUM OF ACTIVITY OF VARIOUS ANTIBIOTICS

| | ACTIVITY OF | | | | | |
ORGANISM	CHLORAM-PHENICOL	TETRA-CYCLINE	AMPI-CILLIN	CEPHALO-THIN	KANA-MYCIN	POLY-MYXIN
Escherichia coli	A	A	A	B	A	A
Klebsiella-Aerobacter	B	B	C	B	A	A
Proteus mirabilis	B	D	A	A	B	D
Proteus, indole +	C	C	D	D	A	D
Paracolon	B	B	B	B	A	A
Pseudomonas	D	D	D	D	D	A
Staphylococcus aureus (Penicillin G resistant)	A	B	D	A	A	D

Abbreviations: A, effective against 75 to 100% of strains tested; B, effective against 50 to 75% of strains tested; C, effective against 10 to 50% of strains tested; and D, effective against less than 10% of strains tested.

occurs, except in patients with Hodgkin's disease. In one study, only 5.4 per cent of febrile episodes could be attributed to the cancer itself (Browder, Huff, and Petersdorf, 1961).

Leukemic patients with granulocytopenia who have persistent fever in spite of antibiotic therapy present a perplexing problem. These patients usually die of *Pseudomonas* sp. or other gram-negative bacilli or fungal infections in spite of antibiotic therapy. It is advisable to consider changing antibiotics if the patient's condition is deteriorating and no organism has been isolated. Occasional patients are infected with organisms resistant to the antibiotic combinations mentioned above, such as indole-positive *Proteus* spp., and *Serratia marcescens*. Kanamycin is the drug of choice for many of these infections. Renal toxicity is a common complication of prolonged therapy with polymyxin B and kanamycin, but occurs much less frequently in children than in adults. It is important to continue culturing specimens from patients with persistent fever even though an etiological agent has been isolated. The frequent occurrence of multiple organism infections has been stressed.

At the present time, amphotericin B is the only antifungal agent available for systemic therapy, and it also has considerable renal toxicity. Since most systemic fungal infections are not diagnosed before death, an extensive experience with this drug has not been accumulated in cancer patients. Unfortunately, it has not been very effective in the management of disseminated candidiasis and aspergillosis. Amphotericin B is active against cryptococcosis, but patients with cancer usually do not respond as well as others when treated with it. Occasionally clinical evidence suggests the diagnosis of systemic candidiasis, yet the organism cannot be isolated from multiple blood cultures. If *Candida* spp. is isolated from multiple sites (throat, urine, and stool) and if the patient is deteriorating in spite of antibacterial antibiotics and cannot be subjected to intensive diagnostic procedures, therapeutic trial with amphotericin B is justified.

In several studies of serious bacterial and fungal infections in leukemic patients with granulocytopenia, the major factor in recovery from infection was improvement in the granulocytopenia (Bodey, Nies, and Freireich, 1965; Bodey, 1966a; Bodey, Wertlake, Douglas, and Levin, 1965). This usually was achieved by inducing remission with chemotherapy. Therefore, it is probably wisest to delay chemotherapy during infectious episodes only in those patients who have adequate numbers of circulating granulocytes. In infected patients with severe granulocytopenia, chemotherapy is unlikely to have a major detrimental effect and may be beneficial by inducing remission.

An effective method of providing granulocytes to deficient patients is by transfusion of plasma rich in white cells from chronic myelogenous leukemia donors (Freireich *et al.*, 1964). By the use of plasmapheresis, a median dose of 5.8×10^{10} granulocytes can be obtained. Transfused granulocytes have been observed in bone marrow aspirates and in exudates obtained by means of the skin window technique. Of 81 white blood cell transfusions given to febrile patients, 54 per cent were followed by return of the temperature to normal (Morse *et al.*, 1966). Seven of 13 episodes of *Pseudomonas* sp. septicemia were cured when granulocyte transfusions were used in conjunction with antibiotics (Freireich *et al.*, 1964). Occasional patients received a bone marrow graft from these transfused cells; the graft maintained a normal level of circulating granulocytes for more than one month (Levin *et al.*, 1963).

Future Prospects for the Prevention and Control of Infection

A major obstacle in the management of infection in cancer patients is the difficulty in identifying sites of infection and etiological agents during many febrile episodes. It is often difficult to differentiate between areas of bronchopneumonia and pulmonary metastases in children with solid tumors. Patients with acute leukemia have frequent febrile episodes as a result of infection without demonstrable signs or symptoms. Some of these patients develop chronic pulmonary infiltrates which fail to respond to antibiotic therapy. Often the patients are unable to produce sputum, and extensive diagnostic procedures are precluded by the presence of thrombocytopenia. Fungal, viral, and protozoal agents are not isolated readily; even *Candida* spp., which are cultured readily from the throat or stool, are seldom isolated from the blood of patients with disseminated candidiasis. Hopefully, new serologic techniques will facilitate the diagnosis of some infections. Taschdjian *et al.* (1967) have developed a precipitin test for the serodiagnosis of disseminated candidiasis. Serial determinations of antibody titers may be helpful in establishing the diagnosis of some infections such as cytomegalic inclusion disease (Duvall *et al.*, 1966).

The role of *Mycoplasma* spp. and L-forms of bacteria as infectious agents in cancer patients needs to be determined. *Mycoplasma* sp. have been cultured from the bone marrow of patients with acute leukemia (Barile *et al.*, 1966), but the significance of this finding is not known.

L-forms of bacteria have been demonstrated as the cause of some cases of obscure fever. They are viable, reproducible bacterial variants which are deficient in cell wall. Consequently, they can survive in the presence of some antibiotics like penicillin whose antibacterial effect is directed against cell wall synthesis, even though the parent organism was sensitive to these antibiotics. In seven of eight problem cases of fever, L-forms were cultured repeatedly from the patient's blood (Mattman and Mattman, 1965). Their role in obscure fever in cancer patients has not been defined.

More effective methods of treatment are needed for patients with altered host defenses. With currently available antibiotics, only gram-positive coccal infections can be controlled uniformly in these patients. With the prompt use of the semisynthetic penicillins, even staphylococcal infections can be cured routinely (Bodey, 1966b). However, gram-negative bacilli infections and especially *Pseudomonas* sp. infections have not responded well to antibiotic therapy. Gentamycin, a new aminoglycoside antibiotic with a broad range of activity, has proved effective against *Pseudomonas* sp. infections in burn patients (Stone and Kolb, 1967). This antibiotic is bactericidal and should be effective in patients with altered host defenses although initial preliminary studies have not been promising. A new semisynthetic penicillin, carbenicillin, has been found to have some activity against *Pseudomonas* sp. in vitro. The antibiotic has been used in patients with *Pseudomonas* sp. infections in Great Britain with very encouraging results (Brumfitt, Percival, and Leigh, 1967). Although only marginally active, the antibiotic is very nontoxic and can be administered safely in high doses. In combination with other antibiotics, it may prove very effective in the management of *Pseudomonas* sp. infections in patients with impaired host defenses. Hopefully, new antifungal agents will soon become available which will be more effective and less toxic than amphotericin B.

In addition to the development of more effective antibiotics, research is being conducted on the replacement of those factors which are deficient in cancer patients and are necessary to combat infection. As mentioned previously, it has been possible to combat infection by the transfusion of granulocytes from chronic myelogenous leukemia donors into granulocytopenic recipients. Current research at this institution is directed to the harvesting of granulocytes from the peripheral blood of normal donors by the use of a white blood cell separator. This unit consists of a centrifuge which removes leukocytes and returns the erythrocytes and plasma to the donor.

Another avenue of approach is the prevention of infection by the elimination of exogenous and endogenous organisms from the susceptible patient. A protected environment and prophylactic, oral nonabsorbable antibiotics are being studied as a means of preventing infection in cancer

TABLE 8.—ORAL, NONABSORBABLE ANTIBIOTIC REGIMEN USED
FOR PATIENTS IN THE PROTECTED ENVIRONMENT

ANTIBIOTIC	DOSAGE	ADMINISTRATION
Paromomycin sulfate	500 mg.	Every four hours
Polymyxin B sulfate	70 mg.	Every four hours
Vancomycin hydrochloride	250 mg.	Every four hours
Amphotericin B	100 mg.	Every four hours

patients. The protected environment, known as the Life Island*, consists of a bed enclosed in a plastic canopy (Fig. 4). Air entering the unit passes through high-efficiency filters which remove all viable particles. All items entering the unit, including food, are sterilized. An effective antibiotic regimen is shown in Table 8. Patients undergoing cancer chemotherapy have been studied for up to 216 days. Experience with children in this unit has been limited. Although the use of this unit and an antibiotic regimen has not completely eliminated the risk of infection in the patients studied, it has produced a significant reduction.

At the present time, laminar air flow rooms, which will serve a similar

Fig. 4.—View of Life Island unit showing console and pass-through locks.

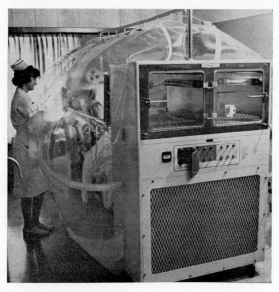

*T. M. Matthews Research, Incorporated, Alexandria, Virginia.

purpose, are being installed at Anderson Hospital. These rooms provide a continuous flow of filtered air in a laminar distribution, and as long as personnel remain downstream from the patient, there is little chance of transferring organisms to him. However, special dress will be required when personnel come in contact with the patient. Prophylactic antibiotics will be used in these rooms as in the Life Island unit. Sterilization of all items entering the rooms, including food, will be routine. The major advantage of a laminar air flow room is that it is not as confining. Hopefully, this type of protected environment will prove acceptable to pediatric patients.

Summary

Infection is a major complication in patients with malignant disease, especially lymphoma and leukemia. Infections are usually caused by gram-negative bacilli; of these, *Pseudomonas* sp. infections are the most common. Staphylococcal infection, once a major problem, has ceased to be a significant cause of death. Fungal infections are observed with increasing frequency and are often difficult to diagnose. Those factors which predispose the cancer patient to infection include granulocytopenia, impaired function of lymphocytes and the reticuloendothelial system, deficiencies in antibody production, and treatment with antitumor agents and adrenal corticosteroids. Since infections in patients with impaired host defenses may be rapidly fatal, antibiotic therapy must be instituted promptly. Broad spectrum antibiotic coverage is necessary until the etiological agent has been isolated. For the best treatment, repeated cultures should be taken from the patients during febrile episodes. Hopefully, current research will lead to more rapid and better methods of diagnosis and more effective management of infection in the cancer patient. A protected environment and oral, nonabsorbable antibiotics appear to be useful in reducing the risk of infection in susceptible subjects.

REFERENCES

Abbatt, J. D., and Lea, A. J.: Leukaemia and pulmonary tuberculosis. *Lancet,* 2:917-918, November 9, 1957.

Aisenberg, A. C.: Manifestations of immunologic unresponsiveness in Hodgkin's disease. *Cancer Research,* 26:1152-1164, June 1966.

Baker, R. D.: Leukopenia and therapy in leukemia as factors predisposing to fatal mycoses. *American Journal of Clinical Pathology,* 37:358-373, April 1962.

Barile, M. F., Bodey, G. P., Snyder, J., Riggs, D. B., and Grabowski, M. W.: Isolation of *Mycoplasma orale* from leukemic bone marrow and blood by direct culture. *Journal of the National Cancer Institute,* 36:155-159, January 1966.

Bodey, G. P.: Fungal infections complicating acute leukemia. *Journal of Chronic Diseases,* 19:667-687, June 1966a.

———: Infectious complications of acute leukemia. *Medical Times,* 94:1076-1085, September 1966b.

Bodey, G. P., Buckley, M., Sathe, Y. S., and Freireich, E. J: Quantitative relationships between circulating leukocytes and infection in patients with acute leukemia. *Annals of Internal Medicine,* 64:328-340, February 1966.

Bodey, G. P., Nies, B. A., and Freireich, E. J: Multiple organism septicemia in acute leukemia. Analysis of 54 episodes. *Archives of Internal Medicine,* 116:266-272, August 1965.

Bodey, G. P., Wertlake, P. T., Douglas, G., and Levin, R. H.: Cytomegalic inclusion disease in patients with acute leukemia. *Annals of Internal Medicine,* 62:899-906, May 1965.

Browder, A. A., Huff, J. W., and Petersdorf, R. G.: The significance of fever in neoplastic disease. *Annals of Internal Medicine,* 55:932-942, December 1961.

Brumfitt, W., Percival, A., and Leigh, D. A.: Clinical and laboratory studies with carbenicillin. A new penicillin active against *Pseudomonas pyocyanea. Lancet,* 1:1289-1293, June 17, 1967.

Casazza, A. R., Duvall, C. P., and Carbone, P. P.: Summary of infectious complications occurring in patients with Hodgkin's disease. *Cancer Research,* 26:1290-1296, June 1966.

Donovan, A. J.: Reticuloendothelial function in patients with cancer. Initial observations. *American Journal of Surgery,* 114:230-238, August 1967.

Duvall, C. P., Casazza, A. R., Grimley, P. M., Carbone, P. P., and Rowe, W. P.: Recovery of cytomegalovirus from adults with neoplastic disease. *Annals of Internal Medicine,* 64:531-541, March 1966.

Forkner, C. E., Jr., Frei, E., III, Edgecomb, J. H., and Utz, J. P.: *Pseudomonas* septicemia. *American Journal of Medicine,* 25:877-889, December 1958.

Freireich, E. J, Levin, R. H., Whang, J., Carbone, P. P., Bronson, W., and Morse, E. E.: The function and fate of transfused leukocytes from donors with chronic myelocytic leukemia in leukopenic recipients. *Annals of the New York Academy of Sciences,* 113:1081-1089, February 28, 1964.

Groch, G. S., Perillie, P. E., and Finch, S. C.: Reticuloendothelial phagocytic function in patients with leukemia, lymphoma and multiple myeloma. *Blood, The Journal of Hematology,* 26:489-499, October 1965.

Han, T., Sokal, J. E., and Neter, E.: Salmonellosis in disseminated malignant diseases. A seven-year review (1959-1965). *New England Journal of Medicine,* 276:1045-1052, May 11, 1967.

Hendry, W. S., and Patrick, R. L.: Observations on thirteen cases of *Pneumocystis carinii* pneumonia. *American Journal of Clinical Pathology,* 38:401-405, October 1962.

Hersh, E. M., Bodey, G. P., Nies, B. A., and Freireich, E. J: Causes of death in acute leukemia: A ten-year study of 414 patients from 1954-1963. *Journal of the American Medical Association,* 193:105-109, July 12, 1965.

Hersh, E. M., Carbone, P. P., and Freireich, E. J: Recovery of immune responsiveness after drug suppression in man. *Journal of Laboratory and Clinical Medicine,* 67:566-572, April 1966.

Hersh, E. M., Carbone, P. P., Wong, V. G., and Freireich, E. J: Inhibition of the primary immune response in man by anti-metabolites. *Cancer Research,* 25:997-1001, August 1965.

Hersh, E. M., and Freireich, E. J: Host defense mechanisms and their modification by cancer chemotherapy. In *Methods in Cancer Research,* Vol. 4, New York, New York, Academic Press, Inc., 1968, pp. 355-451.

Hersh, E. M., and Oppenheim, J. J.: Impaired in vitro lymphocyte transformation in Hodgkin's disease. *New England Journal of Medicine*, 273:1006-1012, November 4, 1965.

————: Inhibition of in vitro lymphocyte transformation during chemotherapy in man. *Cancer Research*, 27:98-105, January 1967.

Hersh, E. M., Wong, V. G., and Freireich, E. J: Inhibition of the local inflammatory response in man by antimetabolites. *Blood, The Journal of Hematology*, 27:38-48, January 1966.

Hirschberg, N.: Phagocytic activity in leukemia. *American Journal of the Medical Sciences*, 197:706-711, May 1939.

Hutter, R. V. P., and Collins, H. S.: The occurrence of opportunistic fungus infections in a cancer hospital. *Laboratory Investigation*, 11:1035-1045, November 1962.

Jaffé, R. H.: Morphology of the inflammatory defense reactions in leukemia. *Archives of Pathology*, 14:177-203, August 1932.

Levin, R. H., Landy, M., and Frei, E., III: The effect of 6-mercaptopurine on immune response in man. *New England Journal of Medicine*, 271:16-22, July 2, 1964.

Levin, R. H., Whang, J., Tjio, J. H., Carbone, P. P., Frei, E., III, and Freireich, E. J: Persistent mitosis of transfused homologous leukocytes in children receiving antileukemic therapy. *Science*, 142:1305-1311, December 6, 1963.

Lowther, C. P.: Leukemia and tuberculosis. *Annals of Internal Medicine*, 51:52-56, July 1959.

Mattman, L. H., and Mattman, P. E.: L forms of *Streptococcus fecalis* in septicemia. *Archives of Internal Medicine*, 115:315-321, March 1965.

Mitus, A., Enders, J. F., Craig, J. M., and Holloway, A.: Persistence of measles virus and depression of antibody formation in patients with giant-cell pneumonia after measles. *New England Journal of Medicine*, 261:882-889, October 29, 1959.

Morse, E. E., Freireich, E. J, Carbone, P. P., Bronson, W., and Frei, E., III: The transfusion of leukocytes from donors with chronic myelocytic leukemia to patients with leukopenia. *Transfusion*, 6:183-192, May-June 1966.

Pinkel, D.: Chickenpox and leukemia. *Journal of Pediatrics*, 58:729-737, May 1961.

Robinson, H. J.: Adrenal steroids and resistance to infection. *Antibiotica et chemotherapia*, 7:199-240, 1960.

Schumacher, H. R., Ginns, D. A., and Warren, W. J.: Fungus infection complicating leukemia. *American Journal of the Medical Sciences*, 247:313-323, March 1964.

Silver, R. T.: Infections, fever and host resistance in neoplastic diseases. *Journal of Chronic Diseases*, 16:677-701, July 1963.

Stone, H. H., and Kolb, L.: Gentamicin sulfate in the treatment of extra-urinary infections due to gram-negative bacteria. *Southern Medical Journal*, 60:142-144, February 1967.

Taschdjian, C. L., Kozinn, P. J., Okas, A., Caroline, L., and Halle, M. A.: Serodiagnosis of systemic candidiasis. *Journal of Infectious Diseases*, 117:180-187, April 1967.

Wertlake, P. T., and Winters, T. S.: Fatal toxoplasma myocarditis in an adult patient with acute lymphocytic leukemia. *New England Journal of Medicine*, 273:438-440, August 19, 1965.

Vincristine Sulfate in the Management of Wilms' Tumor[*]

MARGARET P. SULLIVAN, M.D.,

W. W. SUTOW, M.D., AND

GRANT TAYLOR, M.D.

Department of Pediatrics, The University of Texas M. D. Anderson Hospital and Tumor Institute at Houston, Houston, Texas

IN 1956, the Pediatric Division of the Southwest Cancer Chemotherapy Study Group (SWCCSG) initiated a screening program for new chemotherapeutic agents to be used in the management of childhood tumors. In accordance with protocol provisions, H. C., a two-year-old boy with recurrent pulmonary metastases from Wilms' tumor, following treatment with total thorax irradiation and dactinomycin, was given vincristine sulfate which was then a new agent. Beginning December 3, 1961, vincristine sulfate was given in the dosage of 0.02 mg./kg. of body weight, intravenously, daily for five days. Subsequently, a dosage of 0.05 mg./kg., was given intravenously, weekly for 11 weeks. Significant regression of tumor occurred with no evidence of tumor growth for the next two and one half months.

The group screening study showed complete regression of measurable metastatic masses in eight (67 per cent) of the 12 evaluable patients receiving vincristine; an additional child exhibited a partial response (Sutow, Thurman, and Windmiller, 1963). The onset of antitumor effect occurred before the third week in 75 per cent of the children. The duration of response ranged from three to 28 weeks (median, eight weeks). In two instances, toxicity necessitated some modification of the treatment regimen.

[*]Presented in part at the Vincristine Symposium, St. Jude Children's Research Hospital, Memphis, Tennessee, January 27, 1967.

This study identified vincristine sulfate as a potent antitumor agent in the management of Wilms' tumor, free of serious myelosuppressive effects and lacking in cross resistance with other agents known to be effective for Wilms' tumor, namely, dactinomycin and irradiation. This study also indicated that vincristine sulfate should effect only temporary tumor regression when used alone in the management of visible metastases. The need for surgical intervention and/or irradiation therapy at the peak of drug action was obvious.

Pulmonary Metastases

In an effort to explore the clinical potentials of vincristine, a comparative study was designed by the SWCCSG wherein patients with measurable pulmonary metastases were assigned to one of two treatment groups, vincristine alone or vincristine sulfate plus irradiation to the metastases. The previously described vincristine dosage was employed, and drug administration was discontinued after the eighth week. Irradiation therapy was given daily through each of two parallel opposed fields. The dose rate was 150 rads daily for a total tumor dose of 1,200 to 1,500 rads. Preliminary evaluation of the data for children with pulmonary metastases shows similar response rates for the drug and combination regimens, i.e., 75 per cent and 77 per cent, respectively. The duration of the responses is also similar in the two treatment groups. Recurrence of pulmonary metastases was found to be almost inevitable in children receiving vincristine sulfate alone. Only one of 10 children (10 per cent) given drug alone could be considered a "possible cure," whereas five of 13 (38 per cent) receiving combination therapy appeared to be possible cures. No evidence of synergism, such as intensification of skin reaction, was seen with combination therapy. The conclusion reached was that therapeutic effects of the two modalities were additive.

A logical extension of these clinical investigations has been the initiation of a comparative study of the efficacy of vincristine plus irradiation and dactinomycin plus radiation in the treatment of patients with pulmonary metastases. Because the toxicities of vincristine and dactinomycin are dissimilar, it has been possible to include a third treatment group, vincristine and dactinomycin plus irradiation as shown in the schema (Fig. 1). Children who have had prior therapy with either chemotherapeutic agent receive the alternate drug or the combination.

Drug dosage schedules employed are as follows: (1) vincristine when given alone, 2 mg./square meter body surface area, intravenously, weekly for eight to 12 weeks; (2) dactinomycin when given alone, 75 μg./kg. of

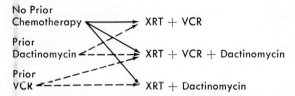

Fig. 1.—Schema showing three different therapy regimens for pulmonary metastases from Wilms' tumor: (1) vincristine plus irradiation, (2) dactinomycin plus irradiation, and (3) vincristine and dactinomycin plus irradiation. Abbreviations: XRT, radiation therapy; VCR, vincristine sulfate.

body weight, intravenously, total dose in three to five days, repeated every two months for three courses; (3) combination therapy: vincristine, 2 mg./square meter of body surface area, intravenously, weekly for eight weeks; and dactinomycin, 15 μg./kg. of body weight, intravenously, daily for five days, monthly for two courses.

Both lungs and the mediastinum are irradiated by means of parallel, opposed, anterior and posterior fields. Both fields are treated daily. The tumor dose rate is 150 rads daily to a total dose of 1,200 to 1,500 rads.

It is anticipated that therapeutic effects of combination drug therapy will at least be additive in the group receiving both vincristine and dactinomycin. Synergism is possible because this effect has been noted in a murine leukemia system. This study has not produced sufficient data to warrant preliminary analysis.

Primary Therapy

In 1962, The University of Texas M. D. Anderson Hospital and Tumor Institute at Houston initiated a pilot study using vincristine sulfate as an adjuvant in the primary treatment for Wilms' tumor in an effort to prevent or successfully treat occult metastatic disease. In this group of patients, nephrectomy was followed by irradiation of the tumor bed with doses varying from 2,500 to 4,500 rads. In addition, the patients received vincristine sulfate in standard doses for a period of 12 weeks, as shown in the schema (Fig. 2). Several of the patients had nephrectomy or both nephrectomy and radiation prior to referral to Anderson Hospital. The

Fig. 2.—Schema illustrating the adjunctive role of vincristine in primary therapy for Wilms' tumor. Abbreviations: XRT, radiation therapy; VCR, vincristine sulfate.

```
                          XRT to tumor bed
        Nephrectomy ———►         +
                          VCR weekly for 12 doses
```

TABLE 1.—PRESENCE OF UNFAVORABLE PROGNOSTIC FACTORS IN CHILDREN WITH WILMS' TUMOR RECEIVING PRIMARY MULTIMODAL THERAPY

PATIENT	UNFAVORABLE FACTORS PRESENT	DEFINITION OF FACTORS
#1	H	A. Age over two years.
#2	A, D	B. Invasion of vasculature.
#3	B, C, E, F	C. Invasion of adjacent nonresectable organs or structures.
#4	A, I	D. Metastases to lymph nodes or in lymphatic channels.
#5	D	E. Invasion of renal pelvis and/or ureter.
#6	B, E	F. Rupture of tumor capsule.
#7	A, B, D, G	G. Invasion of adjacent resectable organs.
#8	A	H. Metastases to bone marrow.
#9	A, B, I	I. Multiple nodules in resected kidney.
#10	A, B	

series, which was reported in 1965, now contains 10 patients (Sutow and Sullivan, 1965). Eight of the 10 children (80 per cent) remain free of neoplastic disease; one child died of metastatic pulmonary and liver disease 14 months after nephrectomy. The second child who had serial intravenous pyelograms, developed Wilms' tumor in the remaining kidney when she was well beyond her "period-of-risk" and died four years and seven months after nephrectomy. Four other children have completed their period-of-risk; eight (80 per cent) have survived two years or more from the time of nephrectomy. Survival times of the living children range from four months to five years and five months (median, four years and three months). The survival in this group is particularly impressive in view of the unfavorable factors found singly or in combination in all of the children (Table 1). These factors included: age over two years, invasion of blood vessels, invasion of adjacent nonresectable organs or structures, metastases to lymph nodes or in lymphatic channels, invasion of renal pelvis and/or ureter, rupture of tumor "capsule," invasion of adjacent resectable organs, metastases to bone marrow, and multiple nodules in resected kidney.

An excerpt from the referral letter, dated March 23, 1965, regarding patient 9 who was then 30 months of age illustrates the unfavorable prognostic factors found in these patients:

"It was decided to attempt removal of as much of the tumor as possible from the vena cava, as this might make future radiation therapy more successful. Therefore, the vena cava was ligated inferiorly at the end of the intravenous tumor and cut, and the vessel freed superiorly to the renal veins. Here the vena cava was severed obliquely so that the left renal vein and the vena cava inferior to it were removed, but the right renal vein left attached to the remaining vena

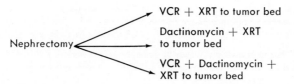

Fig. 3.—Schema showing the three treatment regimens in use in a study comparing the effectiveness of vincristine and dactinomycin as adjuvants in the primary therapy for Wilms' tumor. Abbreviations: VCR, vincristine sulfate; XRT, radiation therapy.

cava. There was absolutely no bleeding from either the right renal vein or the end of the vena cava.

"The gray tumor plug in the renal vein was teased out, and brisk bleeding occurred. The tumor did not appear to be adherent to the intima. An attempt was made to remove the tumor from the end of the vena cava, and a large amount was removed with a sponge forceps. However, in the thoracic portion of vena cava it felt to be adherent to the intima, and would not come loose well. The vena cava was cleaned out well up into the thoracic portion, but at no time was any back bleeding noted. The end of the vena cava was closed with continuous simple sutures of silk 00000. . . ."

In this small group of patients, the effectiveness of vincristine as an adjuvant appears similar to the effectiveness of dactinomycin. Using dactinomycin, Farber (1966) has achieved an 89 per cent two-year survival without metastases among 53 children who were treated at his institution from the time of diagnosis. Among the 54 patients whose therapy had been initiated elsewhere, two-year survival without metastases fell to 39 per cent.

A group study is now underway comparing the effectiveness of the two drugs, vincristine and dactinomycin, as adjuvants. Patients are randomized among the three treatment regimens shown in the schema in Figure 3. Dosage schedules are identical with those used in the study of pulmonary metastases. If the drug effects are truly additive, the cure rate in children receiving both drugs should approach 100 per cent. Fourteen patients now have been entered on this study.

The Nonresectable Primary

Vincristine sulfate also has proved to be a very valuable agent in the clinical management of the patients with a nonresectable primary lesion (Fig. 4). Four children at this hospital, whose lesions were judged nonresectable on admission, were given two to four doses of vincristine sulfate in lieu of irradiation therapy (Sullivan, Sutow, Cangir, and Taylor, 1967). Nephrectomy was followed by irradiation of the abdominal tumor

VCR,   XRT to tumor bed
2 - 4 ⟶ Nephrectomy ⟶   +
doses   VCR weekly to complete 12 doses

Fig. 4.—Schema showing the role of preoperative vincristine in the therapy for inoperable Wilms' tumor. Abbreviations: VCR, vincristine sulfate; XRT, radiation therapy.

bed and of the thorax—if pulmonary metastases were evident—and by completion of the series of 12 weekly vincristine injections. Tumors in these four children were deemed nonresectable because of size, posterior fixation, or fixation to other organs. The degree of preoperative, vincristine sulfate-induced tumor regression which was achieved is illustrated in Figure 5. While nonresectable primary tumor is reduced to resectable proportions, effective treatment is given for occult or demonstrable metastases, as shown by the reduction in mediastinal width, disappearance of left apical mass and significant reduction in size and density of the nodule in the left lateral lung field in Figure 6. Ease of administration and promptness of therapeutic effect confer additional advantages over traditional preoperative irradiation therapy. The treatment plan is rigorous, as illustrated by the complications seen in the four children in the series (Table 2). Fever occurred in all four children after the second injection of vincristine sulfate, but none had clinical or laboratory evidence of infection. Tumor regression was obvious at this time, and fever was assumed to be related to the breakdown of tumor cells. Gross and histo-

Fig. 5.—Photos of abdomen of patient with Wilms' tumor. A, before initiation of chemotherapy, November 17, 1966; B, after four doses of vincristine sulfate, December 2, 1966.

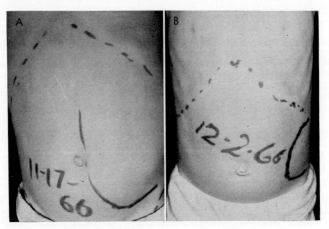

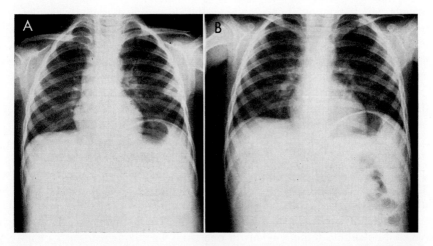

Fig. 6.—Roentgenograms of chest of patient with Wilms' tumor. **A**, November 16, 1966, shows widening of mediastinum and metastatic nodules in left apex and left lateral chest prior to vincristine sulfate therapy. **B**, follow-up film, December 5, 1966, shows almost complete resolution of metastatic nodules after preoperative vincristine sulfate therapy.

logical study of the surgical specimens showed significant necrosis and hemorrhage. In one instance, these changes were so extensive that it was difficult to identify viable tumor and establish the histological diagnosis.

Some degree of hematopoietic depression was seen in each child. This complication occurred late in the treatment regimen as the series of 12 injections of vincristine sulfate and the irradiation of the abdominal tumor bed were being completed. In comparison with most chemotherapeutic

TABLE 2.—COMPLICATIONS IN TREATMENT PROGRAM FOR INOPERABLE WILMS' TUMOR

COMPLICATION		NO. OF PATIENTS
Fever		4
Marrow depression		4
Hb < 10 gm./100 cc.	4	
Plat < 100,000/mm.^{3}	2	
WBC < 2,000/mm.^{3}	1	
Intestinal disorders		3
Intussusception	1	
Postradiation obstruction	1	
Ileus	1	

Abbreviations: Hb, hemoglobin; Plat, platelets; WBC, white blood cells.

agents, vincristine sulfate has minimal myelosuppressive effects. Radiation therapy undoubtedly contributed greatly to the myelosuppression encountered. Depression of all the formed elements of the peripheral blood occurred in a child whose entire abdomen was irradiated because of a suspected tumor implant from previous biopsy. One of the two children receiving irradiation to the entire thorax as well as the abdominal tumor bed developed anemia and thrombocytopenia; the other child developed anemia and moderate leukopenia. Mild anemia was the only hematopoietic side effect seen in the child whose radiation therapy was limited to the abdominal tumor bed. In each case, recovery from the myelosuppressive side effects of therapy was complete. Supportive therapy, other than whole blood transfusions, was not required. Neither child with thrombocytopenia required platelet transfusions.

Disordered peristalsis and obstipation are recognized side effects of vincristine sulfate therapy. Ileus in one child was thought to be a manifestation of vincristine sulfate toxicity, and the patient responded to the symptomatic measures usually employed in this clinical situation. Because jejunal intussusception is extremely rare, the role of chemotherapy in this unusual postoperative complication can be questioned. Plane and upright x-ray films of the abdomen showed only the changes associated with small bowel obstruction, and exploration of the abdomen showed adhesive bands in the area of intussusception. Bowel obstruction in the child receiving radiation to the entire abdomen was thought to be a reaction to radiation.

The rigors of the treatment program have been justified by the outcome of therapy to date. All four patients in this group are living with no evidence of metastatic disease; survival time from nephrectomy ranges from 11 to 28 months (median, 21 months).

The Nonresectable Liver Metastasis

Two children have presented with nonresectable metastatic disease limited to one lobe of the liver. In each child, vincristine sulfate resulted in sufficient decrease in tumor mass to permit lobectomy on the involved side.

Conclusion

In a period of almost six years, it has been possible to demonstrate that vincristine sulfate, when used in treating patients with Wilms' tumor, has a very potent antitumor effect and may be employed effectively as (1) an adjuvant to irradiation in the management of nonresectable metastatic disease, particularly pulmonary, (2) an adjuvant to primary therapy (nephrectomy plus radiation to tumor bed) for the successful management of occult metastatic disease, and (3) a means of rendering some nonresectable primary and metastatic masses amenable to surgical resection.

Studies are in progress which should demonstrate whether vincristine sulfate or dactinomycin is the superior adjuvant. The data obtained also should indicate whether simultaneous use of the two agents as a "dual adjuvant" will contribute to the curability of patients with this tumor.

REFERENCES

Farber, S.: Chemotherapy in the treatment of leukemia and Wilms's tumor. *Journal of the American Medical Association,* 198:826-836, November 21, 1966.

Sullivan, M. P., Sutow, W. W., Cangir, A., and Taylor, G.: Vincristine sulfate in management of Wilms's tumor. Replacement of preoperative irradiation by chemotherapy. *Journal of the American Medical Association,* 202:381-384, October 30, 1967.

Sutow, W. W., and Sullivan, M. P.: Vincristine in primary treatment of Wilms's tumor. *Texas State Journal of Medicine,* 61:794-799, November 1965.

Sutow, W. W., Thurman, W. G., and Windmiller, J.: Vincristine (Leurocristine) sulfate in the treatment of children with metastatic Wilms's tumor. *Pediatrics,* 32: 880-887, November 1963.

Multimodal Treatment
for Wilms' Tumor

RICHARD G. MARTIN, M.D.

*Department of Surgery, The University of Texas M. D. Anderson Hospital
and Tumor Institute at Houston, Houston, Texas*

MULTIMODAL TREATMENT for malignant diseases is not new. Over the years it has come to be a basic principle in the management of almost all types of cancer. For a long time, surgical procedures were the main form of therapy. Then radiation began to be used therapeutically, and the elaborate techniques that are available today were developed. Chemotherapy is the newest treatment modality and the one that has not reached its ultimate potential, mainly because there are currently very few chemotherapeutic agents that can produce the desired effects.

Because surgical procedures are the oldest of the treatment modalities, it is only natural that physicians should have believed once that all tumors must be excised for cure. Once the accepted surgical procedure was performed, the physician believed that very little could be done if the patient developed a local recurrence or a metastatic lesion. With the development of roentgen rays and modern techniques of administration, irradiation came to be considered adequate therapy for certain tumors. Some physicians then realized that possibly these two modalities could be used together, either preoperatively or postoperatively. With the introduction in the last few years of a number of chemotherapeutic agents and with the knowledge that certain of these agents cause tumors to regress, the possibility that drugs could be used for widespread metastatic disease was recognized. No longer is it acceptable for the physician caring for a patient with malignant disease to be satisfied to remove the kidney in this instance, and to do nothing more.

When, how, and where the three modalities discussed fit into the treatment of the patient with cancer depend on the philosophy of the physician. His philosophy should be based on a knowledge of the advantages of the various modalities, their limitations, and the nature of the patient's disease. Even after the basic plan is formulated and the method is outlined, one still wonders why some patients, especially those who are never expected to survive do so well, while some, whose seemingly small lesions have been adequately excised, do so poorly. At the present time, one can merely say that certain tumor host factors are not understood.

Before discussing the basic plan that has evolved at The University of Texas M. D. Anderson Hospital and Tumor Institute at Houston for the management of Wilms' tumor, I believe that it is necessary to review briefly the histology of this lesion. Grossly, Wilms' tumors usually are large, rapidly growing lesions which develop in the renal parenchyma and sometimes reach sizes as large as 20 to 40 cm. in diameter. Because of their rapid growth, they often become necrotic in the center. Although encapsulated, they frequently burst if handled roughly, spilling tumor cells throughout the area. Another characteristic of this tumor is that it tends to invade the veins. It is not uncommon to see a tumor thrombus of the renal vein growing into the vena cava. Metastasis is by the blood stream and the lymphatics. The most common sites of metastases are lung, liver, lymph nodes, and bone. Wilms' tumor is a true kidney tumor in that all elements of the kidney, glandular and stromal, are involved. Because of this multielemental composition, one would expect radiation therapy and chemotherapy to attack successfully some of the elements and thus shrink the tumor, but not necessarily to destroy the entire lesion because the remaining elements might be insensitive to the therapeutic modalities used.

At this point, I would like to discuss some of the special features of each of the three modalities mentioned which will have a bearing on the formulation of a multimodal treatment program for Wilms' tumors.

Surgical Therapy

The first modality is surgical therapy. For this approach to be successful, the surgeon must remove the entire lesion without breaking it. Wilms' tumors are often large, friable, and vascular with enormous blood supplies. To attack these lesions, one must have adequate exposure, and this can only be achieved by a transabdominal incision and at times, only by a thoraco-abdominal incision. These methods allow one to attack the renal vessels before handling the tumor and in this way to prevent blood stream metastasis. Frequently, there are cases in which the renal vein is thrombosed, with tumor extending into the vena cava; this sometimes necessitates removal of a portion of the vena cava. At times, the lesion even extends across the midline and is too large for the surgeon to remove successfully. Occasionally, cells invade the collecting system and move down the ureter in the urine. Cytologic examinations of the urine are usually unreliable although positive results are very significant. These studies do, however, force one to keep in mind that the collecting system is an avenue of spread. Cells have been known to lodge in the bladder and to form a focus of metastasis. Metastatic lesions, when solitary or localized to a single area or organ, sometimes can be excised. This fact should be kept in mind when metastatic lesions do not regress with irradiation or chemotherapy.

X-ray Therapy

X-rays are not specific for certain types of tissue. All tissues exposed will receive some damage depending on their sensitivity. It is therefore necessary that the dosage be limited to a tolerance which is accepted by the exposed normal tissues and the body as a whole. Fortunately, certain types of Wilms' tumor cells seem to be quite sensitive to irradiation. As mentioned earlier, Wilms' tumor is usually made up of both glandular and stromal elements of the kidney; thus, if adequate doses are given regression in tumor size is usually demonstrable. However, one must keep in mind that the patients are young, their growth is by no means complete, and their tissues are very sensitive to radiation. Irradiation to the spine and other organs may cause severe damage. In addition, after certain doses of x-ray therapy, surgical procedures are harder to perform. Healing is much slower, and the complication rate increases. If the tumor does recur in the area previously irradiated, further irradiation in that area is frequently impossible, and the vascular supply to the area often is damaged so that effective chemotherapy is impossible. When irradiation is given to metastatic sites in the lung, permanent damage to the organ can occur if the doses are not controlled properly.

Chemotherapy

All chemotherapeutic agents are toxic. Here again, because of the nature of the modality and its systemic use, all tissues are exposed. This may be an advantage over x-ray therapy and it also may be a disadvantage. The advantage is that if loose cells are circulating throughout the body or multiple foci are present in metastases, they can be managed with a systemic approach. For large local areas without widespread metastases, systemic chemotherapy may be a disadvantage compared to localized

TABLE 1.—WILMS' TUMOR, SUMMARY OF SURVIVORS (I)

NUMBER	NAME	AGE	SEX	TREATMENT	LENGTH OF SURVIVAL
1.	Y.B.	13 mo.	F	Left nephrectomy (lateral)	10 yr. (Living tumor free)
2.	J.L.	3 yr.	M	Left nephrectomy	6 yr. (Living tumor free)
3.	J.S.	8 yr.	M	Left nephrectomy, XRT Lung metastases (1½ yr.) Excised 2 nodules, 1956	13 yr.
4.	J.S.	2.5 yr.	M	Right nephrectomy (spilled) Act. D, 3,500 rads	9 yr.
5.	T.G.	3 yr.	M	Right nephrectomy (spilled) 4,200 rads, Act. D	8 yr.
6.	D.R.	3 yr.	F	Right nephrectomy, 3,420 rads Mediastinum 3,000 rads Act. D	7 yr.
7.	L.W.	4 yr.	F	1,000 rads, preoperative XRT Left nephrectomy, 2,550 rads XRT	7 yr.
8.	S.S.	7 yr.	F	Right nephrectomy, XRT Exploratory laparotomy, Act. D XRT 2,000 rads Act. D VCR Left liver lobectomy, 1962	7 yr. after nephrectomy 5 yr. after left liver lobectomy
9.	R.M.	14 mo.	M	Left nephrectomy, 3,000 rads Act. D	2 yr. (Living tumor free)

10.	J.T.	16 mo.	F	Right nephrectomy, 3,600 rads VCR	5 yr.
11.	J.G.	6 mo.	M	Right nephrectomy, 2,985 rads Act. D	5 yr.
12.	L.G.	22 mo.	F	Right nephrectomy (proximal to ureter) 3,500 rads VCR	5 yr.
13.	R.H.	3 yr.	F	Left nephrectomy, 3,295 rads VCR 1963 Right abdominal mass, 1965 hypertension Exploratory laparotomy, Right Wilms' tumor VCR, act. D 750 rads XRT Died	5 yr. 2 yr.

Abbreviations: XRT, radiation therapy; VCR, vincristine sulfate.

x-ray therapy. Another advantage of chemotherapy is that it does not hinder the performance of further surgical procedures. One must be careful, however, that the patient's platelet and blood count levels remain within normal limits, and this may involve time. Dr. Sullivan outlined the use of vincristine sulfate in the management of Wilms' tumor. As she stated, vincristine is a toxic agent which affects the peripheral nerves, the blood cells, and the gastrointestinal tract.

Multimodal Treatment Plan

Let us now look at a multimodal treatment for patients with Wilms' tumor and the rationale behind it. When first seen, our patients usually have large abdominal tumors or they have had a nephrectomy. Technically it would be easier if their tumors could be reduced in size before nephrectomy. X-ray therapy has been used for this purpose; however, this modality has certain disadvantages, especially in the treatment of young patients. Therefore, a definite diagnosis of Wilms' tumor must be made before irradiation. Radiation therapy unknowingly has been given to patients with polycystic kidneys.

To diagnose a Wilms' tumor is not always easy. A needle biopsy is not advocated because of the likelihood of tumor growing in the needle site. Cytological examination of the urine is not reliable. Intravenous pyelography and angiography are probably the most dependable of the diagnostic tests; however, angiography is not without some danger.

If vincristine—which is a toxic agent—is given preoperatively, less harm probably is done to the patient should the lesion fail to be a Wilms' tumor. Therefore, as Sullivan has mentioned, vincristine often is started before the nephrectomy. When the tumor has begun to regress a nephrectomy is performed; a transabdominal approach is used and the renal pedicle is attacked first. Knowing that even though the capsule has not been broken, there may be some local lymphatic spread or live tumor cells may have been left in the tumor bed, x-ray therapy is routinely given, usually in a dose of about 3,000 r. Also, because it is known that Wilms' tumor spreads systemically through the blood stream, a systemic agent such as actinomycin D or vincristine is given in an attempt to destroy any viable cells that might be present in the lung, liver, or bone. All patients are followed carefully. If metastases do occur, they are managed by chemotherapy and/or local x-ray, if feasible. Irradiation to the lung field is included. If the lesions are localized and do not regress, surgical excision should be attempted whenever possible.

TABLE 2.—WILMS' TUMOR, SUMMARY OF SURVIVORS (II)

NUMBER	NAME	AGE	SEX	TREATMENT	LENGTH OF SURVIVAL
1.	W.W.	2 yr.	M	Right nephrectomy (vein) 3,500 rads, VCR 1,440 rads, lungs, 1963 VCR	4.5 yr.
2.	S.L.	8 wk.	F	Left nephrectomy, 3,000 rads VCR	4.5 yr.
3.	M.F.	4 yr.	F	Left nephrectomy, 5,000 rads in air 100 rads, lungs VCR 1,500 rads, chest	4 yr.
4.	W.T.	21 mo.	M	Left nephrectomy (vein) 3,000 rads, VCR	4 yr.
5.	D.G.	3 yr.	F	Preoperative XRT 1,030 rads (vena cava + nodes) Right nephrectomy 3,040 rads, VCR	3.5 yr.
6.	D.S.	3 yr.	M	Right nephrectomy, XRT 3,400 rads VCR	3 yr.
7.	J.G.	2.5 yr.	M	Left nephrectomy (section of vena cava) 2,530 rads XRT VCR	2.5 yr.
8.	A.G.	21 mo.	M	Left nephrectomy VCR, exploratory laparotomy Act. D, VCR	2 yr.
9.	S.M.	3 yr.	F	Tumor + lung metastases, VCR Left nephrectomy, XRT 3,000 rads 1,500 rads to lungs Lungs clear for 2 yr.	2 yr.
10.	R.Y.	3 yr.	M	VCR left nephrectomy XRT 3,475 rads Widening of mediastinum Excision of thymus	2 yr.
11.	D.M.	8 yr.	F	Exploratory laparotomy, mass across midline, VCR Right nephrectomy, segmental resection of ileum, XRT 3,475 rads VCR	1 yr.

(Continued)

TABLE 2 (Cont.)

NUMBER	NAME	AGE	SEX	TREATMENT	LENGTH OF SURVIVAL
12.	L.M.	3 yr.	F	Left nephrectomy, pulmonary metastases 3,000 rads XRT 1,270 rads VCR	1 yr.
13.	C.A.	9.5 yr.	M	Left nephrectomy, 3,130 rads VCR, lung metastases VCR, act. D, 1,220 rads	2 yr. 1 yr.
14.	D.W.	10 yr.	M	Left nephrectomy, 3,000 rads 1965, mass right lung, 2,500 rads Mass lungs, 1,200 rads 2/1967 liver metastases, VCR 3/1967 right liver lobectomy VCR (foot drop)	42 mo. 8 mo.
15.	K.K.	5 yr.	M	Left nephrectomy (vein) 4,500 rads, VCR Exploratory laparotomy, intestinal obstruction VCR	5 mo.

Abbreviations: XRT, radiation therapy; VCR, vincristine sulfate; act. D., actinomycin D.

For patients with large abdominal masses and distant metastases, an attempt is made to shrink the original tumor mass and the metastases by using vincristine before the nephrectomy, and then x-ray therapy and chemotherapy postoperatively to attack the tumor bed and the metastatic sites as well.

Figure 1 illustrates two of the multimodal approaches used at Anderson Hospital in the management of Wilms' tumor. Tables 1, 2, and 3 summarize the results of these approaches and thereby to show the rationale for multimodal treatment.

TABLE 3.—STATISTICS ON 70 PATIENTS WITH WILMS' TUMOR AT ANDERSON HOSPITAL

Average survival time before death—13 months
Five-year survival rate—13/46 or 28.2%
Two-year survival rate—12/21 or 57.1%*
Number of operative deaths—1

*Most of these patients should live at least five years.

```
VCR                                              XRT to tumor bed
2-4      - - - - - - - - - - nephrectomy - - - - - - - - - -        +
doses                                            VCR weekly to complete 12 doses
```

```
                                      XRT to tumor bed
Nephrectomy  - - - - - - - - - -          +
                                      VCR weekly for 12 doses
```

Fig. 1.—Schema of two multimodal approaches for the management of Wilms' tumor.

Summary

The following points about multimodal treatment should be emphasized. (1) It is no longer adequate to manage malignant diseases with only one modality, especially in the case of Wilms' tumor; all three therapeutic modalities—operation, irradiation, and chemotherapy—have much to offer the patient. (2) It is necessary to follow closely all patients with malignant disease. If they develop local recurrence or distant metastases, one of the three modalities discussed should be used immediately. (3) The histology and natural history of Wilms' tumor lends itself well to multimodal attack. (4) Through the use of a multimodal treatment program for Wilms' tumor, our results over the past years have improved significantly.

Current Concepts in the Management of Neuroblastoma*

WILLIAM G. THURMAN, M.D.C.M., AND

MILTON H. DONALDSON, M.D.

*Department of Pediatrics, University of Virginia School of Medicine,
Charlottesville, Virginia*

The Clinical Problem

A RECENT SURVEY of death certificates in eight states for the two-year period ending January 1, 1967, revealed that the incidence of neuroblastoma exceeded the incidence of Wilms' tumor and that neuroblastoma has become the most common solid tumor in childhood (Valdean and Thurman, personal communication). The clinical presentation of children with this lesion is highly variable. Presenting symptomatology can include pallor, listlessness, shortness of breath, diarrhea, pain in a bone, pain in the abdomen, orbital swelling, paralysis, malnutrition, vomiting, and a number of other symptoms. An abdominal mass rarely is described by parents of the children as a clinical finding. Physical examination may provide an answer readily, but definitive studies often are needed to establish a diagnosis. The lack of a high index of suspicion can mean the difference between survival and death, so the ubiquitous nature of this tumor must be emphasized constantly to all those caring for children. Continuing educational efforts have made both the medical profession and the lay public "leukemia-conscious", but this degree of awareness has not extended to the solid tumors in general. The clinical syndrome of chronic diarrhea associated with ganglioneuroma and/or neuroblastoma now has replaced

*This study was supported in part by the National Cancer Institute (CA 08223), the American Cancer Society, the Children's Bureau (Project # 613), and the United Fund, Blacksburg, Virginia.

Some of this material is reproduced from Acute Leukemia and Pediatric Malignancies (Thurman, 1968).

presentation with orbital swelling as the symptom complex most often considered and recognized by the medical profession, but the diagnosis still is delayed too often to insure a better survival rate. Until early diagnosis is the rule rather than the exception, the prognosis for children with neuroblastoma will continue to be relatively poor.

An Evaluation of Therapy

One of our most significant problems is the collection of evaluable data to establish prognosis. This problem has made assessment of success with a given mode of therapy difficult, and it is probably the reason for the variable degrees of success reported by investigators. Known factors influencing prognosis include: (1) age at diagnosis, (2) degree of cell differentiation, (3) extent of disease spread at operation, (4) presence of skeletal metastases, (5) presence of bone marrow metastases, and (6) race. The successful staging of Hodgkin's disease, as reflected in survival rates and therapy decisions, has led us to consider the staging of neuroblastoma. This staging would provide an opportunity to compare results from one series of patients with results in another and hopefully would make therapy decisions both simple and adequate.

James (1967) and others have proposed various classifications, and I would suggest the staging table given in Table 1 as a reasonable compromise. Any such proposal has weaknesses, but this staging reflects our experience with age, with all degrees of cell differentiation, and with the biochemical aspects of neuroblastoma. In our opinion, there is a treatment and a survival difference between patients with bone marrow metastases and those with bone metastases, but our opinion is not shared by many others. Adoption of such a proposal is essential to an adequate evaluation of therapy if one child or a group of children is to be compared with others.

TABLE 1.—STAGING FOR NEUROBLASTOMA
(Excludes all children under one year of age)

Stage I	Localized and totally resectable*
	a. Well-differentiated b. Undifferentiated
Stage II	Regional, nonresectable
	a. Well-differentiated b. Undifferentiated
Stage III	Generalized, with bone marrow involvement
Stage IV	Generalized, with bone involvement

*Automatically reclassified to stage II if catecholamine excretion remains high three months after removal.

Current Therapy

There have been 28 well-documented cases of neuroblastoma in which spontaneous remission has occurred. Nevertheless, the vast majority of children with this tumor have a rapid downhill course; in one study, 50 per cent were dead at the end of seven months and 75 per cent were dead at the end of one year (Burgert and Mills, 1966). The reason for the high number of early deaths is, of course, that distant metastases are present at the time of original diagnosis and that complete surgical excision, still the procedure of choice in therapy, is rarely possible. Radiation therapy often is limited by the extent of metastatic involvement. Thus, with the limited application of surgical therapy and radiotherapy in the management of neuroblastoma in children, attention presently is focused on the chemotherapeutic approach.

The high probability of early metastases should not discourage a surgical approach unless bone radiographs, bone marrow studies, or lymph node biopsies furnish positive evidence of metastatic disease. If metastases are present, surgical therapy should be reconsidered if there is an adequate response to radiotherapy and/or chemotherapy.

The statement still persists in the literature that neuroblastoma, regardless of the degree of cell differentiation, is usually radioresistant. This has not been our experience nor has it been the experience of others (Phillips, personal communication). There is little question that small tumor doses are ineffective; but, in our opinion, every child with incomplete surgical removal or with evidence of local or regional extension should be treated with a minimum tumor dose of 3,000 rads. Operation and radiotherapy in combination have not been as successful in the management of this tumor as they have in other solid tumors, but they do constitute the treatment of choice until more definitive data on chemotherapy are forthcoming.

The chemotherapeutic management of neuroblastoma has undergone many changes as scientists and physicians have searched for the ideal agent; but experimentation continues, as it has from the beginning, primarily by means of trial and error methods. Of historical interest is the 1950 report from Bodian in London which advocated the first use of massive vitamin B_{12} in the management of neuroblastoma (Bodian, 1963). The rationale behind this therapy was that B_{12}, because it is an essential factor for the normal maturation of hematopoietic cells, might speed maturation of neuroblastic tissue toward the more benign ganglioneuroma. Of the 165 cases in Bodian's series, 32 of the children were considered to be in clinical remission, and 28 lived for periods of two to 12 years on 1 mg. of vitamin B_{12} extract intramuscularly on alternate days for at least the first two years. Bodian used no controls, alternating case methods, or statistical evaluation in his study, and his results never have been substantiated in this country.

The potentialities of the alkylating agent cyclophosphamide (Cytoxan) in the treatment of patients with neuroblastoma were described in a study published by the Pediatric Division of the Southwest Cancer Chemotherapy Study Group (Thurman, Fernbach, and Sullivan, 1964). This study reported both objective and subjective improvement for periods ranging from one to 20 months in 79 per cent of the children treated. Of the 19 children who responded, seven had evidence of metastases to bone marrow and eight had definite signs of bone involvement.

Sullivan (1965) subsequently reported that Cytoxan was suitable for long-term sustained therapy in children and had the additional advantage of rendering nonresectable primary tumors resectable if therapy was continued for an adequate period of time.

The most successful treatment of patients with disseminated neuroblastoma today is with combination therapy. The advantages of the concurrent use of cyclophosphamide and vincristine sulfate are: (1) each given separately has some therapeutic effect on the tumor, (2) the mechanism of action is different in each, and (3) the limiting toxic effect of cyclophosphamide (bone marrow depression) differs from that of vincristine. Thus, the additive effect can be achieved without additional toxicity. James, Hustu, Wrenn, and Pinkel (1965) treated nine consecutive children, age three weeks to 11 years, with a combination regimen of these two drugs. Of these patients, four had evidence of marrow involvement and four had bone metastases, as shown by roentgenography. Vincristine sulfate was given intravenously in dosages of 1.5 mg./square meter the first day and every two weeks thereafter. Cyclophosphamide was injected intravenously on day eight and every two weeks thereafter in dosages of 300 mg./square meter. After its injection, 150-250 cc. of 5 per cent glucose in water was administered to promote diuresis and to lessen the possibility of toxic cystitis. All nine children had objective regression of tumor size, which is defined as a 50 per cent reduction of palpable or radiologically demonstrable tumor mass. Five of the children (including two with evidence of bone marrow metastases) experienced complete disappearance of all evidence of tumor. Two others responded to such an extent that the residual tumor could be resected, and two with tumor cells in the bone marrow achieved complete remission. Toxic effects in this group were mild and transient. They included alopecia, nausea and vomiting, depression of deep tendon reflexes, transient thrombocytopenia, and leukopenia. This therapy did not impede the growth of the children. Even with continual use of drugs for 12 months, they exhibited steady increases in height and weight. This combination of drugs used in alternate weeks has increased survival time in patients with disseminated neuroblastoma, more than has Cytoxan used alone.

Other chemotherapeutic agents also are under study, and several have shown some effectiveness against neuroblastoma. Two of these are dauno-mycin and imidazole. Data are still insufficient, but nothing indicates an improvement over the survival rate produced by cyclophosphamide and vincristine.

Perhaps, faced with the absence of the ideal chemotherapeutic agent for the management of disseminated neuroblastoma, our methods of administration should be changed in order to attack the tumor more effectively. Modifications might include (1) regional chemotherapy by perfusion or continuous infusion techniques, (2) an extensive combination of active chemotherapeutic agents in a specific dosage and regimen of therapy, (3) the combination of chemotherapeutic agents with other forms of treatment, e.g. radiation, to potentiate the effects of the drugs, and (4) the so-called drug adjuvant therapy in which a chemical agent is used adjunctively during the primary curative attack on the tumor.

Of these methods, the drug adjuvant therapy appears to be the most promising at this time. It employs the use of antineoplastic drugs to destroy neoplastic cells left after surgical or radiation therapy, to systemically attack occult tumor cell aggregates outside the primary tumor targets, and to inhibit metastatic colonization by any circulating tumor cells. To discuss the effectiveness of adjuvant drugs, one must be aware of the considerable evidence suggesting that the per cent reduction in neoplastic cells destroyed by a given chemotherapeutic agent remains relatively constant regardless of the number of cells present; this is the phenomenon of first order kinetics in radiobiology. Thus, the number of neoplastic cells destroyed remains relatively constant for a given dose of a given drug. In this first order destruction of neoplastic cells, an agent that produces a 99 per cent kill rate should produce virtually total cure in all animals in which 10^1 cells are present, a substantial cure when 10^2 cells are present, but almost no cure when 10^3 or more cells are present. Thus, the effectiveness of a chemotherapeutic agent as an adjuvant depends upon how many cancer cells are present and how effective the adjuvant is in eradicating these cells.

An important consideration in the use of adjuvant therapy is the presence of neoplastic cells in wound washings and the peripheral blood at the time of primary surgical therapy. It has been proposed that such "free-floating" cells have compromised viability and may be more susceptible.

If this is true, it seems likely that adjuvant therapy which is begun at the time of operation and continued postoperatively would be most effective. However, there are other factors to consider in the postoperative patient. In the two to four weeks after the patient has undergone operation, chemotherapeutic agents should be administered in modified doses because of the adverse effect which many agents have on wound healing and because of the risk of infection and hemorrhage as a result of bone marrow suppression. Since most tumor cells in human beings have a doubling time of about one to three months, there could be a delay in intensive postsurgical use of chemotherapy until wound healing is complete, with at most a twofold increase in the number of cancer cells. After this delay, adjuvant chemotherapy should be given intensively. The steep dose-response curve for most of these agents in man, plus the fact that in experimental systems a twofold difference in dose may cause as much as a tenfold difference in neoplastic cell destruction, strongly support the use of the maximum dosages without toxic effects.

How long adjuvant therapy is to be given is another factor to be considered. Any decision must be based, at least in part, on the stage of the mitotic cycle in which the neoplastic cells are. Evidence currently suggests that methotrexate and 5-flourouracil inhibit cells primarily during deoxyribonucleic acid synthesis and that the vinca alkaloids (vincristine and vinblastine) inhibit cells immediately before and during cell division. It would seem most desirable to continue treatment with these drugs for at least the estimated average generation time of cells during which most of them would be in their "drug-sensitive" stage. For this reason, repetitive courses of two to three months are necessary to produce maximal response. However, with the long duration of treatment, side effects and marrow suppression become more significant problems.

REFERENCES

Bodian, M.: A clinico-pathological study of tumors in the sympathetic nervous system in childhood. *Twenty-eighth Annual Report of the British Empire Cancer Campaign (1950)*, p. 160, 1951.

————: Neuroblastoma—an evaluation of its natural history and the effects of therapy, with particular reference to treatment by massive doses of vitamin B_{12}. *Archives of Disease in Childhood*, 38:606-619, December 1963.

Burgert, E. O., Jr., and Mills, S. D.: Chemotherapy of malignant lesions unique in children. *Mayo Clinic Proceedings*, 41:361-367, June 1966.

James, D. H., Jr.: Letter to the Editor. *Journal of Pediatrics*, 71:764, November 1967.

James, D. H., Jr., Hustu, O., Wrenn, E. L., Jr., and Pinkel, D.: Combination chemotherapy of childhood neuroblastoma. *Journal of the American Medical Association*, 194:123-126, October 11, 1965.

Phillips, R. F.: Personal communication.

Sullivan, M. P.: Curable metastatic tumors of childhood. *Texas Journal of Medicine,* 61:800-805, November 1965.

Thurman, W. G.: *Acute Leukemia and Pediatric Malignancies,* Philadelphia, Pennsylvania, Lea and Febiger, 1968, 248 pp.

Thurman, W. G., Fernbach, D. J., and Sullivan, M. P.: Cyclophosphamide therapy in childhood neuroblastoma. *New England Journal of Medicine,* 270:1336-1340, June 18, 1964.

Valdean, M., and Thurman, W. G.: Personal communication.

Radiotherapy for Wilms' Tumor and Neuroblastoma*

G. J. D'ANGIO, M.D.

*Department of Radiology, University of Minnesota Hospitals,
Minneapolis, Minnesota†*

THE CHILD with a Wilms' tumor characteristically is well. The presence of a mass often is discovered by the mother while bathing or dressing the child or by the physician on a well-baby visit. The child usually is two to three years of age and has no urinary problems (Gross, 1953). Occasionally, hematuria is the presenting complaint. This is of help in the differential diagnosis because neuroblastomas seldom produce this sign. Neuroblastoma occurs in younger children, *i.e.,* the peak incidence is during the first two years of life, and becomes progressively less common during the first decade (Gross, Farber, and Martin, 1959). The neuroblastoma tends to be more centrally located, is fixed, and often extends across the midline. Unlike children with Wilms' tumor, those with neuroblastoma frequently seem chronically ill when first seen. This is because of the propensity of the neuroblastoma to metastasize widely early in its evolution.

Clinical Evaluation

Careful physical examination is followed by clinical, laboratory, and roentgenographic studies. The former two are discussed elsewhere in these proceedings. This report will focus on roentgenographic studies.

*This investigation was supported in part by U. S. Public Health Service grants Nos. CA 5190 and CA 08832.
†Present address: Memorial Hospital for Cancer and Allied Diseases, New York, New York.

183

PLAIN FILMS

ROENTGENOGRAMS OF THE CHEST AND SKELETON.—The presence of pulmonary metastases in a child with a mass in the flank virtually establishes the diagnosis of Wilms' tumor. Pulmonary metastases are rare in patients with neuroblastoma; they are identified roentgenographically in less than 10 per cent of the children before autopsy (D'Angio, unpublished data). On occasion, neuroblastomatous metastases in ribs and pleural sites, when seen end-on, can give the appearance of intrapulmonary lesions. Suitable lateral and oblique projections indicate their proper location. Skeletal involvement without pulmonary metastases in a child with a flank tumor is most consistent with a diagnosis of neuroblastoma. Wilms' tumor almost invariably involves the lungs first before becoming demonstrable in the skeleton; there are only rare exceptions to this general rule.

Both tumors calcify, the neuroblastoma much more frequently than the Wilms' tumor. Differentiation is often easy, however, because the

Fig. 1.—Retrograde pyelogram shows a Wilms tumor. A calcified intrarenal mass is present on the right. The calcification is distributed peripherally in plaques, in an eggshell configuration. It differs from the diffuse speckled mineral deposit in patients with neuroblastoma (see Fig. 6).

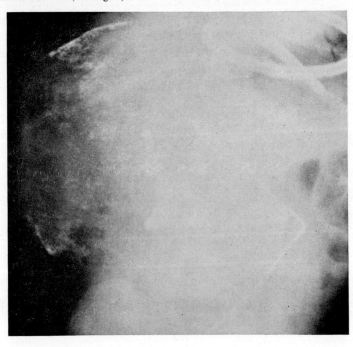

neuroblastoma tends to have a speckled and diffuse calcification within the tumor mass whereas the Wilms' tumor calcifies in an eggshell (peripheral) configuration (Fig. 1). The neuroblastoma often metastasizes to the liver, causing massive enlargement of this organ. Curiously, such metastases do not calcify. When roentgenograms demonstrate a calcified liver mass, the diagnosis is more likely to be a primary hepatoma or another tumor, such as a hemangioma. Differentiation often can be made by analysis of the pattern of calcification or by angiographic studies, as well as on clinical grounds.

CONTRAST STUDIES

EXCRETORY UROGRAM—INFERIOR VENA CAVAGRAM.—Delineation of the kidneys, ureters, and bladder can be obtained with a simultaneous inferior vena cavagram (Fig. 2). This is obtained readily by introducing the contrast material through an ankle vein. Delineation of the inferior

Fig. 2.—Inferior vena cavagram shows a Wilms tumor. The contrast material outlines a small inferior vena cava and demonstrates an intraluminal filling defect (arrow) that completely obstructs the vessel. Abundant collateral venous drainage via the paravertebral plexus is seen.

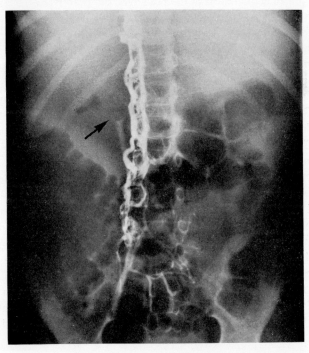

vena cava provides the surgeon with important evidence about the extent of the tumor. For example, propagation of tumor from the renal vein into the inferior vena cava sometimes can be seen, or protrusion of the neuroblastoma around the inferior vena cava encasing that vessel or displacing it from its usual location can be demonstrated. The surgeon thus is alerted to the need for a more extensive dissection and a more complicated resection than is required for the average case.

The excretory urogram is of value for many reasons (Hope and Koop, 1962). It establishes the presence or absence of a second kidney. Roentgen differentiation between neuroblastoma and Wilms' tumor is often relatively easy. The Wilms' tumor is an intrinsic mass splaying the collecting system over its surface whereas the neuroblastoma arises in the pararenal area and characteristically displaces the kidney inferiorly and laterally, but without evident intrinsic distortion of the calyces. In patients with Wilms' tumor, both kidneys should be studied carefully for evidence of bilateral involvement. The appearance is sometimes difficult to differentiate from bilateral multicystic disease; similarly, a multicystic or hydronephrotic kidney sometimes cannot be distinguished from a Wilms' tumor on an excretory urogram.

Lymph nodal masses at some distance below the primary tumor occasionally produce deviation in the course of the ureter (Fig. 3).

The neuroblastoma often will extend across the midline and displace both kidneys laterally. This can be confused with a Wilms' tumor within a renal anomaly, such as a discoid or horseshoe-type kidney.

A large mass in association with a nonfunctioning kidney can represent hydronephrosis; when the diagnosis is Wilms' tumor, this combination of findings sometimes is associated with infiltration of the ureter by the neoplasm. On such occasions, tumor propagation down the ureter to involve the bladder is possible. Cystoscopy to identify tumor deposits is advocated. The entire ureter and a portion of the bladder should be resected in patients with demonstrable bladder metastases.

LYMPHANGIOGRAPHY.—This study usually is not performed in children with either neuroblastoma or Wilms' tumor. Gasquet et al. (1968) have reported their experience with a series of children, including several with neuroblastoma, who were studied by lymphangiography. This technique has been of assistance to the French investigators in delineating the extent of lymph nodal involvement and thus in giving a more complete assessment of the child before definitive therapy is undertaken.

ANGIOGRAPHY.—Aortography or selective angiography may be of great value in differentiating between Wilms' tumor and a hydronephrotic kidney, or between bilateral multicystic kidney disease and bilateral

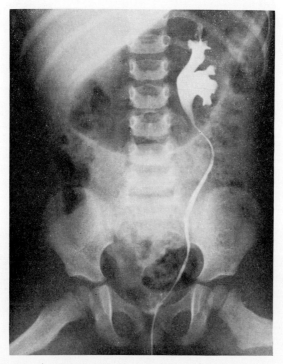

Fig. 3.—Retrograde pyelogram. Deviation of the left ureter laterally at the level of the third, fourth, and fifth lumbar vertebrae is clearly apparent.

Wilms' tumor (Schweisguth, personal communication; Wallace, see pages 79-103, this volume). Studies of this kind can add important information about the size and ramifications of neuroblastomatous masses or about the cause for liver enlargement in patients with hepatomegaly. Many other applications can be envisioned depending on individual patient requirements.

NUCLEAR MEDICINE

Valuable information about the presence of liver or brain metastases often can be obtained most readily by using techniques of nuclear medicine. Important data regarding hepatic damage caused by irradiation of the right hemiabdomen is being accumulated in several clinics in the form of sequential liver scans (Fellows, Vawter, and Tefft, 1968; Loken, see pages 105-113, this volume). Changes in the scan are clearly detectable before biochemical liver function studies become abnormal (Fig. 4). At

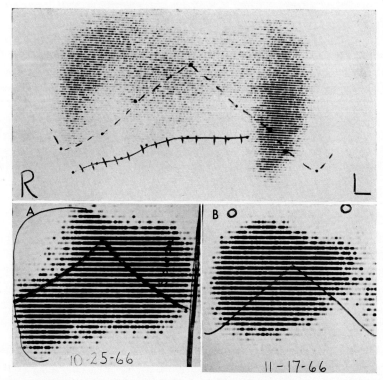

Fig. 4 (above).—Technetium[99m] liver scan. There is irregular visualization of the right lobe of the liver. The edges of the defect are relatively sharp and conform to the radiotherapy portal used in managing the bed of a right-sided Wilms tumor postoperatively. The spleen is enlarged and contains more of the radionuclide than usually is seen. The combination of observations suggests the presence of portal hypertension. This was confirmed by catheter determinations. Upper interrupted line indicates costal margins; lower hatched line is the surgical scar.

Fig. 5 (below).—Hepatoma of right lobe of liver is demonstrated in colloidal gold[198] liver scans. **A,** before operation. There is absence of uptake in a portion of the right lobe of the liver. The expected normal contour is indicated by the curvilinear black line laterally. **B,** three weeks after removal of 80 per cent of the liver. Rapid regeneration has restored the hepatic volume to normal or nearly so. The liver contour is abnormal in that it extends below the costal margin centrally, but there is no evidence of tumor. A scan 10 days earlier showed a smaller liver of similar configuration.

the University of Minnesota, differential counts also are recorded at several sites over the liver and the spleen. Changes in the relative accumulation of the isotope on sequential studies can be shown. Attempts are being made to correlate these changes with recovery, reduction in portal hypertension, and other functional, dynamic alterations in the postradiation period.

Liver scans also are useful in following regeneration of the liver after partial hepatectomy (Fig. 5), *e.g.* to remove metastases.

It should be possible to exploit the functional capacity of the neuroblastoma by tagging suitable precursors and detecting concentrations of labeled metabolites in tumor sites. If the differential in activity were sufficiently high, therapy conceivably could be localized within the tumor. Following a suggestion made by C. Bohuon, a patient with widely disseminated neuroblastoma at the University of Minnesota Hospitals has been studied by means of Selenium[75] methionine. Specific localization of the radionuclide within tumor sites was achieved. Further laboratory and clinical investigations are in progress. (See Loken [pages 105-113, this volume] for a discussion of the diagnostic and therapeutic applications of radionuclides.)

BIOCHEMICAL STUDIES

The value of estimates of the urinary content of the catecholamines is discussed elsewhere in these proceedings. Investigators generally agree that assays of the entire spectrum of norepinephrine degradation products are necessary. Voorhess (1968) finds that determination of the total norepinephrine fraction according to her method of assay is the single most helpful determination.

A rapid, reliable "spot test" would be of great value is sorting out patients with equivocal physical and roentgen findings. LaBrosse (1968) has made a good beginning along these lines. Although a positive LaBrosse spot test is helpful, a negative determination does not necessarily indicate the absence of catecholamines.

BONE MARROW EXAMINATION

Routine bone marrow studies in children with solid tumors almost invariably have negative results unless there is prior roentgen evidence of bone involvement. Patients suspected of harboring a neuroblastoma are exceptions to this rule; in them, routine bone marrow examinations are of undisputed value because extensive deposits can be found without any roentgen sign. Such a finding is of importance in determining therapy and prognosis.

Tumors in Other Sites

NEUROBLASTOMA

Neuroblastoma can occur wherever sympathetic ganglia exist. Primary sites include the region of the organs of Zuckerkandl, Jacobson's organ,

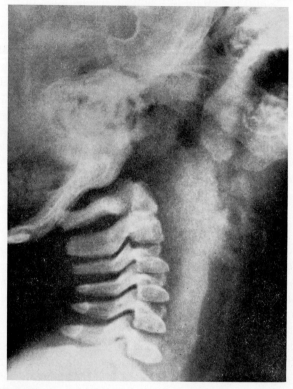

Fig. 6.—Neuroblastoma arising in the neck. The tumor is positioned behind the larynx, trachea, and esophagus, producing anterior displacement of these structures. Speckled calcification is visible within the tumor. Compare this figure with Figure 1.

or more commonly the paraspinal regions along the axis. Thus, tumors can be found intrathoracically or in the neck (Fig. 6) as well as lower in the lumbar area. It is advisable to obtain oblique views of the spine whenever paraspinal primary lesions are encountered. Many of these neoplasms are "dumbbell" in shape and protrude into the spinal canal. Surprisingly large intraspinal protrusions may be present without neurological signs or symptoms.

There is a category of tumor which is seldom encountered and is difficult to designate histopathologically. Typically, the patient is older than the child with neuroblastoma, is often in his teens, and his signs and symptoms frequently simulate those of a herniated intervertebral disc. There often is no paravertebral mass. Roentgen studies sometimes show involvement of the adjacent vertebral body or the pedicles. At operation, the tumor is found to be extradural but intraspinal; it sometimes extends through the intervertebral foramen into the adjoining soft tissues, but without tumefaction. The clinical evolution of this neoplasm is more like that of Ewing's tumor than like that of neuroblastoma. Metastases to the lungs are common and skeletal involvement is often asymmetrical; in these two characteristics, this lesion differs from neuroblastoma which tends to develop diffuse, symmetrical bony lesions without pulmonary deposits. The histological appearance of the tumor mimics in some ways that of the poorly differentiated forms of neuroblastoma, so that this diagnosis frequently is made. This rare neoplasm is perhaps an embryonal tumor and not a neuroblastoma. Estimation of the urinary catecholamine levels would be of value in the attempt to categorize better the nature of tumors such as these.

Wilms' Tumor

Embryonal neoplasms, very similar to Wilms' tumor on histopathological examination, can occur retroperitoneally in other sites and in the liver. Indeed, when a renal Wilms' tumor is found together with a solitary embryomatous hepatic nodule, two separate primary tumors may be present.

Therapy

The initial evaluation of the patient as outlined above usually can be accomplished in 24 to 48 hours, during which time the patient can have his hemoglobin level and blood volume restored to normal, if necessary, and other preoperative measures can be instituted. There is thus no reason to delay surgical exploration in the average uncomplicated case.

Consultation in the operating room among the surgeon, the pediatric chemotherapist, and the radiotherapist is very rewarding. Joint decisions can be reached about extension or curtailment of the surgical maneuver. The margins of the tumor can be demonstrated; the radiotherapist may request the margins and any doubtful zones of extension to be identified by metallic clips for future roentgenographic visualization. In addition, a decision can be reached regarding preservation of the ipsilateral kidney in patients with pararenal neuroblastoma. These tumors often seem well encapsulated, but actually tend to be widely infiltrative. It therefore is usually inadvisable to attempt to separate, by sharp dissection, a suprarenal primary neuroblastoma from the adjoining kidney because of the risk of leaving nests of malignant cells attached to the renal capsule. If postoperative radiotherapy is contemplated, no attempt at preservation of the kidney should be made unless the organ is clearly uninvolved and can be repositioned well outside the tumor bed. Sometimes the structures at the renal pedicle have been stretched and elongated by the mass and permit surgical replacement of the kidney to a lower retroperitoneal site. Another possibility is the transplantation of the patient's own kidney to the iliac fossa in the manner of renal transplants from homologous donors. Obviously, tolerance would be no problem. If there is any doubt regarding these points, it is wise to remove the kidney with the tumor.

It often is useful to mark, with silver clips, the line of resection in patients who are undergoing partial hepatectomy for the removal of neoplastic foci. The relative position of one clip to another can be determined on subsequent roentgenograms. Liver regeneration will cause an initial shift; but thereafter, the pattern should remain constant. Focal displacement of the markers suggests recurrent tumor. Postoperative precaution-

Fig. 7.—Wilms' tumor metastatic to the left lobe of the liver, postresection. The margins of the resection have been marked with metallic clips. A, before radiation therapy. B, after radiation therapy. Note that the clips have coalesced; this indicates suppression of hepatic regeneration (see Fig. 5) and the absence of tumor regrowth.

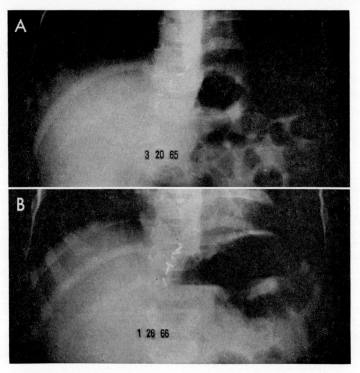

ary irradiation of the resection margin suppresses liver regeneration, and the clips will appear to coalesce (Fig. 7). When a major portion of the liver has been removed, irradiation should not be given unless clearly necessary. Suppression of cellular renewal eventually will lead to hepatic insufficiency of greater or lesser degree if the child survives to grow and develop.

RADIATION THERAPY

GENERAL PRINCIPLES.—Meticulous care and exquisite accuracy are the prerequisites for optimal pediatric radiotherapy. The guiding rule should be that all the tissue at risk must be included in the treatment field, but no more than that. To be as economical as possible regarding the volume irradiated, one should use external heavy metal blocks to shape fields appropriately. Portal films for accurate beam direction and Cobalt[60] teletherapy or equivalent beams should be employed.

WILMS' TUMOR.—It is standard practice in many centers to start postoperative radiotherapy shortly after the time of operation (Gross, 1953). The first treatment usually is given on the same day or the day after operation. While there is no urgency about the delivery of the first dose, there is, at the same time, no need to delay treatment in the average case. Radiotherapy is well tolerated by children in the immediate postoperative period and the therapy does not interfere with wound healing. There need not be any hesitancy, however, in delaying radiotherapy for 24 to 72 hours if the child should be agitated after anesthesia or if vital signs have not returned to normal.

Opposing anterior and posterior fields are used. The size is governed by the findings on the preoperative roentgenographic studies. The field usually is extended across the midline to include the entire vertebral body. This is to assure an even suppression of growth rather than an asymmetrical growth disturbance and inevitable scoliosis (Neuhauser, Wittenborg, Berman, and Cohen, 1952).

Radiotherapists experienced in handling children often only pretend to deliver a first treatment to accustom the child to the procedure and to reassure him about the nature of radiation therapy. In any case, the first dose usually is half the scheduled daily dose. Some children are unusually sensitive to radiation therapy, and excess nausea and vomiting can be avoided by giving such a preliminary half dose. This is an especially useful maneuver in those children who are receiving concomitant actinomycin D (AMD), because the chemical can produce reactions that mimic radiation sickness and thus can confuse the issue.

TABLE 1.—MIDPLANE DEPTH DOSES DELIVERED IN THE MANAGEMENT
OF WILMS' TUMOR AND NEUROBLASTOMA IN CHILDREN OF
DIFFERING AGES (250-KILOVOLT TECHNIQUES)

AGE	DOSE
Less than 12 months	1,800 rads
12 to 18 months	2,000—2,400 rads
19 to 30 months	2,400—3,000 rads
31 to 42 months	3,000—3,500 rads
43 to 60 months	3,500—4,000 rads

At the University of Minnesota, the radiotherapy dose is adjusted according to age. Table 1 indicates the dosage regimen employed. This convention is based on empirical observations which are supported by preliminary laboratory evidence suggesting that age factors affect tumor growth rates (D'Angio and Sillesen, 1966).

The doses quoted are in rads and apply when 250-kilovolt equipment is used. A correction, the so-called quality factor (Q.F.), is necessary for Cobalt[60] teletherapy. The Q.F. employed at the University of Minnesota is 0.85. Thus, to obtain equivalent doses for megavoltage or Cobalt[60] teletherapy units, we divide the doses in Table 1 by 0.85.

Some investigators have questioned the validity of routine postoperative radiation therapy in children with Wilms' tumor (Schneider, 1958). Schneider (1958) and Garcia, Douglass, and Schlosser (1963) have attempted to devise staging systems for the Wilms' tumor and have suggested that radiation therapy should be given only to those patients with more advanced stages of local involvement. One can question easily the necessity of irradiating the tumor bed postoperatively in patients found to have well-encapsulated tumors within the renal substance, without invasion of the capsule or the renal parieties and without evidence of lymph node involvement on ipsilateral node dissection. Some centers, including the University of Minnesota, do not give radiotherapy to infants under one year of age with this favorable combination of findings because the prognosis is known to be especially good in this age group after surgical excision even without AMD (Gross, 1953). The few babies who have been treated in this way have done well.

Distant involvement, and not local recurrence in the tumor bed, seems to be the usual cause for failure in children of any age with early Wilms' tumor. Whether this is true and whether routine postoperative irradiation contributes to the result remain to be shown. Retrospective studies of data available in departments of pathology would be helpful in designing prospective clinical investigations to test the necessity for routine postoperative radiation therapy. Conclusive data are needed urgently if the best chance for survival with the lowest iatrogenic complication rate is to be offered to these children.

Complicated Cases.—Individual consideration is required for the treatment of children with tumors that rupture prior to or during operation, those with metastases at the time of original diagnosis, those with bilateral tumors, and those in several other complicated clinical situations. Methods of procedure have been given in detail elsewhere (D'Angio, 1968).

Preoperative Radiation Therapy.—Preoperative irradiation can be extremely useful under special circumstances, but is not advocated routinely (D'Angio, 1968). Schweisguth and her colleagues (personal communication) are studying the value of routine preoperative irradiation. Their experience indicates that the correct preoperative diagnosis can be made by modern roentgen techniques with only a small percentage of error, and that the surgical intervention is facilitated by prior irradiation. Liquefaction of the tumor and rupture during subsequent removal has not been a problem for these investigators.

Chemotherapy.—This subject is covered elsewhere in these proceedings. The agents of choice are AMD and vincristine sulfate. There is clinical evidence (Farber, 1966) of the usefulness of AMD alone or in combination with radiotherapy in controlling Wilms' tumor. AMD can be given safely by experienced chemotherapists. Neither the radiotherapist nor the chemotherapist should hesitate to combine chemotherapy and radiotherapy. Even large field irradiation, such as the inclusion of the whole thorax and most of the abdomen in a single field, is tolerated satisfactorily by children requiring combination AMD and radiation therapy (D'Angio, 1968).

NEUROBLASTOMA.—The role of routine postoperative radiation therapy in children with neuroblastoma is debated by pediatric oncologists. The advocates (Gross, Farber, and Martin, 1959; Wittenborg, 1950; Wyatt and Farber, 1941) stress the radiosensitivity and radiocurability of these lesions and attribute survival to the cancericidal properties of radiation therapy. Others, notably Koop (1964; 1968), emphasize the tendency of this tumor to regress spontaneously or with the assistance of incomplete surgical therapy, perhaps coupled with chemotherapy. They also recall the deleterious effects of radiotherapy.

The policy adopted at the University of Minnesota is based on the pioneering work of Wyatt and Farber (1941), Gross (1953), Wittenborg (1950), and their numerous collaborators.

Children with tumors confined to the primary site and to adjacent lymph node echelons, whether of flank or paravertebral origin, are treated like those with Wilms' tumor. Infants with primary suprarenal tumors and bulky liver metastases, but without other involvement, have an unusually favorable prognosis (Gross, Farber, and Martin, 1959; Wittenborg, 1950). The treatment portal includes all the involved structures; midplane doses of 1,200 rads are given. The lower dose is administered because of the demonstrated efficacy of this dose regimen, and because both kidneys must be included in the field. Late radiation nephritis is a possible complication (O'Malley, D'Angio, and Vawter, 1963).

Tumors that appear unresectable technically at the time of original exploration sometimes can be converted to an operable state by a preliminary course of radiation therapy with or without chemotherapy. The "second look" follows after a period of six weeks to three months if the child remains free of metastatic involvement in the interval.

Metastatic Neuroblastoma.—Prompt and gratifying relief of painful skeletal metastases can be provided by single midplane doses of 300 rads. Especially troublesome, painful, or disfiguring secondary deposits can be brought under more prolonged control by the delivery of higher doses; for example, 2,000 rads delivered in one and a half weeks.

Chemotherapy.—This modality is discussed in more detail elsewhere in these proceedings. The alkylating agents and periwinkle alkaloids are particularly useful. Anemia or pancytopenia in patients with known bone marrow involvement is an indication of the need for chemotherapy rather than a contraindication to such treatment. The blood counts often rise promptly after a course of nitrogen mustard, for example, because the bone marrow is cleared of the neoplastic infiltrates.

Prognosis

WILMS' TUMOR

The effect of age on the prognosis for children with Wilms' tumor has been recognized. It is a well-known fact that infants have a better prognosis than older children (Gross, 1953). Garcia, Douglass, and Schlosser (1963) have reported other factors which influence prognosis. Farber (1966) recently has reported the best over-all results yet obtained in patients with Wilms' tumor. Eighty-one per cent of patients (55 of 68 children) treated under his direction survived two years or longer. This figure includes patients who had metastases at the time of diagnosis and those who developed secondary deposits after primary therapy.

METASTASES.—Children with metastatic deposits in the lungs, liver, bone, lymph nodes, omentum, and peritoneum can be saved by aggressive combined attacks by the surgeon, radiotherapist, and chemotherapist.

Thus, in patients reported by Farber (1966), 18 of 31 children (58 per cent) who developed metastases at some time during the course of the illness survived for two years or longer. Involvement of the brain and scattered metastases in the liver or the skeleton represent more difficult problems. Children with these complications rarely survive for long periods of time.

NEUROBLASTOMA

The prognosis for patients with neuroblastoma depends on many factors including age and location of the primary site. The worst prognosis is in the older child with a pararenal primary tumor (Gross, Farber, and Martin, 1959). The survival rate in children under two years of age is approximately 50 per cent compared with an over-all survival rate of about 35 per cent (Gross, Farber, and Martin, 1959). Survival is approximately twice as good in patients with primary tumors in the thorax or the pelvis as in those with pararenal primary lesions (Gross, Farber, and Martin, 1959).

METASTASES.—Diffuse involvement of the liver, skin, lymph nodes, or bone marrow (without roentgenographically visible bony metastases) can be controlled in some patients (Gross, Farber, and Martin, 1959; Reilly, Nesbit, and Krivit, 1968; Wittenborg, 1950). Skeletal involvement which is demonstrable roentgenographically carries a very poor prognosis, and patients with this complication rarely survive (Dargeon, 1960; Reilly, Nesbit, and Krivit, 1968).

Favorable results in some patients can be attributed only to spontaneous regression (Everson and Cole, 1966). This tendency seems to be enhanced by surgical, radiotherapeutic, or chemotherapeutic treatment, or a combination of all three.

Subsequent Care

Frequent examinations and assiduous supervision are essential if success is to be achieved. For patients with Wilms' tumor in particular, early detection of metastatic involvement can mean the difference between success or failure in treatment. Biochemical assays in the follow-up period for patients with neuroblastoma are very useful (Voorhess and Whalen, 1964). Changes in the levels of the specific metabolites can be used to gauge whether the disease is quiescent or recrudescent.

Physical examinations, which should include blood pressure determinations, are scheduled at two- to four-month intervals for the first 18 months after treatment and for one-and-a-half additional years thereafter on a semiannual basis. Patients with radiation nephritis can develop hypertension before signs of renal impairment become obvious (O'Malley, D'Angio, and Vawter, 1963). Chest films and skeletal surveys are obtained at these visits for patients with the neuroblastoma. Skeletal surveys are scheduled less frequently for children with Wilms' tumor. Kidney function assays are obtained at the time of physical examination, and excretory urograms are scheduled at least once a year for the first two years after treatment. The irradiated sites should be examined roentgenographically every year for an indefinite period of time. This is to detect not only bone growth abnormalities, but also secondary bone tumors induced by the irradiation (Cohen and D'Angio, 1961).

Late complications can develop after an astonishingly long period of time (O'Malley, D'Angio, and Vawter, 1963). These encompass growth disturbances (Neuhauser, Wittenborg, Berman, and Cohen, 1952), oncogenesis (Cohen and D'Angio, 1961; O'Malley, D'Angio, and Vawter, 1963; Tefft, Vawter, and Mitus, 1968), functional impairment (O'Malley, D'Angio, and Vawter, 1963), and gonadal effects (D'Angio and Tefft, 1967). Gonadal effects include somatic underdevelopment, impaired fertility, and genetic damage (D'Angio and Tefft, 1967). It is especially tragic to succeed in controlling the tumor only to lose the patient in later years because of a treatment complication (O'Malley, D'Angio, and Vawter, 1963; Tefft, Vawter, and Mitus, 1968). Early detection may help to avoid such eventualities. Thus, I cannot stress too strongly that the individual should be followed for life.

Summary

Various aspects of the diagnosis and therapy of children with Wilms' tumor and neuroblastoma are discussed. Radiotherapeutic details are emphasized.

Acknowledgments

The author acknowledges with gratitude the assistance of Dr. M. Loken, under whose direction the nuclear medicine studies at the University of Minnesota are performed, and the kindness of Drs. W. Krivit, M. Nesbit, R. Benjamin, and E. N. Manoles in allowing the use of data from certain of their patients.

REFERENCES

Cohen, J., and D'Angio, G. J.: Unusual bone tumors after roentgen therapy of children: Two case reports. *The American Journal of Roentgenology, Radium Therapy and Nuclear Medicine*, 86:502-512, September 1961.

D'Angio, G. J.: Radiation therapy in Wilms' tumor. *Journal of the American Medical Association*, 204:987-988, June 10, 1968.

D'Angio, G. J., and Sillesen, K.: The influence of age on murine tumor growth rate and survival. (Abstract) *Proceedings of the American Association for Cancer Research*, 7:16, April 1966.

D'Angio, G. J., and Tefft, M.: Radiation therapy in the management of children with gynecologic cancers. *Annals of the New York Academy of Sciences*, 142:675-693, May 10, 1967.

Dargeon, H. W.: *Tumors of Childhood. A Clinical Treatise*. 1st edition. New York, New York, Paul B. Hoeber, Inc., 1960, 476 pp.

Everson, T. C., and Cole, W. H.: *Spontaneous Regression of Cancer*. Philadelphia, Pennsylvania, W. B. Saunders Co., 1966, 560 pp.

Farber, S.: Chemotherapy in the treatment of leukemia and Wilms' tumor. *Journal of the American Medical Association*, 198:826-836, November 21, 1966.

Fellows, K. E., Jr., Vawter, G. F., and Tefft, M.: Hepatic defects following abdominal irradiation in children: Detection by Au-198 scan and confirmation by histologic examination. *The American Journal of Roentgenology, Radium Therapy and Nuclear Medicine*, 103:422-431, June 1968.

Garcia, M., Douglass, C., and Schlosser, J. V.: Classification and prognosis in Wilms' tumor. *Radiology*, 80:574-580, April 1963.

Gasquet, C., Schweisguth, O., Debrun, G., Grosdemange, M., and Markovits, P.: Lymphangiography in malignant diseases in children. *The American Journal of Roentgenology, Radium Therapy and Nuclear Medicine*, 103:1-12, May 1968.

Gross, R. E.: *The Surgery of Infancy and Childhood: Its Principles and Techniques*. 1st edition. Philadelphia, Pennsylvania, W. B. Saunders Company, 1953, 1,000 pp.

Gross, R. E., Farber, S., and Martin, L. W.: Neuroblastoma sympatheticum. A study and report of 217 cases. *Pediatrics*, 23:1179-1191, June 1959.

Hope, J. W., and Koop, C. E.: Abdominal tumors in infants and children. In W. Cornwall, Ed.: *Medical Radiography and Photography*. Rochester, New York, Eastman Kodak Company, 1962, Vol. 38, pp. 6-57.

Koop, C. E.: Current management of nephroblastoma and neuroblastoma. *The American Journal of Surgery*, 107:497-501, March 1964.

————: The surgical management of children with neuroblastoma. *Journal of Pediatric Surgery*, 3:(Conference on the Biology of Neuroblastoma), Part II, 178-179, February 1968.

LaBrosse, E. H.: Biochemical diagnosis of neuroblastoma: Use of a urine spot test. *Proceedings of the American Association for Cancer Research*, 9:39, March 1968.

Loken, M.: Evaluation of neoplasia in childhood using techniques in nuclear medicine. In *Neoplasia in Childhood* (The University of Texas M. D. Anderson Hospital and Tumor Institute, Twelfth Annual Clinical Conference, 1967). Chicago, Illinois, Year Book Medical Publishers, Inc., 1968, pp. 105-113.

Neuhauser, E. B. D., Wittenborg, M. H., Berman, C. Z., and Cohen, J.: Irradiation effects of roentgen therapy on the growing spine. *Radiology*, 59:637-650, November 1952.

O'Malley, B., D'Angio, G. J., and Vawter, G. F.: Late effects of roentgen therapy given in infancy. *The American Journal of Roentgenology, Radium Therapy and Nuclear Medicine*, 89:1067-1074, May 1963.

Reilly, D., Nesbit, M. E., and Krivit, W.: Cure of three patients who had skeletal metastases in disseminated neuroblastoma. *Pediatrics*, 41:47-51, January 1968.

Schneider, M.: Renal embryoma. In F. Buschke, Ed.: *Progress in Radiation Therapy*, New York, New York, Grune and Stratton, 1958, pp. 180-191.

Schweisguth, O.: Personal communication.

Tefft, M., Vawter, G., and Mitus, A.: Second primary neoplasms in children. *The*

American Journal of Roentgenology, Radium Therapy and Nuclear Medicine, 103:800-822, August 1968.

Voorhess, M. L.: The catecholamines in tumor and urine from patients with neuroblastoma, ganglioneuroblastoma and pheochromocytoma. *Journal of Pediatric Surgery,* 3:(Conference on the Biology of Neuroblastoma), Part II, 147-148, February 1968.

Voorhess, M. L., and Whalen, J. P.: Role of catecholamine excretion in diagnosis and treatment of neuroblastoma: Report of two cases. *Radiology,* 83:92-97, July 1964.

Wallace, S.: Diagnostic radiologic techniques. In *Neoplasia in Childhood* (The University of Texas M. D. Anderson Hospital and Tumor Institute, Twelfth Annual Clinical Conference, 1967). Chicago, Illinois, Year Book Medical Publishers, Inc., 1968, pp. 79-103.

Wittenborg, M. H.: Roentgen therapy in neuroblastoma: A review of seventy-three cases. *Radiology,* 54:679-688, May 1950.

Wyatt, G. M., and Farber, S.: Neuroblastoma sympatheticum. Roentgenological appearances and radiation treatment. *The American Journal of Roentgenology, Radium Therapy and Nuclear Medicine,* 46:485-496, October 1941.

Chemotherapeutic Management of Childhood Rhabdomyosarcoma*

W. W. SUTOW, M.D.

Department of Pediatrics, The University of Texas M. D. Anderson Hospital and Tumor Institute at Houston, Houston, Texas

THE EFFECTIVE TREATMENT OF THE CHILD with rhabdomyosarcoma requires the planned, persistent, and combined efforts of the surgeon, the radiotherapist, and the chemotherapist. In this paper, the potentialities of chemotherapy in the therapeutic attack will be explored. The choice of drugs, the schedules of administration, and the rationale for therapy presented are based on clinical experience with 78 children with rhabdomyosarcoma at The University of Texas M. D. Anderson Hospital and Tumor Institute at Houston.

Clinical Experience

Between 1954 and the fall of 1967, 78 children with rhabdomyosarcoma were treated at this institution. The age range of these children was one month to 15 years 11 months, with a median age of 5 years 7 months. The sex ratio was 36 boys to 42 girls (Table 1). The excess of girls is attributable to four cases of sarcoma botryoides of the vagina. Seventy-two of the children were Caucasians and six were Negroes. Histologically, 56 (or 74 per cent) of the lesions were classified as embryonal rhabdomyosarcomas, and 20 (or 24 per cent) were classified as alveolar rhabdomyosarcomas (Table 2). The microscopic findings on which the diagnoses were made have been described by Albores-Saavedra, Butler, and Martin (1965). A number of the cases summarized here were included in that review. In one child, the diagnosis was both alveolar and embryonal rhabdomyosarcoma. In another child, the tumor was rhabdomyosar-

*This study was supported in part by grant CA-3713 and by Public Health Service Research Career Award CA-2501 from the National Cancer Institute.

TABLE 1.—RHABDOMYOSARCOMA IN CHILDREN:
PATIENT CHARACTERISTICS

Number of patients	78
Ratio of males to females	36/42
Ratio of Caucasians to Negroes	72/6
Age	
Median	5 yr. 7 mo.
Range	5 mo. to
	15 yr. 11 mo.

TABLE 2.—RHABDOMYOSARCOMA IN CHILDREN:
PRIMARY SITE AND HISTOLOGICAL TYPE

PRIMARY SITE	EMBRYONAL	ALVEOLAR
Head and neck*	36	12
Extremities	3	5
Body wall†	2	2
Genitourinary tract	6	1
Retroperitoneal tissues	2	0
Unknown site	2	0
Sarcoma botryoides	5	0
TOTAL	56	20

Not included in tabulation:
*Scalp (one), type unspecified.
†Flank (one), both embryonal and alveolar.

coma of an unspecified type. Five of 56 embryonal rhabdomyosarcomas were categorized as sarcoma botryoides. Excluded from Table 1 were the children with a diagnosis of unclassified sarcoma, even those for whom rhabdomyosarcoma was one of the possibilities.

The most common sites of origin for rhabdomyosarcoma were in the head and neck area (Table 2). Forty-nine of the 78 lesions, or 64 per cent, occurred there. The other primary sites included the extremities (10 per cent), the genitourinary system, whose lesions included sarcoma botryoides of the vagina (14 per cent), the body wall (6 per cent), and the retroperitoneal tissues (2 per cent). In two patients (2 per cent), the primary site was not determined. Of the 49 tumors that originated in the head and neck area, one was a sarcoma botryoides involving the larynx. The rest arose from the orbit, nasopharynx, and other structures in this anatomic location.

The clinical factors which significantly influenced the three-year survival rates were: site of primary lesion, extent of disease, age of child, histological type of tumor, and program of treatment. Primary tumor involving the orbit carried the best prognosis, with a three-year survival rate of 84 per cent in 15 patients. Three of five children with sarcoma botryoides were long-term survivors. About half the children with rhabdomyosarcoma of the genitourinary tract (other than sarcoma botryoides of the vagina) were living three years from the time of diagnosis. Of 24 children with extensive regional or metastatic disease at time of diagnosis, 39 per cent survived one year, 9 per cent lived two years, and none have survived three years. Similar life-table analyses of the 54 children with localized disease at time of diagnosis showed the one-year, two-year, and three-year survival rates to be 82 per cent, 63 per cent, and 56 per cent, respectively. The 45 children younger than seven years of age had a significantly higher three-year survival rate than did the 33 children older than seven years at time of diagnosis (51 per cent compared to 24 per cent).

With regard to the influence of the lesion's histological type, the children with sarcoma botryoides had the highest three-year survival rate (60 per cent) and those with the alveolar rhabdomyosarcoma had the lowest (25 per cent). The median survival of 51 children with embryonal rhabdomyosarcoma other than sarcoma botryoides was 21.2 months, with a projected three-year survival rate of 45 per cent.

Results of Treatments

The treatments given to the 78 patients were classified according to the three standard modalities—surgical therapy, radiation therapy, and chemotherapy. They were classified further as either definitive or palliative. A treatment was considered definitive when the clinical situation justified, and the therapy constituted, an intensive effort to eradicate all known foci of tumor. Anything less was considered palliative treatment. Significant chemotherapy required the use of adequate doses of actinomycin D, vincristine sulfate, and cyclophosphamide either singly or in various combinations. For the purposes of this evaluation, the use of chemical agents other than the three mentioned was considered to be simply palliative.

Table 3 shows the types of treatment used and the outcome in 60 of the 78 children treated before 1965. Using 1965 as the cutoff date meant that actual and not projected three-year follow-ups could be evaluated. Eighteen survivors lived three years or longer after diagnosis with no evidence of disease. The relation of survival to type of therapy can be seen. Several factors seemed to be implicated. The preponderance of survivors in the group receiving surgical therapy is explained, to a considerable degree, by the fact that most of the children undergoing operation were young and had localized disease of the histologically more favorable

TABLE 3.—RHABDOMYOSARCOMA IN CHILDREN: TREATMENT REGIMENS (THROUGH 1964)

DEFINITIVE SURGICAL THERAPY	DEFINITIVE RADIATION THERAPY	SIGNIFICANT CHEMOTHERAPY
		yes (9) ******
	yes (15)	
		no (6) ***
yes (32)		
		yes (3) ***
	no (17)	
		no (14) *****
		yes (3)
	yes (8)	
no (28)		no (5) *
	no (20)	

Each star (*) represents one three-year survivor. The number of patients in each treatment category is shown in parentheses.

type. In the early years of the study, chemotherapy was considered the treatment of choice only in problem cases in which the adequacy of surgical extirpation was in question. In spite of this fact, the data show some association of chemotherapy with favorable outcome. Thus, 75 per cent of the long-term survivors received chemotherapy as compared to 40 per cent who did not.

Twenty-four children with widespread or metastatic disease at time of diagnosis did not survive more than three years. The data indicated, however, that the 18 children who received chemotherapy lived longer than did the six children who did not (median survivals were 10.9 months and 3.7 months, respectively).

Chemotherapy Schedules

For lesions in accessible anatomic sites, operation is the definitive treatment of choice (Bardwil and MacComb, 1964; Martin, Butler, and

Albores-Saavedra, 1965). Irradiation becomes the definitive mode of therapy when the lesion(s) cannot be extirpated entirely. The rationale for full utilization of chemotherapy in the treatment of children with rhabdomyosarcoma includes the following:

1. The projected over-all three-year survival rate in this series of 78 cases was only 40 per cent. If this figure were representative of the results obtained in other clinics, the over-all treatment failure rate would be about 60 per cent. Any means, therefore, of improving the survival rate should be explored. Efforts should be concentrated particularly on clinical situations in which poor prognostic factors are present.

2. Clinical data from the Anderson Hospital series suggest that the addition of chemotherapy in the treatment of children with extensive disease has increased the duration of survival.

3. Both surgical extirpation and radiation are target-limited modes of therapy. A number of autopsy examinations have shown local tumor control, but with widespread dissemination of metastases.

4. Definite antitumor effect has been demonstrated by several drugs, particularly vincristine, actinomycin D, and cyclophosphamide (Haddy, Nora, Sutow, and Vietti, 1967; Sutow et al., 1966; Tan et al., 1960).

5. The probability of total tumor eradication with a given drug is greater with a smaller target cell population. Thus, the use of drugs is

TABLE 4.—DOSAGE SCHEDULE AND MAJOR TOXICITY OF DRUGS

DRUG	DOSAGE SCHEDULES	MAJOR TOXICITY
A. Cyclophosphamide	(a) 2.5 to 5.0 mg./kg. daily p.o. or	1. Severe gastrointestinal symptoms
	(b) 15 to 30 mg./kg. once weekly, p.o. or i.v.	2. Bone marrow depression
		3. Chemical cystitis
B. Vincristine sulfate	2.0 mg./square meter weekly i.v. for 8-12 weeks	1. Severe gastrointestinal symptoms, including obstipation and ileus
		2. Progressive neuropathy
C. Dactinomycin (actinomycin D)	Total: 75 μg./kg. per course	1. Severe gastrointestinal symptoms
	(a) In small children 15 μg./kg./day i.v. × 5	2. Severe local reaction in irradiated sites
	(b) In larger children, 200 to 300 μg./day i.v. until total cumulative dose is given	3. Thrombocytopenia

Abbreviations: p.o., orally; i.v., intravenously.

optimal when the residual tumor cell population has been reduced to a minimum by operation and irradiation (Wilcox *et al.,* 1965).

6. The conditions desirable for effective chemotherapy can be satisfied. Rhabdomyosarcoma can be considered a chemosensitive tumor. Effective chemical agents are available. Other effective treatment modalities can be used.

The chemotherapy schedules shown below and currently used at Anderson Hospital have evolved from the cumulative experience summarized. The schedules are based on the administration of the combination of three drugs—vincristine, actinomycin D, and cyclophosphamide (abbreviation for the combination, VAC)—in conjunction with surgical therapy and/or radiotherapy. Each of the drugs has shown definite antitumor activity in children with rhabdomyosarcoma. Each acts on tumor cells by a different mechanism. No cross resistance has been demonstrated clinically. The major toxic manifestations of the agents do not overlap. It is presumed that the total antitumor activity will be at least a summation of the independent actions of the drugs. Table 4 outlines the dosages used and the major-dose limiting toxic manifestations of each agent.

Schedule A (Fig. 1) illustrates the use of VAC therapy in association with operation and postoperative irradiation. As soon as the clinical condition of the patient stabilizes after the primary operative procedure, chemotherapy with actinomycin D and vincristine is begun. The adminis-

Fig. 1.—Schema for schedule A combination therapy. Drugs and irradiation are used postoperatively. Abbreviations: *XRT,* irradiation; *DACT,* dactinomycin.

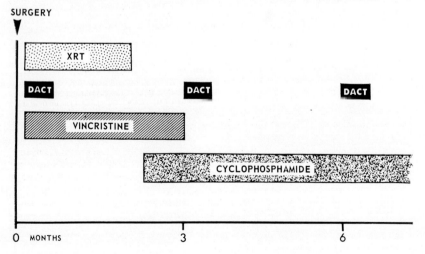

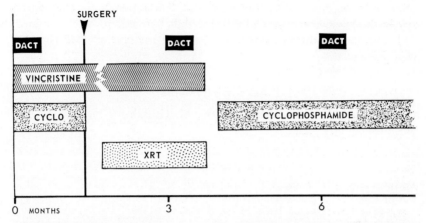

Fig. 2.—Schema for schedule B combination therapy. Preoperative chemotherapy is followed by postoperative drug and radiation treatments. Abbreviations: *DACT,* dactinomycin; *CYCLO,* cyclophosphamide; *XRT,* irradiation.

tration of the two drugs will overlap with the initiation of irradiation. Cyclophosphamide is not given until radiotherapy is completed in order to avoid excessive marrow depression. After irradiation is completed and the condition of the patient's blood stabilizes, cyclophosphamide is started. Courses of actinomycin D are given at three-month intervals for one year. Vincristine is continued for a total of 12 weekly injections. Cyclophosphamide is scheduled for a minimum of two years in the absence of tumor recurrence or metastases. If radiotherapy is not given, all three drugs are used simultaneously.

Schedule B (Fig. 2) shows the application of combination chemotherapy in a situation that is not immediately amenable to definitive surgical therapy or irradiation. After the diagnosis is established by means of biopsy, chemotherapy is started. When regression has been achieved and the tumor is considered operable, chemotherapy is interrupted temporarily while the surgical procedure is performed. If postoperative irradiation is used, cyclophosphamide administration is withheld until radiotherapy is completed. The doses of the drugs and duration of each drug treatment are the same as those outlined in Schedule A.

Summary

The clinical features noted in 78 children with rhabdomyosarcoma have been reviewed. The factors associated with three-year survival in these children were age at diagnosis, extent of disease, type of tumor, site of primary lesion, and program of treatment. The rationale for chemotherapy in the management of childhood rhabdomyosarcoma was examined, and schedules of drug treatment currently in use at Anderson Hospital were presented.

Acknowledgments

Appreciation is expressed to Dr. K. M. Griffith for his assistance in biostatistical analyses.

REFERENCES

Albores-Saavedra, J., Butler, J. J., and Martin, R. G.: Rhabdomyosarcoma: Clinico-pathologic considerations and report of 85 cases. In *Tumors of Bone and Soft Tissue* (The University of Texas M. D. Anderson Hospital and Tumor Institute, Eighth Annual Clinical Conference, 1963). Chicago, Illinois, Year Book Medical Publishers, Inc., 1965, pp. 349-366.

Bardwil, J. M., and MacComb, W. S.: Sarcomas of the head and neck with special references to rhabdomyosarcomas. *The American Journal of Surgery,* 108:476-479, October 1964.

Haddy, T. B., Nora, A. H., Sutow, W. W., and Vietti, T. J.: Cyclophosphamide treatment for metastatic soft tissue sarcoma. Intermittent large doses in the treatment of children. *American Journal of Diseases of Children,* 114:301-308, September 1967.

Martin, R. G., Butler, J. J., and Albores-Saavedra, J.: Soft tissue tumors: Surgical treatment and results. In *Tumors of Bone and Soft Tissue* (The University of Texas M. D. Anderson Hospital and Tumor Institute, Eighth Annual Clinical Conference, 1963). Chicago, Illinois, Year Book Medical Publishers, Inc., 1965, pp. 333-347.

Sutow, W. W., Berry, D. H., Haddy, T. B., Sullivan, M. P., Watkins, W. L., and Windmiller, J.: Vincristine sulfate therapy in children with metastatic soft tissue sarcoma. *Pediatrics,* 38:465-472, September 1966.

Tan, C. T. C., Golbey, R. B., Yap, C. L., Wollner, N., Hackethal, C. A., Murphy, M. L., Dargeon, H. W., and Burchenal, J. H.: Clinical experiences with actinomycins D, KS$_2$, and F$_1$ (KS$_4$). *Annals of The New York Academy of Sciences,* 89: 426-444, October 5, 1960.

Wilcox, W. S., Griswold, D. P., Laster, W. R., Jr., Schabel, F. M., Jr., and Skipper, H. E.: Experimental evaluation of potential anticancer agents. XVII. Kinetics of growth and regression after treatment of certain solid tumors. *Cancer Chemotherapy Reports,* 47:27-39, August 1965.

Rhabdomyosarcoma in Children: Treatment and Results*

ROBERT D. LINDBERG, M.D.

Department of Radiotherapy, The University of Texas M. D. Anderson Hospital and Tumor Institute at Houston, Houston, Texas

RECENTLY THERE HAVE BEEN a number of publications on the management of rhabdomyosarcoma. Most of them discuss rhabdomyosarcoma in the general population rather than in the pediatric age group, *i.e.*, children less than 15 years of age. Edland (1967) showed that patients with rhabdomyosarcomas arising in the head and neck area are curable by large doses of irradiation combined with chemotherapy. The complications of such radical radiotherapy in the pediatric age group may be formidable.

An important fact must be brought out concerning the histology of all soft tissue sarcomas and rhabdomyosarcoma in particular. Suit and Lindberg (1968) recently found a number of cases in which the pathological diagnosis was changed after treatment was completed. These changes point out the difficulty that the pathologist has in specifying the exact histology of certain tumors.

The problems involved in the treatment of children with rhabdomyosarcoma are multiple. How does the age of the patient influence the radicality of the surgical procedure and/or radiotherapy? What is the role of chemotherapy? Should systemic chemotherapy be used prophylactically to "prevent" distant metastasis? Is there a treatment of choice for children with rhabdomyosarcomas? To provide the answers for these questions, a review of the records of all patients with rhabdomyosarcoma seen at The University of Texas M. D. Anderson Hospital and Tumor Institute at Houston was undertaken.

---

*This investigation was supported in part by grants CA 06294 and CA 05654 of the National Cancer Institute, National Institutes of Health, United States Public Health Service.

TABLE 1.—Rhabdomyosarcoma in Children:
1955 through October 1966
Distribution by Age

Sex	0 through 5 Yr.	6 through 10 Yr.	11 through 14 Yr.	Total
Male	8	3	4	15
Female	10	4	5	19
Total	18	7	9	34

Case Material

The records of patients with a histological diagnosis of rhabdomyosarcoma seen between 1948 and October 1966 were analyzed. During that 19-year period, 72 patients presented with previously untreated lesions and no evidence of distant metastasis on admission. Thirty-four of these were 14 years of age or younger, and they comprise the case material in this presentation. There was a slight predominance of females over males in all age groups, but this difference does not appear to be important. More than 50 per cent of the patients (18 of 34) were five years of age or younger (Table 1). There were 30 Caucasians and four Negroes (two males and two females). The degree of surgical disturbance of the primary lesion prior to admission was variable. Twenty-one patients had biopsy only, three had no surgical procedure of any kind, and 10 had local excisions. The group with local excisions is included with the untreated patients because local excision is not considered a definitive procedure. Histologically, the lesions were divided according to Horn and Enterline's (1958) classification as follows: embryonal, 23 tumors; and alveolar, which carries the worst prognosis, eight tumors. The histological subtype of the three remaining lesions was not specified. No pleomorphic rhabdomyosarcomas were noted.

The location of the primary lesion was tabulated. Of the 34 lesions, 27 arose in the head and neck area, with nine in the orbit and six in the nasopharynx. The other seven lesions were scattered throughout the remainder of the body.

Results of Treatment

The absolute survival rate for all children treated for rhabdomyosarcoma are presented in Table 2. The percentage of patients surviving free of disease does not vary significantly from the first through the fifth year, 50 and 41 per cent, respectively. This is because of the rapid onset of primary recurrences after treatment and the early manifestation of distant

TABLE 2.—RHABDOMYOSARCOMA IN CHILDREN:
1955 THROUGH OCTOBER 1966
SURVIVAL OF 34 PATIENTS WITH PRIMARY LESIONS

YEARS AFTER TREATMENT	NO. OF PATIENTS	NED—PER CENT	
1	34	17	50.0
2	28	11	39.3
3	26	11	42.3
4	22	11	50.0
5	17	7	41.2

Abbreviation: NED, no evidence of disease.

metastases. Eight of the ten primary lesions recurred within five months after completion of treatment; the ninth recurred at eight months (the patient was salvaged by repeated surgical procedures), and the tenth recurred at 12 months. Of the 14 patients who developed distant metastases, nine showed evidence of these deposits within six months of the primary treatment; and 13 of the 14, within one year. The fourteenth patient showed distant metastasis 22 months after the primary treatment. Therefore, the one-year survival rate for rhabdomyosarcomas in children can be used to evaluate the efficacy of the various treatment modalities.

The cases were analyzed according to the histology of the primary lesion, the patient's age and sex, the degree of surgical intervention prior to admission, the location of the primary lesion, and the treatment modalities used. One important parameter in the prognosis is the histological type of the rhabdomyosarcoma. The alveolar type carries the worst prognosis (Table 3). Patients 10 years of age or less have a better prognosis than do those in the older age group (Table 4). The distribution of the alveolar lesions according to the age of the patients is as follows: four patients were less than six years old, three were from six through 10

TABLE 3.—RHABDOMYOSARCOMA IN CHILDREN:
1955 THROUGH OCTOBER 1966
INFLUENCE OF HISTOLOGY

	EMBRYONAL	ALVEOLAR	NOT STATED
NED	12	2	3
P	6	3	
DM	5	3	
TOTAL	23	8	3

Abbreviations: NED, no evidence of disease; P, primary failure; DM, distant metastasis only.

TABLE 4.—RHABDOMYOSARCOMA IN CHILDREN:
1955 THROUGH OCTOBER 1966
INFLUENCE OF AGE

	0 THROUGH 5 YRS.	6 THROUGH 10 YRS.	11 THROUGH 14 YRS.
NED	10	4	3
P	3	2	4
DM	5	1	2
TOTAL	18	7	9

Abbreviations: NED, no evidence of disease; P, primary failure; DM, distant metastasis only.

TABLE 5.—RHABDOMYOSARCOMA IN CHILDREN:
1955 THROUGH OCTOBER 1966
INFLUENCE OF PREVIOUS SURGICAL PROCEDURES

	NONE	BIOPSY	EXCISION
NED	2	10	5
P		6	3
DM	1	5	2
TOTAL	3	21	10

Abbreviations: NED, no evidence of disease; P, primary failure; DM, distant metastasis only.

years old, and one was 12 years old. The highest incidence of embryonal lesions was in the oldest age group (seven of nine patients over 10 years old). Thus, the age of the patient as a factor influencing prognosis is independent of the histological type of the lesion. The sex of the patient does not influence the prognosis. Seven of 15 males are living free of disease, whereas 10 of 19 females are living free of disease. This difference is not significant. One important consideration is the extent to which surgical disturbance prior to admission influences the prognosis. As noted in Table 5, the proportion of patients free of disease is the same irrespective of the degree of surgical intervention before admission. Also, the incidence of distant metastasis is not influenced by the degree of surgical interference prior to definitive treatment.

The influence of the location of the primary disease on prognosis is shown in Table 6. Forty-four per cent of patients with head and neck lesions survived at least one year free of disease. There is, however, a marked variation in survival rates when individual sites within the head and neck area are considered. Orbital lesions carry the best prognosis; in this series, eight of nine patients are free of disease, and one died because of primary recurrence. Nasopharyngeal lesions carry the worst prognosis;

TABLE 6.—RHABDOMYOSARCOMA IN CHILDREN:
1955 THROUGH OCTOBER 1966
RESULTS BY LOCATION OF PRIMARY LESION

	Orbit	Nasopharynx	Other Head and Neck Sites	All Head and Neck Sites	Other Sites
NED	8		4	12	5
P	1	5	3	9	
DM		1	5	6	2
Total	9	6	12	27	7

Abbreviations: NED, no evidence of disease; P, primary failure; DM, distant metastases only.

all six patients died of disease, five of primary failure and one of distant metastases. Primary sites other than the head and neck area appear to carry a good prognosis, but the number of cases involved is too small to be significant.

The results of treatment then were analyzed according to the various modalities used. The data are presented in Table 7. A cursory examination of this table indicates that the combination of radiation therapy, surgical therapy, and chemotherapy gives the best prognosis; all six patients so treated are free of disease. This fact may be somewhat misleading unless the location of the primary lesion is considered. Patients presenting with primary lesions of the nasopharynx have a uniformly poor prognosis regardless of the treatment modality used. Four patients with nasopharyngeal lesions were treated by combined radiation therapy and chemotherapy. In three, the tumor dose was limited to 5,000 rads in five weeks; and all three patients died because of lack of control of primary disease. In one patient, the tumor dose was carried to 6,000 rads in seven weeks and was combined with actinomycin D and vincristine sulfate. The

TABLE 7.—RHABDOMYOSARCOMA IN CHILDREN: 1955 THROUGH OCTOBER 1966
RESULTS BY TREATMENT MODALITY

	Surg.	Xrt	Surg. and Xrt	Chemo.	Xrt, Surg., and Chemo.	Xrt and Chemo.	Surg. and Chemo.
NED	2	2	1	1*	6	4	1†
P	4	1		1		3	
DM						8	
Total	6	3	1	2	6	15	1

Abbreviations: Surg., surgical therapy; Xrt, radiation therapy; Chemo., chemotherapy; NED, no evidence of disease; P, primary failure; DM, distant metastases only.
*Local excision prior to admission followed by perfusion; NED at 84 months.
†Primary recurrence; patient was salvaged by additional surgical therapy and had NED at 61 months.

primary disease in this patient was controlled, but he died from distant metastases seven months after treatment was completed. One patient was treated by radiation therapy only; he received a tumor dose of 6,000 rads in eight weeks and died of primary disease 14 months later.

In contrast to nasopharyngeal lesions, orbital lesions carry an excellent prognosis. The nine patients with orbital lesions were treated by three basic techniques: surgical excision, radiotherapy, and a combination of the two modalities. Four patients received combined radiation therapy, surgical therapy, and chemotherapy. Three of the four received preoperative irradiation (a tumor dose of 5,000 rads in five weeks) combined with chemotherapy. The fourth patient received postoperative irradiation combined with chemotherapy. The fifth patient underwent orbital exenteration followed by radiation therapy; the tumor dose was 5,000 rads in five weeks. The sixth patient was treated by radiation therapy only; he received 5,000 rads in four-and-a-half weeks. The seventh patient received radiation therapy (a tumor dose of 6,000 rads in seven weeks) followed by chemotherapy—actinomycin D, vincristine, and Cytoxan sequentially. The two remaining patients were treated by surgical techniques alone. The only failure in the group with orbital lesions was an 11-year-old Caucasian female with an embryonal rhabdomyosarcoma who underwent exenteration and had a primary recurrence three months later.

Twelve other lesions arose in scattered head and neck sites. Seven of the 12 were managed by combined radiation therapy and chemotherapy. The tumor dose varied from 4,500 rads in five weeks to 6,000 rads in six weeks. Chemotherapy consisted of actinomycin D, with or without vincristine. The primary lesion was controlled in all seven patients, but five patients died of distant metastases. One patient was treated by radiation therapy alone (a tumor dose of 6,000 rads in seven weeks) and was free of disease 48 months after treatment. Four patients with primary head and neck lesions were treated by surgical procedures. In one of the four, surgical treatment was combined with actinomycin D. All four patients had primary recurrences; three died of the primary disease, and one was salvaged by three additional surgical procedures and is living and well 61 months after treatment.

Chemotherapy only was used in two patients. One patient with a nasopharyngeal primary lesion received various regimens of chemotherapy and died five months later of primary disease. The other patient receiving chemotherapy only had a primary lesion of the thigh which was excised prior to admission. The lower extremity was perfused with actinomycin D and phenylalanine mustard, and the patient is living and free of disease 84 months after therapy.

Discussion

The data presented demonstrate that rhabdomyosarcomas arising in the head and neck region can present as one of three different clinical entities. First is the nasopharyngeal lesion; because of the lack of and/or vagueness of symptoms, this lesion is usually extensive when first diagnosed. Invasion occurs early: superiorly involving the base of skull, laterally into the paranasal sinuses and orbit, or inferiorly into the oropharynx. Occasionally, the tumor may present in the external ear by extension along the eustachian tube. To be effective the radiation therapy must be radical, *i.e.,* a tumor dose of 6,000 rads in six weeks. One must be prepared to accept the late sequelae of such radical doses of irradiation in children. The addition of chemotherapy, *i.e.,* actinomycin D and vincristine, at the time of radiation therapy, does not permit a lower dose of irradiation (5,000 rads in 5 weeks) to be effective in control of primary lesions in the nasopharynx. Thus, the potential benefit derived from the addition of chemotherapy must be weighed against the increased local reaction which often necessitates a change in time-dose relationship.

The second type of lesion is the orbital primary, which carries an excellent prognosis. Orbital lesions are diagnosed earlier than nasopharyngeal lesions because of their symptomatology. Most are embryonal, *i.e.,* eight of nine in this series. These lesions tend to remain confined, apparently limited by the bony structure of the orbit. Nerves in the orbit may be invaded, but significant extension along the nerves is unusual. Although our series is small, orbital lesions can be controlled by irradiation only or in combination with surgical therapy. Since exenteration is disfiguring, we prefer irradiation alone. A recent report of Cassady and associates from Columbia-Presbyterian Hospital shows that patients with orbital rhabdomyosarcomas are radiocurable (Cassady, Sagerman, and Tretter, 1967). Six of their patients were treated by radiation therapy only, and all have been free of disease from one to four years. These patients received a tumor dose of approximately 5,000 rads in five weeks by means of a single anterior port with 22.5 Mev x-rays. Because of the depth of buildup of the high energy x-rays (22 Mev) the lens received minimal irradiation. Two of six patients developed cataracts, but both have reasonable vision in the affected eye. Thus, the eye can be irradiated without significant sequelae. Concomitant chemotherapy in orbital lesions is not indicated.

The remaining primary lesions in the head and neck region represent the third clinical type. These lesions, diagnosed at various stages, infiltrate along the fascial planes without restraint and metastasize frequently. This diffuse extension accounts for the high recurrence rate after operation (four of four in our series). Because of the general feeling that chemotherapy is beneficial, most of the lesions were managed by a combined modality approach: radiation therapy (a minimum tumor dose of 5,000 rads in five weeks) and chemotherapy (actinomycin D and vincristine). Even though we used generous portals to encompass the disease, some marginal recurrences occurred. Since we do not have a series of patients treated by radiotherapy only, the value of concomitant chemotherapy has not been established.

A total of 14 of 34 patients had distant metastases. Eight patients died of distant metastases only. Six of nine patients dying of primary recurrence also had distant metastases. Of the group of 27 patients with primary head and neck lesions, 12 had distant metastases (44 per cent). Since 41 per cent of all the patients developed distant metastases, the role of systemic chemotherapy must be reconsidered seriously. It has been postulated that systemic chemotherapy given prophylactically may either decrease the incidence of distant metastases or actually eradicate small, unrecognized foci of distant metastases. Twenty-three of the 34 patients received some form of systemic chemotherapy. One additional patient had intra-arterial perfusion only. Ten of the 23 patients (43 per cent) receiving systemic chemotherapy developed distant metastases, compared to four of 11 patients (36 per cent) who did not receive chemotherapy. In addition, all eight patients who died with distant metastases only received a combination of radiation therapy and chemotherapy. Thus, from our data, we conclude that the incidence of distant metastases is not influenced significantly by systemic chemotherapy.

Conclusions

A review of the primary rhabdomyosarcomas in children seen at Anderson Hospital between 1948 and October 1966 has shown the following:

1. Since all primary recurrences and most distant metastases are manifest within one year after treatment, the one-year and five-year survival rates are similar (50 versus 41 per cent).

2. The histology of the lesion and the age of the patient influence the prognosis: embryonal lesions in young patients carry a better prognosis.

3. The prognosis is markedly influenced by the location of the primary lesion, which presents as one of three distinct clinical entities in the head and neck area:

a. Orbital lesions carry a good prognosis. Radiation therapy alone is the treatment of choice. By utilizing special techniques, the eye can be irradiated without significant sequelae. Concomitant chemotherapy is not needed.

b. Nasopharyngeal lesions carry a poor prognosis; radical radiation therapy is the only effective treatment. The benefit of the addition of chemotherapy must be weighed against increased local reactions.

c. The rest of the head and neck lesions can be controlled locally by radiotherapy with the use of wide fields. Surgical resection is of little value (four of four patients had primary recurrences). The value of concomitant chemotherapy has not been established.

4. Systemic chemotherapy does not prevent or eradicate occult foci of distant metastases.

REFERENCES

Cassady, J. R., Sagerman, R. H., and Tretter, P.: Radiation therapy for orbital rhabdomyosarcoma. (In preparation.)

Edland, R. W.: Embryonal rhabdomyosarcoma: Five-year survival of a patient treated by radiation and chemotherapy. *The American Journal of Roentgenology, Radium Therapy and Nuclear Medicine,* 99:400-403, February 1967.

Horn, R. C., Jr., and Enterline, H. T.: Rhabdomyosarcoma: A clinicopathological study and classification of 39 cases. *Cancer,* 11:181-199, January-February 1958.

Suit, H., and Lindberg, R.: Radiation therapy administered under conditions of tourniquet-induced local tissue hypoxia. *The American Journal of Roentgenology, Radium Therapy and Nuclear Medicine,* 102:27-37, January 1968.

Regional Perfusion for Soft Tissue Sarcomas of the Extremities[*]

JOHN S. STEHLIN, JR., M.D.

Department of Surgery, Baylor University College of Medicine,
Houston, Texas

REGIONAL PERFUSION was instituted as a clinical experimental program at The University of Texas M. D. Anderson Hospital and Tumor Institute at Houston in December 1957. In the beginning, little was known about the problems involved. For this reason, the procedure was employed only for locally advanced tumors which required amputation or for disseminated tumors. In our early experience with perfusion for soft tissue sarcomas, we found that about 40 per cent of the tumors, even those which were far advanced, exhibited an impressive response, *i.e.,* they clinically regressed to a pronounced degree. As more was learned about the technique, the local tissue tolerance, the leakage factor, and the drugs and their dosages, the use of perfusion was extended to include lesions with a more favorable prognosis. It seemed that the procedure might be employed as an adjuvant to excision, irradiation, or both, in the treatment of potentially curable patients with soft tissue sarcomas of the extremities. We hoped that the incidence of local recurrence, and perhaps of dissemination, might be reduced by perfusing the affected extremity, preferably before the tumor was excised, and perhaps by combining irradiation with either or both of these procedures. Of paramount importance was the possibility that fewer amputations would be necessary after the use of combined treatment.

The present study was based on the records of 32 patients, six of whom were under 21 years of age and all of whom had histopathologically proved soft tissue sarcoma of an extremity. Omitted from the study was a

---

*This study was supported in part by grant NCI 02620 from The National Cancer Institute, National Institutes of Health, United States Public Health Service.

TABLE 1.—Soft Tissue Sarcomas:
Histopathological Types

Type	Number
Unclassified	4
Rhabdomyosarcoma	3
Synovial sarcoma	9
Liposarcoma	11
Myxosarcoma	1
Fibrosarcoma	2
Leiomyosarcoma	2
Total	32

group of patients with tumors which were originally classified as malignant, though later reviewed by an Anderson Hospital pathologist and classified more appropriately into the category of the nonmalignant variants
such as fibromatosis, nodular fasciitis, proliferative myositis, and chon-
dromatosis. The initial definitive treatment of the 32 patients included
perfusion, with or without irradiation, and with or without simple or
radical local excision of the tumor. Amputation of the involved extremity,
although often indicated according to conventional methods of treatment,
was not employed as initial therapy. None of these patients had clinical
evidence of distant metastasis at the time of perfusion. The response of
all the tumors could be evaluated adequately in terms of both local recurrence and survival. The histopathological types of the tumors in this
study are shown in Table 1. The largest group consisted of the liposarco-
mas and the second largest group, the synovial sarcomas.

Treatment

All of these patients were given perfusion with a combination of phenylalanine mustard and actinomycin-D. Subsequent to perfusion, several
patients received an intra-arterial infusion of methotrexate over a period
of at least one week, together with intramuscular injections of calcium
leucovorin.

The technique of perfusion involves the use of two Sigmamotor pumps
and a small, disposable bubble oxygenator. The oxygenator is primed
with 500 ml. of heparinized blood, and a mixture of 95 per cent oxygen
and 5 per cent carbon dioxide is delivered at a rate of 3 to 5 L. per min-
ute. Immediately before perfusion is started, the patient is given heparin
intravenously, at a dose of 200 units/kg. of body weight. For perfusion
of the entire lower extremity at the level of the trunk, the dose of phe-

nylalanine mustard varies from 1 to 1.5 mg./kg. of body weight; and the dose of actinomycin D varies from 30 to 50 mcg./kg. of body weight. Approximately one half of these two doses is administered at the popliteal level. In perfusion of the entire upper extremity, the dose of phenylalanine mustard does not exceed 75 mg. and that of actinomycin D does not exceed a total of 1 mg.

Preferably, the lower extremity, including the lymph nodes within the femoral triangle, is perfused through the external iliac artery and vein. These vessels are exposed in their extraperitoneal position, and an Esmarch's bandage is applied as a tourniquet around the groin and held in this high position by a Steinmann's pin driven into the crest of the ileum. The upper extremity is perfused either through the highest portion of the brachial artery or through the axillary artery. The brachial artery is exposed through a short longitudinal incision along the medial aspect of the upper arm, whereas the axillary artery is approached through a short infraclavicular muscle-splitting incision.

During the past year, two major alterations in the perfusion technique were made. The first was the addition of hyperthermia with temperatures of perfused blood ranging from 100 to 125 F. (37.7 to 51.6 C.). The temperature of the skin of the extremity was elevated from normal levels to as high as 107 F. (41.6 C.). Second, the duration of the perfusion was increased from 45 minutes to approximately two hours. These additions to the perfusion technique were patterned after the work of Cavaliere *et al.* (1967). Our early results indicate that the two changes have increased materially the effectiveness of perfusion.

Although most soft tissue sarcomas are regarded as radioresistant, 12 patients with these lesions received tumor irradiation with Cobalt[60] in addition to perfusion. The dosage of the majority consisted of an average of 3,000 rads in two treatments; the first treatment was administered on the day before perfusion and the second, immediately after perfusion. Some of these patients were given radiation therapy postoperatively for four to six weeks, in total doses ranging from 5,000 to 6,000 rads. Most of the 12 patients had been treated by some type of excision, varying from incisional biopsy to attempts at local removal of the tumor, before they were referred to us for definitive treatment. For the majority of patients, perfusion, with or without irradiation, was followed in four to six weeks by radical local excision of the remaining tumor or scar at the site of the original excision. For 25 per cent of the patients, however, the location of the primary tumor, *i.e.,* foot, shin, wrist, knee, prevented re-excision without amputation. Thus, this group of patients received only perfusion and irradiation. Some patients with large tumors, for which amputation was clearly indicated, refused amputation; for this reason, they were placed on this clinical experimental program.

The results of this study were evaluated, (1) to determine the degree of control of the local tumor within the extremity and (2) to determine the five-year survival rate. The shortest follow-up was two months and the longest was nine years. Two thirds of the patients underwent surgical therapy at least five years ago.

This combination of therapy without amputation was successful in controlling local disease within the extremity in 22 of the 32 patients (69 per cent (Table 2). No further treatment was required for 18 of the 22. Small local recurrences necessitated additional local excision of the tumors of four of these patients. Early in our experience, amputation of the extremity of one patient was necessary as a result of complications associated with the combination of perfusion and irradiation. The patient received a total of 4,000 rads in two treatments—one, the day of perfusion and the other, the day after. She had a large synovial sarcoma of the sole of the foot. After treatment, the tumor disappeared; because of pain and a draining sinus, however, the foot was amputated. The patient's tumor was such that under normal circumstances, amputation would have been required.

The combination of perfusion, with or without radiation therapy, and with or without local or radical local excision, failed to control the local disease within the extremity in 10 of the 32 patients (31 per cent). The local recurrences in nine of the 10 patients were clinically evident within one year after perfusion. Amputation of the entire extremity or portion of the extremity of six of the 10 patients was necessary to control the local recurrence. In the remaining four, local recurrences appeared coincidentally with disseminated metastases; because of this, and the fact

TABLE 2.—SOFT TISSUE SARCOMAS:
LOCAL CONTROL OF TUMOR

RESULTS	NUMBER OF PATIENTS (Per Cent)
1. Success	22 (69%)
No further treatment	18
Additional excision	3
Amputation (no tumor)	1
2. Failure	10 (31%)
Amputation	6
Co-existing distant metastases	4
TOTAL	32

TABLE 3.—SOFT TISSUE SARCOMAS:
5-YEAR SURVIVAL RATES

LOCAL CONTROL vs. NUMBER OF PATIENTS (Per Cent)	SURVIVAL* PER CENT
1. Success 22 (69%)	84%
2. Failure 10 (31%)	36%
Over-all 32 (100%)	67%
66% of patients operated on more than 5 years ago	

*Calculated by the Berkson-Gage Method.

that no symptoms were associated with the local recurrences, no amputations were performed. The primary tumors of the 10 patients who had local recurrences were located on the foot, shin, knee, groin, and deltoid region. All of these locations lend themselves poorly to wide local excision. The five-year survival rate, as calculated by the Berkson-Gage method, of all 32 patients is 67 per cent. The survival rate of these patients relates to the initial success or failure in controlling the primary tumor. Among those patients whose treatment was successful in controlling the primary tumor (69 per cent), the five-year survival rate was 84 per cent (Table 3). On the contrary, among those whose treatment failed to control the primary tumor within the extremity (31 per cent), the five-year survival rate was 36 per cent. Thus, the initial success or failure to control the local primary tumor by these means serves as an indicator of the survival prospects of the patients.

Discussion

No conclusions can be drawn from this study because the number of patients is too small. Experience with the treatment described, however, leaves us with the distinct impression that combination therapy of this type has merit. The local recurrence rate of 31 per cent in this group of patients, none of whom had a radical amputation as the initial form of definitive therapy, compares favorably with the over-all local recurrence rate of 28 per cent after radical surgical excision at Anderson Hospital. Martin, Butler, and Albores-Saavedra (1965) reported this rate in a paper on soft tissue tumors. They stated that radical treatment often consisted of excision and skin graft or extensive amputations, such as iliosacral disarticulation and interscapulothoracic amputation. They further pointed out that most local recurrences developed in sites where wide radical excisions were impossible, *i.e.,* the head and neck, the trunk, and the retroperitoneal area. This was also true in our series. According to conventional methods, many of the patients in this study undoubtedly would have been treated by radical amputation of the extremity initially. Thus, it appears that the necessity for radical amputation in some of these patients has been obviated.

One major objection to this conservative form of therapy is the possibility that it may adversely affect the patient's prospect of survival. In our opinion, this objection is not justified since our five-year survival rate is 67 per cent, as compared to Martin and co-workers' over-all five-year survival rate of 39.8 per cent. Again, both series comprise only those patients with malignant soft tissue tumors, *i.e.,* those capable of metastasizing. The survival rate for patients receiving the conservative form of therapy appears unusually good. One wonders whether treatment by perfusion and irradiation before excision of the tumors may initiate some immune response within the patients.

If further experience bears out current impression, we believe that the combination of regional chemotherapy, irradiation, and excision will sharply reduce, although not entirely remove, the necessity for amputation of soft tissue sarcomas.

REFERENCES

Cavaliere, R., Ciocatto, E. C., Giovanella, B. C., Heidelberger, C., Johnson, R. O., Margottini, M., Mondove, B., Moricca, G., and Rossi-Fanelli, A.: Selective heat sensitivity of cancer cells: Biochemical and clinical studies. *Cancer,* 20:1351-1381, September 1967.

Martin, R. G., Butler, J. J., and Albores-Saavedra, J.: Soft tissue tumors: Surgical treatment and results. In *Tumors of Bone and Soft Tissue* (The University of Texas M. D. Anderson Hospital and Tumor Institute, Eighth Annual Clinical Conference, 1963). Chicago, Illinois, Year Book Medical Publishers, Inc., 1965, pp. 333-347.

Bone Sarcoma in Children

SIR STANFORD CADE, M.D., D.Sc. (HON.),
F.A.C.S. (HON.)

Formerly of Westminster Hospital, London, England

ALTHOUGH PRIMARY SARCOMA OF BONE is relatively uncommon and annually accounts for only 11 deaths per million (250 deaths per year) in England and Wales, it is of considerable interest to physicians for a number of reasons. The disease affects young age groups almost exclusively; it is of a very high order of malignancy; and only a small percentage of patients can be saved regardless of the method of treatment.

Three main types of bone sarcoma are recognized: (1) osteogenic sarcoma, (2) Ewing's sarcoma, and (3) reticulum cell sarcoma. Each of these types has a characteristic age at onset, natural history, prognosis, and survival rate.

The cardinal manifestations of bone sarcoma are: pain, swelling, and dysfunction, and occasionally fever, anemia, and loss of weight. Pain is the most common presenting symptom. Diagnosis should be, in the first instance, presumptive. Radiological investigation is the next step; roentgenograms are of considerable importance, but do not always provide conclusive information.

Biopsy is essential and can be done by open exploration or by a drill; the latter does not always provide a representative piece of tissue. The potential danger of biopsy resulting in possible dissemination can be lessened by prebiopsy radiotherapy or chemotherapy. For a variety of reasons, my colleagues and I do not rely on frozen-section histology.

Osteogenic Sarcoma

Osteogenic sarcoma is characterized by the presence of osteoid tissue in a pleomorphic stroma composed mainly of spindle cells. It falls chiefly into three histological subgroups: osteoblastic, chondroblastic, and fibroblastic.

225

The roentgenograms vary considerably in appearance; the well-known terms—Codman's triangle, "onion-peel layers," "sun-ray spicules," sclerosis, new-bone formation, and osteolysis—describe the various features, but do not indicate subvarieties.

MANAGEMENT

Since 1931 preoperative radiotherapy followed by elective amputation has been used experimentally at Westminster Hospital, London. This clinical trial justified itself because of the clinical, radiological, and histological evidence that the course of the disease can be influenced by this combined method of treatment.

Preoperative radiotherapy is given by megavoltage x-rays at two to six million electron volts or by means of cobalt units. The dosage goal is 6,000 rads in a period of six weeks. Ablation of the limb is postponed for a time period varying between a few weeks and six or eight months, according to the response to treatment.

It is our practice to ablate the limb by disarticulation at the proximal joint, *i.e.*, at the hip in a patient with a sarcoma of the femur and at the shoulder joint in one with a sarcoma of the humerus. We do not amputate through the affected bone; evidence suggests that the incidence of stump recurrence is thus avoided.

METASTASES

Metastases are almost always blood-borne, although lymph node metastases do occur.

Metastases are found in other bones and in any of the viscera, but the most common site is in the lungs. Pulmonary metastases occur early, mainly within the first eight to 10 months after diagnosis. Pulmonary metastases are, as a rule, multiple and are of the radiological type known as "cannon-ball." Occasionally, a solitary lung metastasis develops; it occurs late, sometimes several years after the onset of the primary tumor. This solitary metastasis may remain stationary for several months or may grow slowly. It can be managed by lobectomy, segmental resection, or pneumonectomy.

Ewing's Sarcoma

Ewing's sarcoma was first described as a definite entity by James Ewing in 1922. It is a round-celled tumor, uniform in structure, with a minimum of stroma. Histologically it resembles metastatic deposits from a primary

TABLE 1.—EWING'S SARCOMA AND METASTASES OF NEURO-
BLASTOMA: A COMPARISON OF FEATURES

	EWING'S SARCOMA	NEUROBLASTOMA
Age	11 to 20 years	Months to 10 years
Metastases	Lungs	Bones (skull)
	Bones	Lymph nodes
	Viscera	Liver
Survival rate	15%	None
Increase in catechol-amine metabolites	None	95%

neuroblastoma. This resemblance produced much controversy and even a denial of the existence of Ewing's sarcoma as a pathological entity. It is, of course, accepted now and, in the opinion of Jaffe (1958), one no longer needs to be on the defensive or feel apologetic about believing in the existence of Ewing's tumor.

The distinguishing features of Ewing's sarcoma and metastases of neuroblastoma are shown in Table 1.

TREATMENT

Treatment of patients with Ewing's sarcoma is primarily by radiotherapy. Because the tumor is of a very high order of radiosensitivity, amputation is not indicated, except electively if local activity persists.

A recent review of Ewing's sarcoma at the Walter Reed General Hospital, Washington, D.C. (Boyer, Bricker, and Perry, 1967), concludes: "Removal of limbs and other portions of the body (in Ewing's sarcoma) has become a needless surgical exercise. Radiation therapy regularly controls the lesion and is the most effective agent for palliation of metastases. Supervoltage radiation is the treatment of choice in all cases."

Reticulum Cell Sarcoma

Recognized as a definite entity by Parker and Jackson in 1939, reticulum cell sarcoma now is believed to be derived from the reticulum cells of the bone marrow. The cells are morphologically identical with those of reticulum cell sarcomas found in the lymph nodes, spleen, and intestinal tract.

Patients with solitary bone lesions of this group have a relatively favorable prognosis. The rate of radiocurability is high. Reticulum cell sarcoma is both radiosensitive and radiocurable. It is an uncommon type of sarcoma, and only 20 patients in this study fall into this group. Four of the 20 who had tumors in the long bones were not subjected to amputation and have remained well, with useful limbs, for periods of eight to 14 years. Of the three patients who underwent amputation, one died five years later from multiple metastases; the other two remain well.

Our experience indicates that primary ablation of a limb in reticulum cell sarcoma of bone is not indicated, and amputation should be reserved for those patients who show tumor reactivation after radiotherapy.

Conclusions

Combined therapy involving radiation and operation has improved the five-year survival rate and spared some patients with early metastatic spread an unnecessary mutilation.

REFERENCES

Boyer, C. W., Jr., Bricker, T. J., Jr., and Perry, R. H.: Ewing's sarcoma: Case against surgery. *Cancer,* 20:1602-1606, October 1967.

Ewing, J.: Review and classification of bone sarcomas. *Archives of Surgery,* 4:485-533, May 1922.

Jaffe, H. L.: *Tumors and tumorous conditions of the bone and joints.* Philadelphia, Pennsylvania, Lea & Febiger, 1958, 629 pp.

Parker, F., Jr., and Jackson, H., Jr.: Primary reticulum cell sarcoma of bone. *Surgery, Gynecology and Obstetrics,* 68:45-53, January 1939.

The Treatment of Retinoblastoma

NORAH DUV. TAPLEY, M.D.

*Department of Radiotherapy, The University of Texas M. D. Anderson Hospital
and Tumor Institute at Houston, Houston, Texas*

IN A HIGH PERCENTAGE OF CASES, retinoblastoma, a rare malignant tumor of the eye in young children, can be controlled and useful vision can be preserved. Successful treatment requires the combined efforts of physicians in several disciplines. After the diagnosis is established by the ophthalmologist, the treatment is selected according to the extent of disease. An ophthalmologist, radiation therapist, surgeon, and pediatrician form the team which shares in the treatment of children with various stages of retinoblastoma. The Retinoblastoma Team at the Institute of Ophthalmology, Columbia-Presbyterian Medical Center, has demonstrated a continually improving control rate in the treatment of 750 patients with unilateral and bilateral retinoblastoma since 1938.

Incidence

The current incidence of retinoblastoma is calculated to be one case per 14,000 births (Francois and Matton-Van Leuven, 1964), a rate indicative of an increase in frequency during the past 20 years. A congenital disease, retinoblastoma occurs as a result of either spontaneous mutation or germinal transmission in families. The appearance of sporadic cases is consistently of much greater frequency than the appearance of familial cases. The genetic mutation for the retinoblastoma characteristic is autosomal dominant, but has a varying rate of penetrance, as evidenced by the inconstant appearance of the disease in offspring of individuals who have had retinoblastoma. The reported incidence of retinoblastoma in these offspring varies from 25 per cent to as high as 75 per cent (Reese, 1954). Retinoblastoma may develop in 4 per cent of siblings in families who have not shown previous evidence of the disease. This fact should prompt careful examination of all siblings of a child with a newly diagnosed retinoblastoma.

Pathology and Routes of Spread

Tumors of the central nervous system and retina are derived from the neuroectoderm. Embryologically, neuroectoderm cells are capable of differentiating into either nerve or supporting tissue. The most undifferentiated tumors of neuroectodermal origin are medulloblastomas and retinoblastomas.

Retinoblastoma develops in the nuclear layers of the retina and is multicentric in origin. Bilateral disease occurs in approximately one third of the patients; and in 84 per cent of diseased eyes, more than one focus of tumor has been described (Reese and Ellsworth, 1964). The tumor may develop in the external nuclear layer and detach the retina lying behind it, or it may originate in the internal layer of the retina and form a mass which projects into the vitreous. The lesion may spread anteriorly with invasion of the ciliary body and the anterior chamber of the globe. The rich blood supply of the choroid permits rapid and extensive growth outside the globe. Optic nerve invasion may occur, and if the eye is to be enucleated, the longest possible segment of the optic nerve should be removed. Invasion of the periglobal soft tissues via the emissary veins of the sclera, which leads to orbital recurrences, may also occur.

In a review of the autopsy reports of 17 patients with retinoblastoma, Merriam (1950) noted that distant metastasis, not intracranial extension, was the cause of death in slightly more than half the patients. Intracranial extension was the only site of tumor dissemination in 47 per cent of those autopsied. In patients showing distant metastases, tumor deposits were found in the bones, viscera, and lymph nodes. In every patient with orbital recurrence, involvement of the cervical lymph nodes was found.

Diagnosis

Retinoblastoma is diagnosed prior to the age of two years in 75 per cent of patients, but has been discovered initially as late as age 52. The few reports of diagnosis at this advanced age describe disease which apparently has undergone spontaneous regression. The lesion, rarely diagnosed before relatively far-advanced disease is present in one or both eyes, is most often first observed by the parents as a peculiar white, or "cat's eye," reflex seen through the pupil of the eye. Strabismus as a result of loss of vision and/or other symptoms of partial blindness may be present before the ocular growth is recognized. Frequently, tumor growth merely is observed and definitive treatment is not instituted until rupture of the globe is imminent or has occurred. Treatment delay permits the continuing destruction of the retina and the possibility of tumor spread beyond the globe. If retinoblastoma is suspected, prompt institution of proper treatment can result in salvation of life and preservation of vision, because the tumor tends to grow initially within the globe.

Irradiation Tolerance of Orbital Tissues

The eye and surrounding structures have a wide range of radiosensitivity and varying degrees of functional impairment result from radiation injury. The skin, bony orbit, and surrounding muscle and connective tissues can tolerate high radiation doses. The resistance of the sclera to irradiation is demonstrated by its tolerance to 30,000 to 40,000 rads delivered with cobalt[60] surface applicator, as described by Stallard in the treatment for malignant melanoma of the choroid (Stallard, 1966). The retina is derived from the neural tube and would be expected to have the same resistance as the central nervous system, which can tolerate doses of 4,500 to 5,000 rads in five weeks. With radiation doses above 6,000 rads, the possibility of damage to the retinal vessels, with hemorrhagic retinitis or hemorrhage into the vitreous as frequent sequelae, increases. If the tumor dose does not exceed 4,500 rads in four weeks, this risk is practically eliminated. The amount of irradiation to the ciliary body which produces obliteration of Schlemm's canal with subsequent glaucoma is not known, but acute glaucoma has occurred in patients with extensive eyelid tumors who received 5,000 rads in six weeks with the entire globe included in the irradiation field.

Chemotherapy

In 1953, Kupfer published the first case report of retinoblastoma treated with the combination of irradiation and nitrogen mustard; he described rapid regression of an extensive lesion. With the recognition that a synergistic or additive effect might result from the concomitant administration of an alkylating agent and irradiation, the Retinoblastoma Team at Columbia-Presbyterian Medical Center initiated a treatment program for patients with bilateral lesions in which they used triethylenemelamine (TEM) and then irradiation of the other eye (Reese, Hyman, Tapley, and Forrest, 1958). A tumor dose much lower than that previously used was considered acceptable because of the added chemotherapy. In patients with limited retinal involvement, a randomized study which used irradiation alone for the control group and irradiation combined with intramuscular TEM for the study group did not demonstrate improved results with the addition of TEM (Tapley, 1964). In this study, the tumor control rate was over 90 per cent for both the experimental and the control patients. A randomized study has not been done in patients with extensive retinal involvement, and the effect of the addition of the chemical on control of advanced disease has not been determined.

Photocoagulation

Destruction of small tumor masses on the surface of the retina and obliteration of nutrient vessels to the tumor are achieved with light coagulation (Höpping and Meyer-Schwickerath, 1964). This technique has been effective in the primary treatment for very small retinal tumors. It is a particularly useful adjuvant treatment for those accessible retinoblastoma lesions which have not responded satisfactorily to irradiation, have regressed slowly, or have shown signs of activity two to six months after the completion of radiotherapy. Selective re-treatment of a limited area of the retina is highly desirable since re-treatment of the entire retina with irradiation usually will produce irreversible damage, and thus necessitate enucleation of the eye.

Staging

The treatment selected for the retinoblastoma patient—either a single modality or several modalities in succession—is based on the extent of disease, stage of involvement of the retina, and influence of stage on prognosis for useful vision (Hyman, Ellsworth, and Reese, 1964). The patient is placed in one of five groups—the very favorable, favorable, doubtful, unfavorable, or very unfavorable—according to the size, location, and number of foci of tumor in the retina (Table 1). The extent of retinal involvement and the location of the tumor are of particular significance with reference to visual acuity because tumors which have destroyed large areas of the retina will produce large defects in the visual field; and if the macula is involved, the area of greatest visual acuity is lost. Lesions located anterior to the equator provide greater possibility for a geographical miss in the attempt to avoid irradiation of the lens than do lesions located posterior to the equator. In the past, the regression or regrowth of these lesions has been difficult to follow adequately but with the advent of the indirect ophthalmoscope, visualization in the region of the ora serrata is easily achieved. Patients in the most unfavorable group for control of disease and preservation of vision are those with tumor involvement of more than half the retina and those with vitreous seeds (small tumor masses floating in the vitreous). The two conditions often occur together.

TABLE 1.—Staging for Method of Treatment and Prognosis

Group 1. Very favorable
    a. Solitary tumor, less than 4 dd. in size, at or behind the equator
    b. Multiple tumors, none over 4 dd. in size, all at or behind the equator

Group 2. Favorable
    a. Solitary lesion, 4-10 dd. in size, at or behind the equator
    b. Multiple tumors, 4-10 dd. in size, behind the equator

Group 3. Doubtful
    a. Any lesion anterior to the equator
    b. Solitary tumors larger than 10 dd. behind the equator

Group 4. Unfavorable
    a. Multiple tumors, some larger than 10 dd.
    b. Any lesion extending anteriorly beyond the ora serrata

Group 5. Very unfavorable
    a. Massive tumors involving over half the retina
    b. Vitreous seeding

All patients seen by the Retinoblastoma Team at Columbia-Presbyterian Medical Center are grouped according to location and extent of tumor in the retina. Treatment is determined by the group in which the patient is placed.

Abbreviation: dd., disc diameter.

Program of Treatment

Unilateral Disease

Approximately two thirds of all retinoblastoma patients have disease limited to one eye, but extensive retinal involvement makes enucleation of the eye necessary. With massive tumor growth, useful vision cannot be preserved even though the lesion is destroyed with irradiation; retinal hemorrhages and detachment are common, and secondary glaucoma may occur. The apparently uninvolved eye must be examined carefully under anesthesia and observation must be continued because tumor may develop in the second eye at a later date.

Very rarely a small tumor may be diagnosed, either in the sibling of a retinoblastoma patient, or because the location of the tumor on the macula has produced early symptoms of visual impairment. These lesions may be managed by the Stallard technique of scleral cobalt[60] applicators or by photocoagulation, but the incidence of new foci of tumor in the untreated retina is high. A sharply defined megavoltage beam through a single lateral field, because of limited side scatter and minimal irradiation to the lens of the involved eye, provides a satisfactory method of treating these rare, unilateral lesions.

BILATERAL DISEASE

For patients in groups 1, 2, and 3 (Table 1), a tumor dose of 3,500 rads in three weeks is given to the posterior retina. Since this treatment is given in nine fractions, it can be equated with a tumor dose of 4,000 rads in three weeks—given in the conventional five times per week fractionation.

Megavoltage irradiation with a well-defined beam is preferred over other types of irradiation because of the limited side scatter and the decreased bone absorption. Optimal external irradiation technique requires accurate localization of the beam to include all of the retina posterior to the equator of the globe. To include as much of the retina as possible, the anterior margin of the beam should pass just posterior to the lens. This provides the best insurance against the appearance of second or multiple tumors after completion of therapy. Stallard, limiting his treatment field to the lesion itself, noted the appearance of multiple islands of retinoblastoma in 26 of 43 patients after initially successful treatment with gamma-ray surface applicators (Stallard, 1955).

A single 4 × 3-cm. temporal port (the 4-cm. diameter oriented in the caudad-cephalad direction) insures that a 0.75-1.0 cm. margin of radiation surrounds the globe, except anteriorly. The anterior edge of the beam is aligned with, or slightly above, the lateral orbital rim and is angled two to three degrees posteriorly to insure passage of the beam posterior to the lens. The height of the cornea above the lateral orbital rim may be determined by an exophthalmometer; this will assist in the location of the anterior margin of the beam with reference to the posterior pole of the lens. Figure 1, a drawing of a coronal section through the orbit, indicates that almost the entire retina will be included in the beam if its anterior margin is positioned slightly above the lateral orbital rim.

If the meticulous efforts made to achieve this positioning are to be effective, maintenance of optimum positioning of the eye with reference to the beam is essential. Satisfactory immobilization can be achieved in most patients. Mild sedation may be used for the particularly apprehensive child at the onset of therapy, but this usually can be discontinued. Repeated anesthesia is undesirable, unnecessary, and of limited value since the eye, unless sutured in position, will wander in the anesthetized patient. If a child is well swaddled and thus provided with a sense of security, if he is not frightened, and if a brightly colored moving object (such as a bird or butterfly mobile) is suspended overhead for gaze fixation, treatment can be accomplished with little, if any, eye movement.

When the lesion is anterior to the equator (group 3), light coagulation

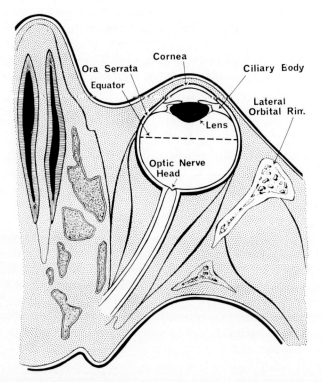

Fig. 1.—Diagram of horizontal section through the eye and adjacent structures. The temporal portal is positioned so that the anterior margin of the irradiation beam extends slightly forward of the equator. This will include most of the retina in the beam and will spare the lens. It is important to remember that lesions located anteriorly, close to the ora serrata, can be irradiated incompletely in the effort to avoid the lens.

is used at the completion of irradiation if significant tumor regression is not evident. When patients in groups 1-3 are examined under anesthesia four to six weeks after completion of radiotherapy, light coagulation is used if tumor shrinkage and calcification are not well defined. In succeeding months, if the tumor still appears active or if regrowth is evident, light coagulation again will be used. For tumor regrowth, re-treatment of the entire retina with external beam irradiation has been demonstrated to produce severe radiation damage and is, therefore, of no value for salvation of vision. If photocoagulation does not control regrowth, enucleation is required.

Group 4 and 5 patients with large tumors and vitreous seeding receive

4,500 rads tumor dose in four weeks (treatment administered in three fractions each week) after intra-arterial TEM. All patients in the unfavorable group and all those with recurrent tumors receive intra-arterial TEM (0.08 to 0.1 mg./kg. of body weight) 24 to 48 hours before initiation of radiation therapy. Photocoagulation is used early in these patients to destroy the tumor's blood supply unless there is significant tumor regression at the conclusion of irradiation.

In those rare patients in whom the disease is limited in both eyes or whose parents refuse to permit enucleation, treatment to both eyes is given with the use of bilateral opposed fields. The tumor dose to the posterior retina is 3,500 rads in three weeks or 4,500 rads in four weeks.

RESIDUAL DISEASE

The term "residual disease" refers to the presence of tumor cells in the cut end of the optic nerve or in the periglobal tissues. The megavoltage photon beam is used to irradiate the orbit via a 3- or 4-cm. anterior field and a 3 × 4-cm. or 4 × 5-cm. lateral field. The tumor dose of 5,000 rads in five weeks is calculated at a depth 2.5 cm. from the eyelid surface and the temporal skin surface. Treatment is administered every day. In patients with residual or recurrent orbital disease, intra-arterial TEM is always given prior to irradiation.

Results of Treatment

The over-all mortality rate in patients with retinoblastoma is approximately 15 per cent; death is a result of intracranial spread or distant metastases, or both. Successful treatment means not only the eradication of tumor for maintenance of life, but also the preservation of useful vision whenever possible. Success or failure figures in the tables of treatment results, therefore, are given in terms of survivors with useful vision. Useful vision encompasses visual acuity from 20/20 to 20/200; the lower limit of visual acuity is included with the recognition that it provides the individual with some visual benefit. The category loss of useful vision (failure) includes patients who are blind because of uncontrolled tumor or irradiation injury to the eye and patients who have died with disease. Loss of vision as a result of irradiation damage is rarely seen with the tumor doses now in use. The failure rate increases significantly in patients with large tumors (group 5) not only because of the increase in deaths caused by disseminated disease, but also because of the total retinal area destroyed by tumor.

TABLE 2.—RESULTS OF TREATMENT IN
PATIENTS WITH BILATERAL RETINO-
BLASTOMA OR ORBITAL DISEASE

GROUP	NO. OF PATIENTS	CONTROL RATE
1	96	77%
2	66	68%
3	67	73%
4	39	49%
5	123	29%
Orbital Disease	74	20%
	465	

This table includes: (1) patients treated prior to
1953 with total tumor doses of over 8,000 r (in some
instances as high as 14,000 r), and (2) patients treated
from 1953 to September 1965, when the dose of external
beam irradiation was decreased sharply and chemotherapy was added selectively.

A total of 750 patients with unilateral and bilateral retinoblastoma
was seen by the Retinoblastoma Team at Columbia-Presbyterian Medical
Center prior to September 1965. The over-all results of treatment of 465
patients (391 with bilateral disease and 74 patients with either residual or
recurrent orbital disease) selected from the total 750 are shown in Table
2. Treatment has included high dose irradiation alone and low dose irradiation with or without adjunctive chemotherapy and photocoagulation.
All patients have been followed for at least 40 months. Almost all recurrences of retinoblastoma are seen within two years after the completion
of treatment. Control of disease has been achieved in approximately three
fourths of the patients in the favorable groups with significantly poorer
results in patients in the less favorable groups.

Table 3 compares the treatment results in 164 patients treated from
1953 to 1960 with those in 175 patients treated from 1958 to 1963. Since
1958, all irradiation has been given with the photon beam of the 22.5
Mev betatron. With megavoltage irradiation, the orbital tissues, bony
orbit, and irradiated skin show minimal late radiation changes. Since
1960, chemotherapy in the form of intra-arterial TEM has been used
only for those patients with extensive involvement of the retina or with
residual or recurrent disease. Improved results are demonstrated in each
group in the more recent series and in the over-all control rate. This
improvement is considered particularly significant in view of the higher
percentage of patients in the doubtful and unfavorable groups treated
from 1958 to 1963 compared with the distribution of patients treated
from 1953 to 1960 and the distribution in the entire series.

TABLE 3.—RESULTS OF TREATMENT IN PATIENTS WITH BILATERAL
RETINOBLASTOMA OR ORBITAL DISEASE (1953–1963)

| | 1953–1960—164 PATIENTS | | 1959–1963—175 PATIENTS | |
GROUP	NO. OF PATIENTS	CONTROL RATE	NO. OF PATIENTS	CONTROL RATE
1	39	85%	20	95%
2	30	60%	29	83%
3	21	52%	33	76%
4	19	68%	17	71%
5	35	23%	59	32%
Orbital Disease	20	20%	17	35%

In 1953, triethylenemelamine (TEM) was added to the treatment for retinoblastoma, and the dose of external beam irradiation was decreased to 3,500 rads in three weeks or 4,500 rads in four weeks. In 1958, the 22.5 Mev photon beam replaced the 250-kilovolt unit for external beam therapy. Since 1960, TEM has been used only for patients staged in groups 4 and 5, for patients with re-growth of retinal tumor, and for those with recurrent or residual orbital disease.

Conclusion

The current treatment for retinoblastoma has developed as a result of the growth characteristics of this tumor and its response to radiation:

(1) It is multicentric in origin, in one or both eyes.

(2) Extension of tumor beyond the cut end of the optic nerve or through the sclera into the periglobal tissue is infrequent.

(3) In patients with bilateral lesions, the rate of tumor growth is usually unequal in both eyes; this condition permits salvation of useful vision in one eye.

(4) Retinoblastoma is sensitive to ionizing radiation and can be controlled with tumor doses of 3,500 rads in three weeks or 4,500 rads in four weeks, with treatment given three times per week.

Acknowledgments

I wish to acknowledge with great appreciation the generosity of the Retinoblastoma Team at Columbia-Presbyterian Medical Center who made available to me the data from the retinoblastoma treatment program. In particular, I wish to thank Drs. Robert Ellsworth, Patricia Tretter, and Algernon B. Reese for sharing their material and current results in the treatment of patients with retinoblastoma.

REFERENCES

Francois, J., and Matton-Van Leuven, M. T.: Recent data on the heredity of retino-blastoma. In Boniuk, M., Ed.: Ocular and Adnexal Tumors. St. Louis, Missouri, The C. V. Mosby Company, 1964, pp. 123-141.

Höpping, W., and Meyer-Schwickerath, G.: Light coagulation treatment in retino-blastoma. In Boniuk, M., Ed.: *Ocular and Adnexal Tumors*. St. Louis, Missouri, The C. V. Mosby Company, 1964, pp. 192-196.

Hyman, G. A., Ellsworth, R. M., and Reese, A. B.: The results of combination therapy of retinoblastoma. A nine year study of 250 cases. *Acta Unio internationalis contra cancrum*, 20:407-410, 1964.

Kupfer, C.: Retinoblastoma treated with intravenous nitrogen mustard. *American Journal of Ophthalmology*, 36:1721-1723, December 1953.

Merriam, G. R., Jr.: Retinoblastoma. Analysis of seventeen autopsies. *Archives of Ophthalmology*, 44:71-108, July 1950.

Reese, A. B.: Frequency of retinoblastoma in the progeny of parents who have survived the disease. *Archives of Ophthalmology*, 52:815-818, December 1954.

Reese, A. B., and Ellsworth, R. M.: Management of retinoblastoma. *Annals of the New York Academy of Sciences*, 114:958-962, April 1964.

Reese, A. B., Hyman, G. A., Tapley, N. duV., and Forrest, A. W.: The treatment of retinoblastoma by x-ray and triethylene melamine. *Archives of Ophthalmology*, 60:897-906, November 1958.

Stallard, H. B.: Multiple islands of retinoblastoma: Incidence rate and time span of appearance. *British Journal of Ophthalmology*, 39:241-243, March 1955.

————: Malignant melanoma of the choroid treated by radioactive applicators. In Fletcher, G. H.: *Textbook of Radiotherapy*. Philadelphia, Pennsylvania, Lea & Febiger, 1966, pp. 307-311.

Tapley, N. duV.: The treatment of bilateral retinoblastoma with radiation and chemotherapy. In Boniuk, M., Ed.: *Ocular and Adnexal Tumors*. St. Louis, Missouri, The C. V. Mosby Company, 1964, pp. 158-170.

The Chemotherapy of Acute Leukemia: A Therapeutic Model for the Management of Childhood Tumors

MYRON KARON, M.D.,*
EMIL J FREIREICH, M.D., AND
GERALD P. BODEY, M.D.

*Department of Developmental Therapeutics, The University of Texas
M. D. Anderson Hospital and Tumor Institute at Houston,
Houston, Texas*

SINCE THE INTRODUCTION OF CHEMOTHERAPY for acute leukemia 20 years ago, the median period of survival of children with this disease has increased four- to sixfold (Frei and Freireich, 1965). In spite of this significant improvement, no treatment program has emerged which can cure the patient with leukemia. Since each new rational approach to the management of a fatal illness is potentially better than those used in the past, the optimal medical care of a child with acute leukemia is synonymous with clinical research. It is the purpose of this paper to review the current status of the treatment of children with leukemia, to stress some of the new therapeutic approaches, and to emphasize the applicability of such approaches to the general problems of childhood neoplasia.

The goal of chemotherapy is the development of curative treatment. Each new therapeutic approach must, therefore, be judged in terms of its effect on the duration of survival. Measurements of this effect are most useful for tumors that quickly cause death. Ironically, as the duration of survival is increased by treatment, the use of this parameter for evaluating new chemotherapeutic agents becomes less practical; longer periods of observation with increased numbers of patients are required. In contrast, a criterion such as per cent reduction of visible tumor might not be ade-

---

*Present address: Division of Hematology, Childrens Hospital of Los Angeles.

quate for measuring cell kill sufficient to affect the duration of survival or it might fail to demonstrate activity in slowly growing tumors (Frei, Karon, Sutow, and Hart, in preparation). Clearly, progress in the field of chemotherapy requires the development of meaningful quantitative criteria of response appropriate to each tumor-host situation. Many of these developments can be illustrated by a consideration of certain aspects of the chemotherapy of acute childhood leukemia.

One of the most important and useful principles in the chemotherapy of acute leukemia is the proposition that an increased period of survival is the result of the duration of remission produced by therapy. The data underlying this assertion are illustrated in Figure 1 (Freireich *et al.,* 1961). The curve with the closed circles represents the months of survival from the beginning of treatment of a group of patients who had one or more complete remission(s). The curve with the triangles represents the months of survival of patients who had no remissions. The curve with the open circles represents the months of survival of patients who achieved remission when the duration of their remission is subtracted.

Fig. 1.—Effect of remission on duration of survival of children with acute leukemia; •, indicates months of survival from beginning of treatment in patients who achieved remission(s); ▲, indicates months of survival for those who did not achieve remission; O, indicates months of survival in patients who achieved remission minus the duration of remission.

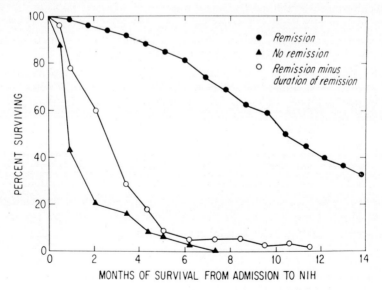

This "corrected" survival curve resembles that of patients who did not achieve remission. The duration of remission, therefore, is responsible for an improved survival rate.

The chemotherapist studying leukemia can investigate new agents in terms of their ability to prolong remission, confident that such measurements are predictive of survival. This fact is especially useful since children with acute leukemia currently have a median survival approaching three years. The relationship between "remission duration" and survival period needs to be investigated directly for other childhood tumors, though *a priori* one would expect the same relationship.

During a complete remission, the child feels perfectly healthy and can return to normal activities. There is an abatement of all symptoms attributable to leukemia. Physical findings disappear and the blood and bone marrow status return to normal. Chemotherapy for leukemia, therefore, produces useful survival time and does not merely extend a period of chronic illness.

Remission Induction

The most useful agents for the induction of remission of acute lymphocytic leukemia are tabulated in Table 1. Prednisone and vincristine sulfate are drugs capable of inducing remission rapidly, almost always within four weeks. Prednisone has no significant bone marrow toxicity. Vincristine is rarely myelosuppressive, but its prolonged use has been associated with peripheral nerve palsies. This complication can largely be avoided by the restriction of drug therapy to a four- to six-week period (Karon *et al.*, 1966).

Methotrexate, 6-mercaptopurine, and Cytoxan produce a lower remission rate. Their use is associated with bone marrow toxicity, as evidenced by leukopenia and thrombocytopenia. All of these agents act on the cell at different metabolic steps. They are not cross resistant in animal tumor systems.

The differences among these drugs in mechanism of action, sites of toxicity, and lack of cross resistance represent a sound basis for combination chemotherapy (Frei and Freireich, 1965). Under such circumstances, each drug can be given in combination at full dosage and maximum effectiveness is assured. Combinations of prednisone with vincristine, 6-mercaptopurine, or methotrexate can yield remission rates of 80 to 90 per cent with no increase in toxicity (Table 2). Combination therapy for remission induction has become the treatment of choice in the untreated

TABLE 1.—REMISSION INDUCTION WITH SINGLE AGENT TREATMENT

AGENT	DOSE (MG./M.²)	RATE (%)	TYPE OF AGENT	TOXICITY	REFERENCE
Prednisone	50/day P.O.	50–60	Adrenal hormone	Cushingoid manifestations	Pearson et al., 1949; Farber et al., 1951; Freireich et al., 1963; Wolff et al., 1967
Vincristine	2/week I.V.	50–60	Plant alkaloid	Paresthesia, paresis, alopecia, constipation	Karon, Freireich, and Frei, 1962; Johnson, Armstrong, Gorman, and Burnett, 1963; Evans, Farber, Brunet, and Mariano, 1963; Karon et al., 1966; Heyn et al., 1966
Methotrexate	3/day P.O.	22	Antimetabolite of folic acid	Bone marrow, mucosal ulcers, G.I.	Farber et al., 1948; Frei et al., 1961
6-Mercaptopurine	90/day P.O.	35	Antimetabolite of hypoxanthine	Bone marrow, G.I.	Burchenal et al., 1953; Frei et al., 1961; Freireich et al., 1963
Cyclophosphamide (Cytoxan)	100/day P.O.	20–30	Alkylating agent	Bone marrow, alopecia, cystitis	Tan et al., 1961; Fernbach, Sutow, Thurman, and Vietti, 1962; Pierce et al., 1966

Abbreviations: M.², square meter of body surface; P.O., orally; I.V., intravenously; G.I., gastrointestinal manifestations.

TABLE 2.—REMISSION INDUCTION WITH COMBINATION TREATMENT

AGENTS	DOSE (MG./M.[2])	RATE (%)	REFERENCE
Pred. + VCR	40/day 2/week	50–60	Frei et al., 1965
Pred. + 6MP	40/day 90/day	80–90	Frei et al., 1965 Fernbach et al., 1966 Krivit et al., 1966
Pred. + MTX	60/day 3.5/day	80	Krivit et al., 1966
Pred. + Cytoxan	60/day 100/day	76	Fernbach et al., 1966

Abbreviations: Pred., prednisone; VCR, vincristine sulfate; 6MP, 6-mercapto-purine; MTX, methotrexate; M.[2], square meter of body surface.

patient with acute lymphocytic leukemia. Combinations of prednisone and/or vincristine with other active new agents are currently under investigation.

These drugs are less effective for the treatment of acute granulocytic leukemia (AGL). Remission rates for children with AGL are usually less than 50 per cent. Promising agents for the treatment of patients with this disease are currently under investigation and include cytosine arabinoside (Nesbit and Hartmann, 1967; Ellison, Carey, and Holland, 1967), 6-mercaptopurine and 6-methyl mercaptopurine riboside in combination (Freireich, Bodey, and Hart, 1967), methylglyoxal-bis-guanylhydrazone (methyl GAG) (Levin, Henderson, Karon, and Freireich, 1965), and daunomycin (Tan et al., 1967).

Remission Maintenance

With such good methods of inducing remissions in patients with acute lymphocytic leukemia, chemotherapists have turned their major attention to ways of prolonging these remissions. The drugs commonly used for remission maintenance are listed in Table 3. Neither vincristine nor prednisone is useful for maintaining remission. 6-Mercaptopurine, Cytoxan, and methotrexate, in contrast, are effective for maintenance. This dichotomy is of practical importance in the evaluation of new agents since the ability of a drug to maintain remission is rarely tested if it cannot induce remissions in late refractory disease. This also draws attention to the fact that there are some drugs, such as vincristine and prednisone, which are uniquely effective for inducing remissions while others are effective primarily for maintaining remissions. Agents which maintain remissions tend to be more myelosuppressive than those which induce remissions.

TABLE 3.—REMISSION DURATION WITH SINGLE AGENT TREATMENT

AGENT(S) USED FOR INDUCTION	AGENT(S) USED FOR MAINTENANCE	NUMBER OF PATIENTS	REMISSION DURATION (WEEKS)	REFERENCE
Pred.	None	126	8–9	Freireich et al., 1963; Wolff et al., 1967
VCR	None	28	6	Karon et al., 1966
Pred.	Pred.		9–12	Hyman et al., 1959
VCR	VCR	36	9	Karon et al., 1966
6MP	6MP	21	21	Frei et al., 1961
Pred.	6MP	28	33	Freireich et al., 1963
Pred. + 6MP	6MP	122	20–24	Fernbach et al., 1966; Saunders, Kauder, and Mauer, 1967
Pred.	Cytoxan	47	12	Hoogstraten, 1962
Cytoxan	Cytoxan		12–15	Fernbach, Sutow, Thurman and Vietti, 1962
Pred. + Cytoxan	Cytoxan	34	20	Fernbach et al., 1966
MTX	MTX daily	17	17	Frei et al., 1961
Pred. + VCR	MTX daily	27	12–13	Selawry, 1965
Pred. + VCR	MTX q. 4 days	22	68	Selawry, 1965

Abbreviations: Pred., prednisone; VCR, vincristine sulfate; 6MP, 6-mercaptopurine; MTX, methotrexate; q., every.

The data in Table 3 illustrate another aspect of chemotherapy: the importance of schedule. For 15 years, daily administration was regarded as the optimum way to use methotrexate. Because of the demonstration in mouse leukemia L1210 that methotrexate was more effective when given on an intermittent schedule (Goldin, Venditti, Humphreys, and Mantel, 1956), a study was undertaken to compare daily with twice weekly use of this agent for remission maintenance (Acute Leukemia Group B, 1965). At equitoxic doses, methotrexate proved to be five times more effective when given intermittently than when given daily. Thus, in the case of methotrexate, extrapolation from studies performed in a mouse model system L1210 to studies performed in man resulted in a significant improvement in antileukemic therapy.

The results of quantitative studies designed to prolong remission duration by the use of combination chemotherapy for maintenance are shown in Table 4. The main rationale for such therapy is to delay the emergence of resistance (Frei et al., 1965). The longest remission duration was achieved with the use of the "total therapy" of Program E. Although Program D did not maintain remissions as long as the intermittent methotrexate schedule (Table 3), it was significantly better than combination therapy with 6-mercaptopurine and methotrexate (Programs A and B)

TABLE 4.—REMISSION DURATION WITH COMBINATION TREATMENT

PROGRAM	AGENT(S) USED FOR INDUCTION	AGENT(S) USED FOR MAINTENANCE	NUMBER OF PATIENTS	REMISSION DURATION (WEEKS)	REFERENCE
A	MTX or 6MP	MTX + 6MP	17	16	Frei et al., 1961
B	Pred. + 6MP	MTX + 6MP	37	27	Frei et al., 1965
C	Pred. + 6MP	6MP alternated with MTX q. mo.	34	26	Frei et al., 1965
D	Pred. + 6MP	6MP alternated with MTX q. 3 mo.	175	44	Zuelzer, 1964
E	Pred. + 6MP	6MP daily VCR, MTX, and Cytoxan q. wk.	28	64	George, Hernandez, Borella, and Pinkle, 1966

Abbreviations: MTX, methotrexate; 6MP, 6-mercaptopurine; Pred., prednisone; q., every.

and alternation between 6-mercaptopurine and methotrexate monthly (Program C). Since daily 6-mercaptopurine maintenance therapy (Table 3) produced periods of remission which were equivalent to those obtained with Programs B and C, and since daily methotrexate maintenance therapy after a prednisone-vincristine induced remission was only minimally effective (Table 3), the simplest explanation for the lack of an additive effect in Programs A, B, or C is that daily methotrexate was ineffective for remission maintenance. The apparent longer duration of remission achieved by oral methotrexate in an earlier program (Table 3) employing methotrexate induction (Frei et al., 1961) might have been a result of the selection of patients who were more sensitive to this agent (Frei and Freireich, 1965). The increased effectiveness of Program D over Program C is probably related to the different lengths of time during which 6-mercaptopurine was used: three months of 6-mercaptopurine is a substantially better consolidation treatment time than is one month. It should be clear from these data that much more needs to be known about the biology of the leukemic tumor in the remission state. One approach to this problem is through the consideration of cell population kinetics.

Recently, Skipper, Schabel, and their collaborators re-explored the chemotherapy of L1210 mouse leukemia in terms of cell kinetics (Schabel and Skipper, 1967). This approach has significantly affected the thinking about the treatment of human beings with leukemia. The most important principles of the mouse model system are as follows: a single viable cancer cell can proliferate to a number lethal to the host which is accurately predicted by the generation time of the tumor cell. The duration of survival of the animal after the inoculation of tumor is related directly to the number of tumor cells in the inoculum. Consequently, the duration of survival after a given antitumor treatment can be used to estimate the number of cells killed by a particular treatment program. The same fraction of the tumor cell population is killed by a given dose of drug regardless of the population's size. The best chance of completely eradicating the tumor, therefore, is to deliver as much chemotherapy as can be tolerated by the host when the tumor is small.

Are there analogies between the L1210 mouse and man? If chemotherapy is discontinued when the patient achieves a complete remission, the disease will reappear rapidly; the average duration of the unmaintained remission is only two to three months. One explanation for recurrence is the regrowth of residual leukemic cells which are present at a concentration lower than that which could be detected by bone marrow examination. Histological examination of patients in hematological remission has demonstrated persistent foci of leukemic cells (Nies et al., 1965; Mathé et al., 1966). One major objective of remission maintenance chemotherapy is the eradication of this residual leukemia.

In November 1962, a study which has received the abbreviated name VAMP (V = vincristine, A = amethopterin, M = 6-mercaptopurine, and P = prednisone) was undertaken in an effort to reach this therapeutic objective (Freireich, Karon, and Frei, 1964). The maximum tolerated dose of vincristine, amethopterin, 6-mercaptopurine, and prednisone in combination was given over a period of 10 days to achieve remission. When the bone marrow had returned to normal, additional 10-day courses of therapy, separated by an interval of 10 to 14 days to allow for recovery from toxicity, were administered. After a median of five consolidation treatments given early in remission, therapy was discontinued. Patients then were followed by monthly examinations of bone marrow and blood. While the VAMP study was in progress, a second study which was called the "BIKE" or bicyclic program was undertaken (Freireich, Karon, Flatow, and Frei, 1965). In this treatment program, remission induction was accomplished with the combination of vincristine and prednisone, and consolidation treatment consisted of a five-day course of the maximum tolerated dose of 6-mercaptopurine and then a single large dose of Cytoxan. This program allowed the use of the full therapeutic dosage of all five compounds of established value in the treatment for acute leukemia. After each drug had been given twice, treatment was discontinued and the patient was observed. The important feature of both of these programs was the effort

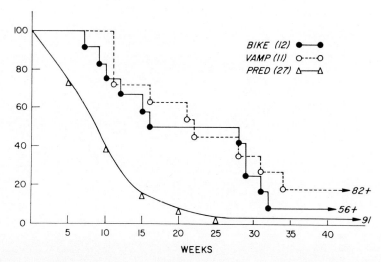

Fig. 2.—The duration of unmaintained remission. The duration of remission is dated from the last day of chemotherapy. The percentage of patients still in remission after discontinuation of therapy is shown. The number of patients in each treatment group is indicated in parentheses. The numbers 82+, 56+, and 91 indicate the number of weeks during which patients still in remission have remained in this condition. Abbreviations: BIKE, bicycle treatment program; VAMP, treatment program using vincristine sulfate, amethopterin, 6-mercaptopurine, and prednisone; PRED, prednisone.

to give maximum tolerated therapy early in remission in an effort to eliminate residual leukemia.

The results of this approach are illustrated in Figure 2 which traces the pattern of recurrence after discontinuation of therapy. The duration of unmaintained remission was similar for both the VAMP and the BIKE programs. Both programs gave unmaintained remissions which were significantly longer than those observed if only prednisone remission induction therapy was given. Twenty of the 23 patients who completed the consolidation treatment after the achievement of complete hematological remission had recurrent leukemia within 35 weeks of the time therapy was stopped. For most of the patients, therefore, eradication of the disease was not accomplished. The longer duration of unmaintained remission, however, does indicate that the amount of residual leukemia was reduced significantly by the consolidation therapy.

By making certain assumptions, one can use the VAMP experience to get an estimation of the reduction in tumor cells by consolidation therapy.

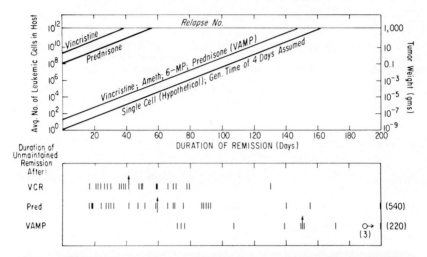

Fig. 3.—Effect of treatment on number of leukemic cells in children with acute lymphocytic leukemia. Abbreviations: Ameth, amethopterin; 6-MP, 6-mercaptopurine; VAMP, combination treatment program using vincristine sulfate, amethopterin, 6-mercaptopurine, and prednisone; Gen., generation; VCR, vincristine sulfate; Pred, prednisone.

These approximations are illustrated in Figure 3. It has been estimated that a child with acute lymphocytic leukemia who weighs 30 kg. has 10^{12} leukemic cells when in full relapse. This is approximately 1 kg., or 3 to 4 per cent of the patient's total body weight. The average doubling time for acute lymphocytic leukemia cells is thought to be approximately four days (Ellison and Murphy, 1964). Simple calculations based on these figures indicate that regrowth from one cell to 10^{12} cells requires 40 doublings. With an average doubling rate of four days, this would take five to six months. The curves for vincristine, prednisone, and VAMP are simply derived by extrapolating backward; a constant generation time is assumed. One should appreciate that this figure for the average doubling time is probably too low since the rate of cell proliferation is not constant and decreases as the tumor size increases (Frindel, Malaise, Alpen, and Tubiana, 1967). This variation is probably the result of an increasing number of cells which leave the proliferative phase and enter a resting stage. Even if these calculations are off by a factor of 10, it should be clear that a reasonable explanation for the prolongation of unmaintained remission after intensive chemotherapy is the reduction of the total body burden of leukemic cells. It can also be seen that the estimated number of residual leukemic cells after remission induction has only been decreased by two to three logarithms.

With the realization that the VAMP program would not eradicate all residual leukemia, another intensive therapy program termed "POMP" (P = prednisone, O = oncovin, M = methotrexate, and P = Purinethol) was undertaken (Henderson, Freireich, Karon, and Rosse, 1966). The POMP program incorporated the two major components of the VAMP and BIKE treatments. There was an induction period during which a five-day combination therapy with prednisone, vincristine, methotrexate, and 6-mercaptopurine was used, followed by nine days of no treatment to observe recovery from any side effects. This program included a median of two remission induction courses followed by four consolidation therapy courses given at two-week intervals. Unlike the two preceding studies, however, a five-day course of combination therapy was given once a month for 12 months before all treatment was discontinued. This monthly maintenance program was given because of the possibility that the failure of the VAMP and BIKE programs might have been caused by a population of cells in the resting phase of the cell cycle which could not be destroyed by the chemotherapy. It was reasoned that such cells might re-enter the proliferative phase during the month when treatment was discontinued and be destroyed by an intensive treatment course.

At this date, it is still too early to make a definitive analysis of the 17 of 32 patients who completed the remission maintenance phase of the POMP program and entered the unmaintained remission phase. Nonetheless, an estimate can be made on the basis of the life-table technique, *i.e.,* even if all the patients currently in remission were to relapse immediately after analysis, the duration of unmaintained remission will be substantially longer than that seen with the VAMP and BIKE treatments. Thus, the present data indicate that the intensive intermittent treatment has further reduced the residual leukemia cell body burden.

One explanation for the prolonged duration of unmaintained remissions is that during the remission induction, consolidation, and maintenance phases, the physician selects out those patients who would have relapsed anyway. This possibility is evaluated in Figure 4. These curves depict the total remission duration achieved with intensive treatment from the onset of remission, including the periods of consolidation and maintenance therapy.

The duration of remission for the VAMP and BIKE programs was similar to that seen in an earlier study with 6-mercaptopurine maintenance chemotherapy after a prednisone-induced remission. The median duration in both programs was approximately 35 weeks. The patterns of

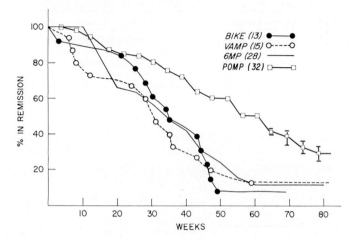

Fig. 4.—The duration of total remission time. The duration of remission is dated from the first complete remission according to bone marrow studies to the recurrence of leukemic cells in the bone marrow aspiration. The number of patients in each treatment group is indicated in parentheses. For the POMP study, the upper and lower limits for the incomplete data are shown after 60 weeks of follow-up. All the other values are completed data. Abbreviations: BIKE, bicycle treatment program; VAMP, combination treatment program using vincristine, amethopterin, 6-mercaptopurine, and prednisone; 6MP, 6-mercaptopurine; POMP, combination treatment program using prednisone, oncovin, methotrexate, and Purinethol.

recurrence after the induction of hematological remission were similar for VAMP and BIKE. Thus, the intensive chemotherapy given during the first 12 to 16 weeks of remission in the BIKE and VAMP programs was as effective as daily oral chemotherapy with 6-mercaptopurine given throughout the remission. Even more important, there was no sudden change in the rate of recurrence after discontinuation of intensive chemotherapy. This indicates that stopping chemotherapy after consolidation does not result in a more rapid rate of disease recurrence than that observed if chemotherapy were continued throughout the duration of remission.

The duration of remission for the POMP program was longer than that for any of the other programs. There was no abrupt change in the pattern of recurrence after 14 months when all treatment was discontinued. These data emphasize the effectiveness of chemotherapy early in remission in prolonging the duration of remission and also demonstrate the value of intermittent treatment for remission maintenance.

It has been shown that profound immune suppression occurs during

TABLE 5.—Duration of Survival

Program		Duration (Months)	Reference
6MP	6MP → MTX		
or →	MTX → 6MP		
MTX	6MP → MTX	10	Frei *et al.*, 1961
VCR	6MP + MTX		
+ →	6MP alt. MTX		
6MP	(q. 4 wk.)	14	Frei *et al.*, 1963
Pred. →	6MP → MTX		
	(q. 6 wk.)	14	Brubaker *et al.*, 1963
Pred.	Pred. Pred.		
+ →	+ → +	17	Saunders, Kauder,
6MP	MTX Cyt.		and Mauer, 1967
Pred.			
+ →	6MP alt. MTX		
6MP	(q. 12 wk.)	17	Zuelzer, 1964
MTX q.i.d.		30–31	Acute leukemia group B, 1965

Abbreviations: 6MP, 6-mercaptopurine; MTX, methotrexate; VCR, vincristine sulfate; alt., alternated with; q., every; Pred., prednisone; Cyt., Cytoxan; q.i.d., four times a day.

intensive combination treatment with POMP. The immunologic responsiveness of the host, however, recovers rapidly within three to five days after the discontinuation of treatment (Hersh, Carbone, and Freireich, 1966). As a result, an intermittent maintenance program permits the patient to have normal host defense for most of the time that he is in remission. This may account, in part, for the enhanced effectiveness of intermittent remission maintenance chemotherapy.

Survival data on the patients who have received BIKE and VAMP chemotherapy are shown in Figure 5 and indicate that 42 per cent of the patients were alive 32 months after treatment began. This figure compares favorably with the duration of survival obtained with other treatment programs (Table 5). The intermittent treatment schedule, therefore, did not compromise the duration of survival. Most patients who relapsed during the period of unmaintained remission had remission reinduced easily and were maintained with the same agents used to produce the original remission.

In our somewhat naive discussion of tumor kinetics, we have made the tacit assumption that anticancer agents have free access to all leukemic cells. There is very good evidence that this is not true, especially when large amounts of tumor are present (Schabel, see pages 61 to 78,

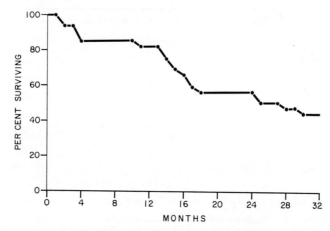

Fig. 5.—Survival time for 32 consecutive patients entered in the VAMP and BIKE studies. The percentage of patients surviving is shown. Survival is dated from the onset of treatment. No patients were excluded from analysis who began treatment programs. Abbreviations: BIKE, bicycle treatment program; VAMP, combination treatment program using vincristine, amethopterin, 6-mercaptopurine, and prednisone.

this volume). In addition to the problems of blood supply, there are pharmacologic barriers which prevent the free access of drugs to the target site (Oliverio and Zubrod, 1965). The central nervous system can harbor leukemic cells which seem immune from direct attack by many agents, presumably because they cannot cross the so-called blood-brain barrier. Other organs, such as the kidneys and glands, offer similar drug-protected havens for the development of leukemic foci.

An intensive chemotherapy program requires an enthusiastic and experienced staff and the availability of measures to combat the complications of bone marrow failure, *i.e.,* hemorrhage and infection. Hemorrhage as a result of thrombocytopenia can now be controlled almost completely by platelet transfusion (Freireich, see pages 125 to 133, this volume). Methods of handling infections which result from granulocytopenia are currently under intensive study (Freireich, Judson, and Levin, 1965). Such measures as strict environmental control in the Life Island or Laminar Air Flow Room (Schwartz and Perry, 1966), aggressive antibiotic treatment, and the development of techniques for granulocyte replacement have shown promise in preliminary studies.

The consideration regarding cell population kinetics and the experience with intensive chemotherapy of childhood acute leukemia can be used to develop useful concepts for a more general approach to childhood cancer. Intensive chemotherapy can drastically reduce the number of tumor cells. Since this reduction is proportional to the initial number of cells, such therapy is most effective when the tumor is small. Consequently, for the responsive tumors, chemotherapy should no longer be relegated to a palliative role late in the course of the illness. The real goal of the multimodal approach to childhood cancer is to achieve maximum tumor reduction by a concerted attack and to continue treatment, especially for the more slowly growing tumors, until maximum therapeutic benefit is achieved. The increased cure rate for patients with Wilms' tumor which has been produced by the use of actinomycin D in combination with operation and radiation (Farber, personal communication) and the impressive results with methotrexate in the management of choriocarcinoma (Hertz *et al.*, 1958) attest to the ability of intensive therapy to cure patients who have cancer at least in selected incidences.

If there are immune mechanisms for tumor control in man, they will be most effective when the tumor size is minimal. Intermittent chemotherapy permits the recovery of host immunological responsiveness. Further progress in chemotherapy for childhood cancer will be made with the discovery of new agents which have unique tumor spectra, different sites of action, and widespread pharmacologic distribution; and with the development of better ways of using currently available agents, ways which are based on considerations of cell population kinetics and host-immune phenomena.

REFERENCES

Acute Leukemia Group B: New treatment schedule with improved survival in childhood leukemia. Intermittent parenteral vs. daily oral administration of methotrexate for maintenance of induced remission. *Journal of the American Medical Association*, 194:75-81, October 4, 1965.

Brubaker, C. A., Wheeler, H. E., Sonley, M. J., Hyman, C. B., Williams, K. O., and Hammond, D.: Cyclic chemotherapy for acute leukemia in children. (Abstract) *Blood, The Journal of Hematology*, 22:820-821, December 1963.

Burchenal, J. H., Murphy, M. L., Ellison, R. R., Sykes, M. P., Tan, T. C., Leone, L. A., Karnofsky, D. A., Craver, L. F., Dargeon, H. W., and Rhoads, C. P.: Clinical evaluation of a new antimetabolite, 6-mercaptopurine, in the treatment of leukemia and allied disease. *Blood, The Journal of Hematology*, 8:965-999, November 1953.

Ellison, R. R., Carey, R. W., and Holland, J. F.: Continuous infusions of arabinosyl cytosine in patients with neoplastic disease. *Clinical Pharmacology and Therapeutics*, 8:800-809, November-December 1967.

Ellison, R. R., and Murphy, M. L.: "Apparent doubling time" of leukemic cells in marrow. (Abstract) *Clinical Research*, 12:284, April 1964.

Evans, A. E., Farber, S., Brunet, S., and Mariano, P. J.: Vincristine in the treatment of acute leukemia in children. *Cancer*, 16:1302-1306, October 1963.

Farber, S.: Personal communication.

Farber, S., Diamond, L. K., Mercer, R. D., Sylvester, R. F., and Wolff, J. A.: Temporary remissions in acute leukemia in children produced by folic acid antagonist, 4-aminopteroyl-glutamic acid (Aminopterin). *New England Journal of Medicine,* 238:787-793, June 3, 1948.

Farber, S., Schwachman, H., Toch, R., Downing, V., Kennedy, B. H., and Hyde, J.: The effect of ACTH in acute leukemia in childhood. (Abstract) In *Proceedings First Clinical ACTH Conference.* Philadelphia, Pennsylvania, The Blakiston Co., 1951, p. 328.

Fernbach, D. J., Griffith, K. M., Haggard, M. E., Holcomb, T. M., Sutow, W. W., Vietti, T. J., and Windmiller, J.: Chemotherapy of acute leukemia in childhood. Comparison of cyclophosphamide and mercaptopurine. *New England Journal of Medicine,* 275:451-456, September 1, 1966.

Fernbach, D. J., Sutow, W. W., Thurman, W. G., and Vietti, T. J.: Clinical evaluation of cyclophosphamide. A new agent for the treatment of children with acute leukemia. *Journal of the American Medical Association,* 182:30-37, October 6, 1962.

Frei, E., III, and Freireich, E. J: Progress and perspectives in the chemotherapy of acute leukemia. In Goldin A., Hawking, F., and Schnitzer, R. J., Eds.: *Advances in Chemotherapy.* New York, New York, Academic Press, Inc., 1965, Vol. 2, pp. 269-298.

Frei, E., Freireich, E. J, Gehan, E., Pinkel, D., Holland, J. F., Selawry, O., Haurani, F., Spurr, C. L., Hayes, D. M., James, G. W., Rothberg, H., Sodee, D. B., Rundles, R. W., Schroeder, L. R., Hoogstraten, B., Wolman, I. J., Traggis, D. G., Cooper, T., Gendel, B. R., Ebaugh, F., and Taylor, R.: Studies of sequential and combination antimetabolite therapy in acute leukemia: 6-Mercaptopurine and methotrexate. *Blood, The Journal of Hematology,* 18: 431-454, October 1961.

Frei, E., III, Karon, M., Levin, R. H., Freireich, E. J, Taylor, R. J., Hananian, J., Selawry, O., Holland, J. F., Hoogstraten, B., Wolman, I. J., Abir, E., Sawitsky, A., Lee, S., Mills, S. D., Burgert, E. O., Jr., Spurr, C. L., Patterson, R. B., Ebaugh, F. G., James, G. W., III, and Moon, J. H.: The effectiveness of combinations of antileukemic agents in inducing and maintaining remission in children with acute leukemia. *Blood, The Journal of Hematology,* 26:642-656, November 1965.

Frei, E., Karon, M., Sutow, W., and Hart, J.: Cell kinetics, criteria for response and chemotherapy of solid tumors. (In preparation.)

Freireich, E. J, Bodey, G. P., Harris, J. E., and Hart, J.: Therapy of acute granulocytic leukemia. *Cancer Research,* 27:2573-2577, December 1967.

Freireich, E. J., Gehan, E., Frei, E., III, Schroeder, L. R., Wolman, I. J., Anbari, R., Burgert, E. O., Mills, S. D., Pinkel, D., Selawry, O. S., Moon, J. H., Gendel, B. R., Spurr, C. L., Storrs, R., Haurani, F., Hoogstraten, B., and Lee, S.: The effect of 6-mercaptopurine on the duration of steroid-induced remissions in acute leukemia: A model for evaluation of other potentially useful therapy. *Blood, The Journal of Hematology,* 21: 699-716, June 1963.

Freireich, E. J, Gehan, E. A., Sulman, D., Boggs, D. R., and Frei, E., III: The effect of chemotherapy on acute leukemia in the human. *Journal of Chronic Diseases,* 14:593-608, December 1961.

Freireich, E. J., Judson, G., and Levin, R. H.: Separation and collection of leukocytes. *Cancer Research,* 25:1516-1520, October 1965.

Freireich, E. J, Karon, M., Flatow, F., and Frei, E., III: Effect of intensive cyclic chemotherapy (BIKE) on remission duration in acute lymphocytic leukemia. (Abstract) *Proceedings of the American Association for Cancer Research,* 6:20, March 1965.

Freireich, E. J, Karon, M., and Frei, E., III: Quadruple combination therapy (VAMP) for acute lymphocytic leukemia of childhood. (Abstract) *Proceedings of the American Association for Cancer Research,* 5:20, March 1964.

Frindel, E., Malaise, E. P., Alpen, E., and Tubiana, M.: Kinetics of cell proliferation of an experimental tumor. *Cancer Research,* 27:1122-1131, June 1967.

George, P., Hernandez, K., Borella, L., and Pinkle, D.: "Total therapy" of acute lymphocytic leukemia in children. (Abstract) *Cancer Research,* 7:23, 1966.

Goldin, A., Venditti, J. M., Humphreys, S. R., and Mantel, N.: Modification of treatment schedules in the management of advanced mouse leukemia with amethopterin. *Journal of the National Cancer Institute,* 17:203-212, August 1956.

Henderson, E. S., Freireich, E. J, Karon, M., and Rosse, W.: High dose combination chemotherapy in acute lymphocytic leukemia of childhood. (Abstract) *Cancer Research,* 7:30, 1966.

Hersh, E. M., Carbone, P. P., and Freireich, E. J: Recovery of immune responsiveness after drug suppression in man. *Journal of Laboratory and Clinical Medicine,* 67:566-572, April 1966.

Hertz, R., Bergenstal, D. M., Lipsett, M. B., Price, E. B., and Hilbish, T. F.: Chemotherapy of choriocarcinoma and related trophoblastic tumors in women. *Journal of the American Medical Association,* 168:845-854, October 18, 1958.

Heyn, R. M., Beatty, E. C., Jr., Hammond, D., Lewis, J., Pierce, M., Murphy, M. L., and Severo, N.: Vincristine in the treatment of acute leukemia in childhood. *Pediatrics* 38:82-91, July 1966.

Hoogstraten, B.: Cyclophosphamide (Cytoxan) in acute leukemia. *Cancer Chemotherapy Reports,* 16:167-171, February 1962.

Johnson, I. S., Armstrong, J. G., Gorman, M., and Burnett, J. P., Jr.: The vinca alkaloids: A new class of oncolytic agents. *Cancer Research,* 23:1390-1427, September 1963.

Karon, M. R., Freireich, E. J., and Frei, E., III: A preliminary report on vincristine sulfate—A new active agent for the treatment of acute leukemia. *Pediatrics,* 30: 791-796, November 1962.

Karon, M., Freireich, E. J., Frei, E., III, Taylor, R., Wolman, I. J., Djerassi, I., Lee, S. L., Sawitsky, A., Hananian, J., Selawry, O., James, D., George, P., Patterson, R. B., Burgert, O., Jr., Haurani, F. I., Oberfield, R. A., Macy, C. T., Hoogstraten, B., and Blom, J.: The role of vincristine in the treatment of childhood acute leukemia. *Clinical Pharmacology and Therapeutics,* 7:332-339, May-June 1966.

Krivit, W., Brubaker, C., Hartmann, J., Murphy, M. L., Pierce, M., and Thatcher, G.: Induction of remission in acute leukemia of childhood by combination of prednisone and either 6-mercaptopurine or methotrexate. *The Journal of Pediatrics,* 68:965-968, June 1966.

Levin, R. H., Henderson, E., Karon, M., and Freireich, E. J: Treatment of acute leukemia with methylglyoxal-bis-guanylhydrazone (methyl GAG). *Clinical Pharmacology and Therapeutics,* 6:31-42, January-February 1965.

Mathé, G., Schwarzenberg, L., Mery, A. M., Catters, A., Schnieder, M., Amiel, J. L., Schlumberger, J. R., Poissor, J., and Wajcner, G.: Extensive histological and cytological survey of patients with acute leukemia in "complete remission." *British Medical Journal,* 1:640-642, March 12, 1966.

Nesbit, J., and Hartmann, J.: Cytosine arabinoside treatment in acute leukemia of childhood. (Abstract) *Cancer Research,* 8:50, 1967.

Nies, B. A., Bodey, G. P., Thomas, L. B., Brecher, G., and Freireich, E. J.: The persistence of extramedullary leukemic infiltrates during bone marrow remission of acute leukemia. *Blood, The Journal of Hematology,* 26:133-141, August 1965.

Oliverio, V. T., and Zubrod, C. G.: Clinical pharmacology of the effective antitumor drugs. *Annual Review of Pharmacology,* 5:335-356, 1965.

Pearson, O. H., Eliel, L. P., Rawson, R. W., Dobrinen, K., and Rhoads, C. P.: Adreno-corticotropic hormone- and cortisone-induced regression of lymphoid tumors in man: A preliminary report. *Cancer,* 2:943-945, November 1949.

Pierce, M., Shore, N., Sitarz, A., Murphy, M. L., Louis, J., and Severo, N.: Cyclophosphamide therapy in acute leukemia of childhood. *Cancer,* 19:1551-1560, November 1966.

Saunders, E. F., Kauder, E., and Mauer, A. M.: Sequential therapy of acute leukemia in childhood. *The Journal of Pediatrics,* 70:632-635, April 1967.

Schabel, F. M., Jr., and Skipper, H. E.: In vivo leukemic cell kinetics and "curability" in experimental systems. In *The Proliferation and Spread of Neoplastic Cells* (The University of Texas M. D. Anderson Hospital and Tumor Institute at Houston, Twenty-first Annual Symposium on Fundamental Cancer Research, 1967). Baltimore, Maryland, The Williams and Wilkins Company, 1968, pp. 379-408.

Schwartz, S. A., and Perry, S.: Patient protection in cancer chemotherapy. *Journal of the American Medical Association,* 197:623-627, August 22, 1966.

Tan, C. T. C., Phoa, J., Lyman, M., Murphy, M. L., Dargeon, H. W., and Burchenal, J. H.: Hematologic remissions in acute leukemia with cyclophosphamide. (Abstract) *Blood, The Journal of Hematology,* 18:808, December 1961.

Tan, C., Tasaka, H., Yu, K. P., Murphy, M. L., and Karnofsky, D. A.: Daunomycin, an antitumor antibiotic, in the treatment of neoplastic disease. *Cancer,* 20:333-353, March 1967.

Wolff, J. A., Brubaker, C. A., Murphy, M. L., Pierce, M. I., and Severo, N.: Prednisone therapy of acute childhood leukemia: Prognosis and duration of response in 330 treated patients. *The Journal of Pediatrics,* 70:626-631, April 1967.

Zuelzer, W. W.: Implications of long-term survival in acute stem cell leukemia of childhood treated with composite cyclic therapy. *Blood, The Journal of Hematology,* 24:477-494, November 1964.

Complications in the Treatment for Acute Leukemia

MARGARET P. SULLIVAN, M.D.

Department of Pediatrics, The University of Texas M. D. Anderson Hospital and Tumor Institute at Houston, Houston, Texas

IMPORTANT COMPLICATIONS occurring during the treatment of children with acute leukemia which are yet to be considered include: (1) autonomous extramedullary disease, (2) hyperuricemia with uric acid nephropathy, and (3) immunosuppression.

Autonomous Extramedullary Leukemic Disease

Effective chemotherapy for the hematologic component of acute leukemia has resulted in the increasing prominence of extramedullary aspects of the disease which are unrelated to the remission status of the marrow. The most frequently recognized sites of autonomous disease during remission are (1) the central nervous system, (2) the kidneys, and (3) the testicles and ovaries. Involvement of the bowel, isolated lymph nodes, liver, and lung is less common.

CENTRAL NERVOUS SYSTEM INFILTRATIONS

Meningeal leukemia now occurs in one fourth to one half of the children with acute leukemia. The affected children exhibit a clinical syndrome characterized by the signs and symptoms of increased intracranial pressure and meningeal irritation. In approximately 40 per cent of the patients, there are additional findings which indicate involvement of other structures such as the dura, hypothalamus, cerebellum, cranial and/or spinal nerves and nerve roots, and peripheral nerves. Examination of the cerebrospinal fluid shows elevation of the pressure and pleocytosis; the protein level may be elevated and the glucose content may be decreased.

259

The cells present are predominantly of the mononuclear type and show the histological characteristics of blast cells.

The gross changes of early involvement are minimal and consist of thickening and opacification of the meninges. Hydrocephalus is found in patients with longstanding or neglected disease. On microscopic study, diffuse infiltrations of the dura, leptomeninges, and perivascular spaces of both the brain and the spinal cord are seen. Infiltrations are noted less commonly in nonneural areas of the brain, which include the area postrema, tuber cinereum, pineal gland, and choroid plexus.

No blood-brain barrier exists for adrenocorticosteroids; and these agents, when administered systemically, will affect meningeal leukemia favorably if resistance has not been established. In critical situations of impending blindness or paralysis, adjuvant steroid therapy may produce more rapid improvement than either irradiation or intrathecal methotrexate alone.

Radiation therapy has proved effective in the control of symptoms of meningeal leukemia and is especially useful when there is involvement of deeper structures of the brain, spinal nerves, or nerve roots. Doses of radiation have varied from 400 to 2,000 r with the duration of symptomatic control ranging from three to four months. A recent study conducted by the Pediatric Division, Southwest Cancer Chemotherapy Study Group showed that a tumor dose of 1,000 rads to both brain and spinal cord was required to normalize the cerebrospinal fluid. Cerebrospinal fluid relapse, however, occurred within one to two months although symptoms often did not reappear for a number of weeks (Sullivan *et al.*, 1966).

The feasibility of intrathecal methotrexate therapy for meningeal leukemia was demonstrated by studies in dogs. A commonly employed dosage schedule calls for injections of methotrexate into the lumbar sac— 0.5 kg./mg. every four to five days—until the cerebrospinal fluid white blood cell count falls to normal levels, *i.e.*, less than 10/mm.[3]. Citrovorum factor can be used simultaneously for protection from systemic toxicity. A good symptomatic response to intrathecal methotrexate therapy may be expected in more than two thirds of the patients. Mean duration of the responses has been reported as two-and-a-half to five months. Remissions, as judged by a normal cerebrospinal fluid white blood cell count, tend to be at least one month shorter than symptomatic responses.

Combination treatment regimens are being devised in an effort to increase the duration of central nervous system remissions. A recently completed Southwest Cancer Chemotherapy Study Group study has shown that the administration of intrathecal methotrexate twice before and once after radiation of the brain and spinal cord produces cerebrospinal fluid remissions in 100 per cent of patients. The mean duration of these remissions, however, does not differ from that obtained with the use of methotrexate alone.

Regardless of the treatment modality employed, meningeal leukemia recurs frequently. At The University of Texas M. D. Anderson Hospital and Tumor Institute at Houston, 43 per cent of the children with acute leukemia have developed recurrences, and multiple recurrences have not been unusual.

Prophylactic intrathecal methotrexate therapy has been given at several centers with the hope of preventing recurrences of meningeal leukemia. A study which uses prophylactic intrathecal methotrexate on a bimonthly basis was initiated recently through our Pediatric Division of the Southwest Cancer Chemotherapy Study Group, but the data are too few at present for any conclusions.

Efforts are now being directed toward the development of compounds which will pass the blood-brain barrier and permit management of meningeal leukemia with systemically administered compounds. Essential physical characteristics of such compounds are (1) nonionization in aqueous solutions at pH 7, and (2) lipid solubility (Rall and Zubrod, 1962). The compound 1,3-bis(2-chloroethyl)-1-nitrosourea (BCNU) possesses these attributes and is effective in controlling L1210 leukemia implanted intraperitoneally or intracerebrally (Rall, Ben, and McCarthy, 1963). Clinical trials with BCNU in patients with meningeal leukemia have shown the compound to be useful in the management of autonomous disease in the central nervous system, but serious toxicity, often of a delayed nature, has restricted its intensive use (Iriarte, Hananian, and Cortner, 1966). Currently we are giving BCNU, 100 mg./square meter, bimonthly to selected children as prophylaxis against recurrent meningeal leukemia.

Interest in meningeal leukemia is high, for it may be that this isolated compartment serves as a reservoir of leukemic cells from which the remainder of the body can be reseeded with leukemic cells which are resistant because of exposure to low drug levels. New techniques for the intrathecal administration of methotrexate are being devised in an effort to achieve the drug concentration and distribution required to effect a meningeal leukemia "cure." At the National Cancer Institute, three children have been treated by ventricular perfusion, with input through a ventricular cannula and output from the lumbar sac. One child died six months after his second perfusion with no evidence of meningeal leukemia (Rubin et al., 1966). A second child, also perfused twice, lived 10 months after perfusion with clear cerebrospinal fluid. The Ommaya reservoir, a device which gives ready access to the ventricular fluid, is now being used to treat children at M. D. Anderson Hospital who have had multiple recurrences of leukemic meningitis. Use of the reservoir has simplified treatment and follow-up monitoring of the ventricular fluid, but the contribution to curability of meningeal leukemia cannot be determined as yet.

RENAL MASSES

Postmortem studies of 124 children who died with acute leukemia at Anderson Hospital have shown some degree of renal enlargement in 60 per cent. Massive enlargement (five to more than 15 times normal weight) occurred in 9 per cent of the children, as shown in Table 1. In most instances, the involvement of the two kidneys was symmetrical with the infiltrates distributed diffusely throughout the cortex and with less intense, or minimal, involvement of the medulla. Associated alterations in renal function are rare in children, but minimal depression of the glomerular filtration rate, renal plasma flow, and maximum tubular excretory capacity for para-aminohippuric acid (Tm_{PAH}) has been noted. Studies at this hospital showed normal renal function tests in five of the children with enlargement of the kidneys. In one child, there was lowering of the Tm_{PAH}; in two children, all three parameters—glomerular infiltration rate, renal plasma flow, and Tm_{PAH}—were reduced greatly.

Decrease in renal size with associated improvement in renal function has been reported after effective systemic chemotherapy and after irradiation of the kidneys. Nine children with leukemic infiltration of the kidneys have been given x-ray therapy for renal masses (Table 2). Only two of these children had significant clinical benefit.

TABLE 1.—KIDNEY WEIGHT AT DEATH OF
124 CHILDREN WITH ACUTE LEUKEMIA

KIDNEY WEIGHT: % OF NORMAL	NUMBER AND % OF PATIENTS
150%	50 (40.3%)
150–249%	46 (37.1%)
250–499%	17 (13.7%)
500–749%	8 (6.5%)
750–999%	1 (0.8%)
1,000–1,499%	1 (0.8%)
1,500%	1 (0.8%)
	124 (100.0%)

TABLE 2.—RESULTS OF RADIATION THERAPY FOR
LEUKEMIC INFILTRATION OF THE KIDNEYS

PATIENT	FIELD		DOSAGE	RESULTS	
	Unilateral	Bilateral		Function	Size
PR		Yes	GD 205 r	Improved	No change
MR	Right		TD 370 r	No change	Decreased
GR	Right		GD 275 r	No change	No change
JC		Yes	GD 450 r	Significant improvement	Decreased
TN		Yes	GD 600 r	Improved	No change
LM		Yes	TD 1,618 rads	Significant improvement	Decreased to normal
LG		Yes	TD 720 rads	No change	No change
RG		Yes	TD 1,000 rads	No change	Decreased
AB		Yes	TD 1,525 rads	No change	Decreased

TESTICULAR INFILTRATIONS

Bilateral, and often asymmetrical, enlargement of the testicles occurs during complete remission as well as during relapse. The postmortem incidence of testicular infiltrations in boys with leukemia at Anderson Hospital is 28 per cent (22/78). No systematic treatment plans have been developed for this complication, which is often left untreated. Orchiectomy, irradiation, and the administration of steroids or Cytoxan have been the treatment modalities most frequently employed. In contrast to the relative frequency of testicular infiltrates, ovarian involvement is uncommon. In both situations, surgical treatment seems preferable to other therapeutic modalities.

The occurrence of autonomous extramedullary disease raises some interesting questions about pathogenesis. The blood-brain barrier may be no more than a contributory factor in the development of meningeal leukemia. The frequency of extramedullary disease in two of the three sites of "immunologic privilege," *i.e.,* central nervous system and testicles, is striking. The occurrence of central nervous system and renal infiltrations in the same patient is noteworthy, but not statistically significant. Among the 13 children with significant enlargement of the kidneys (five to more than 15 times normal weight) at this hospital, nine, or 64 per cent, had central nervous system infiltrates.

Hyperuricemia and Uric Acid Nephropathy

The increased excretion of uric acid in patients with acute leukemia has been recognized for almost a century. During remission induction, hyperuricemia may occur as a direct result of effective therapy. In patients with resistant leukemia, hyperuricemia may reflect overproduction of uric acid, a characteristic of the primary disease which is unrelated to therapy.

Unrelieved serum uric acid levels in excess of 10 mg./100 cc. expose the patient to the risk of uric acid nephropathy. In this clinical situation, uric acid crystals precipitate in the lumina of the distal convoluted tubules and collecting ducts and obstruct urine flow. An internal hydronephrosis results and the condition is manifest clinically by azotemia, electrolyte imbalance, and oliguria.

Hyperuricemia with associated uremia has been reported in a number of leukemic children, but the incidence of uric acid nephropathy is unknown. At Anderson Hospital, two children in the leukemic phase of lymphosarcoma developed fatal uric acid nephropathy during initial remission induction; five other children with resistant leukemia had hyperuricemia with uremia as a part of their terminal illness.

Institutions or physicians involved in the care of large numbers of patients with leukemia and lymphoma should arrange with Burroughs Wellcome and Company for an "on-hand" supply of Zyloprim, allopurinol, (4-hydroxypyrazolo [3,4-d] pyrimidine, HPP) for use in managing hyperuricemia. This remarkable drug, a xanthine oxidase inhibitor, blocks the final metabolic pathways in uric acid formation at the hypoxanthine-xanthine stages.

Allopurinol in doses ranging from 200 to 800 mg. daily for adults and older children and in doses of 50 mg. for children less than eight years of age will relieve hyperuricemia within 24 to 48 hours after therapy is initiated (Yu and Gutman, 1964; DeConti and Calabresi, 1966). During remission induction, allopurinol may be required for five to seven days. Patients with resistant leukemia who have hyperuricemia may be given the drug on a maintenance schedule. Allopurinol toxicity has been minimal; erythematous skin eruptions and transient diarrhea have been reported in single patients.

Patients receiving Purinethol and allopurinol simultaneously should be given Purinethol in one fourth the usual dosage. One of the end products of Purinethol metabolism, 6-thio uric acid, is formed through the action of xanthine oxidase. Inhibition of this enzyme by allopurinol results in significant potentiation of Purinethol activity.

Immunosuppression

All of the five commonly used classes of antileukemic agents inhibit the primary immune response to some extent. There appears to be no interference with pre-existing antibody levels or with an amnestic response. In leukemic children, immunosuppression may be manifest by unusual susceptibility, or response, to viral infections including measles, chickenpox vaccinia, and cytomegalic inclusion disease as well as exotic infections such as *Pneumocystis carinii*. The death of children in complete remission who had cytomegalic inclusion disease led to a longitudinal study of the development of cytomegalovirus complement fixation antibodies* Antibodies were not demonstrable in children with newly diagnosed acute leukemia who were less than 12 years of age (Fig. 1). Within a median time of two months from onset of chemotherapy, 50 per cent of these children showed serologic conversion. Cytomegalovirus inclusion disease infections were asymptomatic in half the serologic converters; the re-

Fig. 1.—Relationship of age to initial cytomegalovirus complement fixation antibody titer and duration of chemotherapy. Abbreviation: CMV CF, cytomegalovirus complement fixation.

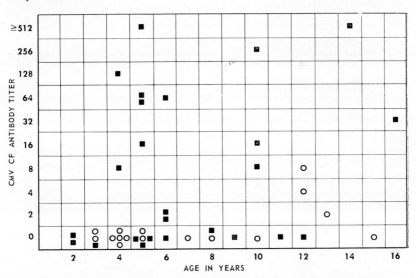

O PATIENT HAVING NO PRIOR THERAPY OR CHEMOTHERAPY FOR ≤ 1 MONTH
■ PATIENT RECEIVING CHEMOTHERAPY MORE THAN 1 MONTH

*Complement fixation antibody titers were determined by Dr. J. B. Hanshaw, Rochester, New York.

mainder had prolonged upper respiratory infections culminating in pneumonitis. Of the children who had received chemotherapy for more than one month at the time of initial testing, approximately 50 per cent showed significant titers. In these children, there was no correlation between clinical events and fourfold titer changes. Information on the extent of immunosuppression in leukemic children and its resultant morbidity and mortality is incomplete. It would appear, however, that intensive treatment programs must employ intermittent schedules to avoid serious risk from immunosuppression.

REFERENCES

DeConti, R. C., and Calabresi, P.: Use of allopurinol for prevention and control of hyperuricemia in patients with neoplastic disease. *New England Journal of Medicine,* 274:481-486, March 3, 1966.

Iriarte, P. V., Hananian, J., and Cortner, J. A.: Central nervous system leukemia and solid tumors of childhood. Treatment with 1,3-bis(2-chloroethyl)-1-nitrosourea (BCNU). *Cancer,* 19:1187-1194, September 1966.

Rall, D. P., Ben, M., and McCarthy, D. M.: 1,3-bis-β-chloroethyl-1-nitrosourea (BCNU). Toxicity and initial clinical trial. (Abstract) *Proceedings of the American Association for Cancer Research,* 4:55, April 1963.

Rall, D. P., and Zubrod, C. G.: Mechanisms of drug absorption and excretion. Passage of drugs in and out of the central nervous system. *Annual Review of Pharmacology,* 2:109-128, 1962.

Rubin, R. C., Ommaya, A. K., Henderson, E. S., Bering, E. A., and Rall, D. P.: Cerebrospinal fluid perfusion for central nervous system neoplasms. *Neurology,* 16:680-692, July 1966.

Sullivan, M. P., Fernbach, D. J., Griffith, K. M., Haddy, T. B., Vietti, T. J., and Watkins, W. L.: Treatment of meningeal leukemia: Intrathecal methotrexate vs. radiation. (Abstract) *Proceedings of the American Association for Cancer Research,* 7:69, April 1966.

Yu, T. F., and Gutman, A. B.: Effect of allopurinol (4-hydroxypyrazole-(3,4-d) pyrimidine) on serum and urinary uric acid in primary and secondary gout. *American Journal of Medicine,* 37:885-898, December 1964.

Hodgkin's Disease in Children

JAMES J. BUTLER, M.D.

*Department of Pathology, The University of Texas M. D. Anderson Hospital
and Tumor Institute at Houston, Houston, Texas*

AMONG THE SEVERAL INVESTIGATORS who have reported studies of Hodgkin's disease in children, there is little agreement on whether the prognosis is better (Kelly, 1965), worse than (Evans and Nyhan, 1964; Pitcock, Bauer, and McGavran, 1959), or the same as (Jackson and Parker, 1944; Jenkin, Peters, and Darte 1967) the prognosis for adults. Only two (Kelly, 1965; Pitcock, Bauer, and McGavran, 1959) of the studies attempt to correlate histological findings and the duration of survival; in one (Kelly, 1965) of the two, the total number of cases of paragranuloma and sarcoma was so small (three of 42) that no conclusions were possible.

The chief purpose of the present study is to determine the distribution of Hodgkin's disease in children, according to the recently proposed histological classification (Lukes *et al.,* 1966), and to relate these findings to the clinical course of the disease and to the duration of survival.

Materials and Methods

All available sections of lymph nodes from children 15 years old or younger whose diagnosis was Hodgkin's disease or malignant lymphoma were reviewed without knowledge of the clinical findings or course of the disease. The children, patients at The University of Texas M. D. Anderson Hospital and Tumor Institute at Houston, were included in the study only if histological material was available.

The presence of typical Reed-Sternberg cells, variants of which are shown in Figure 1, was required for the diagnosis of Hodgkin's disease. The histological classification system followed was that of Lukes and Butler (1966), as modified at the 1965 symposium on Hodgkin's disease held at Rye, New York (Lukes *et al.,* 1966). The four subtypes of Hodgkin's disease, with a brief description of each, are: (1) lymphocytic pre-

267

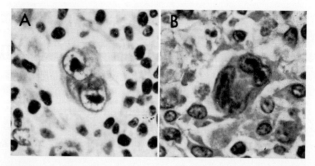

Fig. 1.—Diagnostic Reed-Sternberg cells: A, binucleated variant, and B, lobulated variant (hematoxylin and eosin ×400).

dominance (Fig. 2), in which lymphocytes are prominent, although histiocytes may be the predominant cells. The growth pattern of this type may be nodular or diffuse. (2) nodular sclerosis (Fig. 3), in which bands of collagen of variable thickness partially or completely circumscribe nodules of abnormal lymphoid tissue. The lymphoid tissue exhibits Reed-Sternberg cells, which appear to be situated in lacunae; their nuclei have

Fig. 2 (left).—Lymphocytic predominance type. In this example, lymphocytes predominate; a smaller number of normal histiocytes are also present (hematoxylin and eosin ×150).

Fig. 3 (right).—Nodular sclerosis type. A thick band of collagen surrounds the nodule of abnormal lymphoid tissue (hematoxylin and eosin ×50).

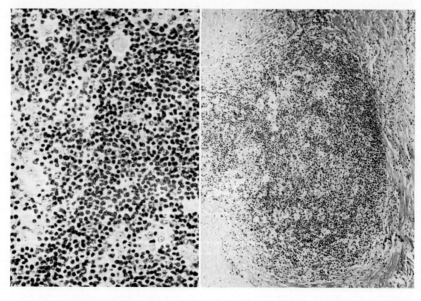

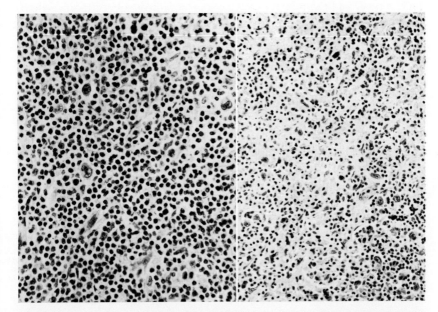

Fig. 4 (left).—Mixed cellularity type. There is a mixture of lymphocytes, normal histiocytes, eosinophils, plasma cells, and abnormal reticulum cells, including two Reed-Sternberg cells in this field, with early fibrous tissue formation (hematoxylin and eosin ×200).

Fig. 5 (right).—Lymphocytic depletion type. The general hypocellularity results primarily from a decrease in lymphocytes. There is an increase in abnormal reticulum cells (hematoxylin and eosin ×100).

prominent lobulations and their nucleoli are frequently smaller than those of Reed-Sternberg cells in other subtypes of Hodgkin's disease. (3) mixed cellularity (Fig. 4), including any of the components found in Hodgkin's disease, *i.e.,* eosinophils, plasma cells, neutrophils, lymphocytes, histiocytes, and Reed-Sternberg cells, as well as a variable degree of fibrosis. This type is an intermediate between the other three types. (4) lymphocytic depletion (Fig. 5), in which the paucity of lymphocytes is accompanied by either a general cellular depletion or a pronounced increase of Reed-Sternberg cells, almost to the exclusion of other cellular types. The variety of this subtype, which exhibits a general cellular depletion has a background of hypocellular connective tissues; this background resembles fibrous tissue, although it contains no collagen and frequently appears to consist of proteinaceous material deposited on the reticular framework of lymph nodes. The number of Reed-Sternberg cells depends on the histological type, and the number of lymphocytes is inversely proportionate to the number of Reed-Sternberg cells.

After the lesions were classified histologically, clinical information was obtained from hospital charts. Clinical staging also was based on the staging agreed upon at the 1965 meeting on Hodgkin's disease at Rye, New York (Rosenberg, 1966). In this scheme, stage I_1 represents disease limited to one anatomic region; stage I_2 is disease limited to two contiguous anatomic regions on the same side of the diaphragm; stage II is disease in more than two anatomic regions or in two noncontiguous regions on the same side of the diaphragm; and stage III is disease on both sides of the diaphragm which does not extend beyond the lymph nodes, the spleen, or Waldeyer's ring. Seven patients had been treated before their admission to this hospital, and thus their disease could not be staged clinically. Ten of the patients had had lower limb lymphangiograms.

With one exception, duration of survival was calculated from the date of biopsy. The one exception, a patient who had a mediastinal mass, was given radiotherapy after a nondiagnostic scalene lymph node biopsy, which was done because of respiratory symptoms. A post-therapy scalene lymph node biopsy was diagnostic of Hodgkin's disease, although subclassification was not possible because of the therapy.

Clinical Findings

The series consisted of 58 children; the oldest was 15 years of age and the youngest was four years. The median age was 10. Of the children, 26 were nine years old or younger; and 32, 11 of whom were girls, were 10 years old or older. Of the 58, 44 (76 per cent) were boys and 14 (24 per cent) were girls. Fifty-four of the children were Caucasians; four, three girls and one boy, were Negroes.

According to the histories, enlarged peripheral lymph nodes were the initial sign of disease in 52 (90 per cent) of the patients. The cervical lymph nodes of 43 patients were enlarged, those of 19 on the right, of 21 on the left, and of three on both sides. The inguinal lymph nodes of six patients were enlarged, those of five on the right and of one on the left. Two patients had enlarged axillary lymph nodes, one on the right side and the other on the left.

Either the children or their parents had observed signs and symptoms of the disease a few days to four years before the diagnosis was established. Fifty-six per cent of the children or their parents had been aware of signs or symptoms for three months or less, and only seven per cent for more than nine months. There was no correlation between the duration of the signs and symptoms and the clinical stage of the disease when the child was first seen at Anderson Hospital. The duration of the signs and symptoms, however, could be correlated with the histological type of the disease and the duration of survival of the patients. Sixty-eight per cent of the children with the nodular sclerosis type of Hodgkin's disease had noted signs and symptoms for three months or less, in contrast to 42 per cent with the mixed cellularity type, 50 per cent with the lymphocytic predominance type, and 33 per cent with the lymphocytic depletion type. The five-year survival rate of patients with signs and symptoms for three months or less was 65 per cent compared to a survival rate of 40 per cent for those with clinical manifestations of the disease for more than three months.

Widening of the mediastinum was the initial finding in six patients. In two patients, an unsuspected mediastinal widening was discovered on routine roentgenography of the chest. Mediastinal widening was found on chest radiograms of four patients—three underwent roentgenographic examination because of a persistent cough and one because of fatigue over a period of several weeks.

When first observed at this hospital, 25 of the 51 untreated patients had mediastinal widening. Seventeen (68 per cent) of the 25 had the nodular sclerosis type, three the mixed cellularity type, and three the lymphocytic depletion type; two had unclassified Hodgkin's disease. The 17 patients with the nodular sclerosis type of disease who had mediastinal involvement constituted 77 per cent of the 22 untreated patients with that type (one patient had been treated previously). Eight of the nine girls with this type had mediastinal tumor. The other girl's disease was confined to the right supraclavicular region.

In eight of 23 patients with the nodular sclerosis type of Hodgkin's disease, the tumor had involved the soft tissues or the lung or had produced compression of the spinal cord. Foci of tumor were observed in the lungs of three patients and were proved histologically in two of the three. In another three patients, histologically proved foci of tumor were present on the anterior chest wall between the infraclavicular fossa and the breast area, without demonstrable underlying intrathoracic disease. One of these patients also had proved tumor in the lung. A mass developed around the knee of still another patient; when excised and examined, it proved to be Hodgkin's disease. Compression of the spinal cord developed in two patients. One was the patient in whom a mass developed around the knee a year earlier. None of the other patients had clinical evidence of tumor in the soft tissues or lungs, or compression of the spinal cord.

The distribution of the disease according to stage is given in Table 1.

TABLE 1.—DISTRIBUTION OF CASES ACCORDING TO
HISTOLOGICAL TYPE AND CLINICAL STAGE*

	No.	%	STAGE I_1	STAGE I_2	STAGE II	STAGE III	NOT STAGED†
Lymphocytic predominance	6	10	6(1)	0	0	0	0
Nodular sclerosis	23	40	5(3)	2(0)	10(1)	5(2)	1(0)
Mixed cellularity	20	34	8(5)	1(0)	3(3)	2(2)	6(4)
Lymphocytic depletions	7	12	2(1)	0	0	5(3)	0
Unclassified	2	4	0	1(0)	0	1(1)	0
TOTAL	58	100	21(10)	4(0)	13(4)	13(8)	7(4)

*The number of children nine years old or younger is in parentheses.
†Treated prior to being seen at this hospital.

All four Negroes had stage III disease when first observed, even though three had had signs or symptoms for two months or less, and the other for less than a year. As indicated in Table 1, the ages of the patients and clinical stages of the disease were related. Patients nine years old or younger constituted the younger age group, and those 10 years old or older constituted the older age group. The proportion of patients with stage I disease was about the same in both groups; stage III disease was more common in the younger group (36 per cent), and stage II disease was more common in the older group (30 per cent). Although only 13 girls were untreated, five had stage III disease; three of the five were Negroes.

Histological Findings

The distribution of patients according to their ages and the histological types of their tumors is given in Table 1. The type of Hodgkin's disease in two patients could not be determined: in one because of the small size of the biopsy specimen; and in another—whose disease was initially confined to the mediastinum—because of prior treatment.

Although the number of patients with the nodular sclerosis type and the number with the mixed cellularity type were almost equal in this series, the age distribution of the two groups differed widely. Of 23 patients with the nodular sclerosis types, 17 were in the older group, as compared to six of the 20 patients with the mixed cellularity type. Eight of the 17 children in the older group with the nodular sclerosis type were girls. Nine of the 14 girls (64 per cent) in the entire series had the nodular sclerosis type.

The only tumors that did not have a definite relationship to the age of

TABLE 2.—HISTOLOGICAL DIAGNOSES

ORIGINAL	NUMBER	REVISED	NUMBER
Lymphocytic lymphoma	3	Lymphocytic predominance	2
		Mixed cellularity	1
Hodgkin's paragranuloma	4	Lymphocytic predominance	2
		Mixed cellularity	1
		Nodular sclerosis	1
Hodgkin's granuloma	39	Lymphocytic predominance	1
		Nodular sclerosis	18
		Mixed cellularity	14
		Lymphocytic depletion	6

the patient were the few of the lymphocytic depletion type. In contrast, five of six patients with the lymphocytic predominance tumors were in the older group.

When Hodgkin's disease extends beyond the lymph nodes, its subclassification as to type is usually not possible. An exception is the nodular sclerosis type involving the lungs, mediastinal connective tissues, and the soft tissues or overlying skin of the chest wall. In these locations, the nodular pattern, with characteristic cells, is generally as prominent as in the lymph nodes.

Table 2 gives the original and revised diagnoses in all patients in whom diagnosis was made before adoption of the present classification, and in whom the subclassification of Hodgkin's disease by the method of Jackson and Parker (1944) was indicated. This table illustrates the relationship between the present classification and that of Jackson and Parker (1944), which is schematically represented in Table 3. The confusion between Hodgkin's disease of the lymphocytic predominance type and lympho-

TABLE 3.—COMPARISON OF HISTOLOGICAL CLASSIFICATION

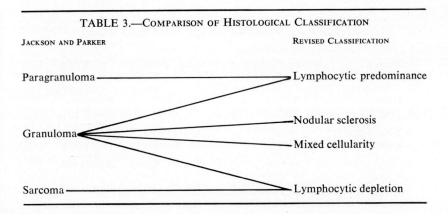

JACKSON AND PARKER — REVISED CLASSIFICATION

Paragranuloma — Lymphocytic predominance

Granuloma — Nodular sclerosis — Mixed cellularity

Sarcoma — Lymphocytic depletion

cytic lymphoma also has been reported by Pitcock, Bauer, and McGavran (1959).

Duration of Survival

The duration of survival according to the clinical stage of the disease is shown in Table 4. As indicated, the survival figures for those who received all of their therapy at Anderson Hospital and those who had previously received treatment elsewhere were essentially identical.

Table 5 gives the duration of survival with respect to the histological types. One of the two boys with the lymphocytic predominance type died of Hodgkin's disease 10.5 years after the diagnosis; the other boy is alive without evidence of the disease 12 years after diagnosis. One of the girls with the nodular sclerosis type who was alive 10 years after diagnosis died of the disease after living an additional 4.5 years. The other three patients are alive and without evidence of disease 10 to 13 years after diagnosis. The one boy with the mixed cellularity type who was living 10 years after diagnosis is still alive an additional 4.5 years without evidence of disease. All of the children with clinical stage II disease who survived three years or longer, and four of the five with clinical stage III disease who survived three years or longer had the nodular sclerosis type.

The relationship between age and duration of survival shown in Table 6 appears to be a real one. It does not seem to be related to the sex of the younger and older groups, since all three girls in the younger group died within less than four years, compared to three of 11 girls in the older group. In addition, the survival rate for boys alone in each of the two age groups is essentially the same as the survival shown in Table 6 for both sexes combined in each age group. The difference in duration of survival is

TABLE 4.—DURATION OF SURVIVAL BY CLINICAL STAGE

	3 YEARS	5 YEARS	10 YEARS
Stage I	18/20(90%)	12/15(80%)	7/9(78%)
Stage I_1	15/17(88%)	10/13(77%)	5/7(71%)
Stage I_2	3/3(100%)	2/2(100%)	2/2(100%)
Stage II	7/12(58%)	3/9(33%)	0/4(0%)
Stage III	5/10(50%)	1/7(14%)	0/2(0%)
Total (staged)	30/42(71%)	16/31(52%)	7/15(47%)
Unstaged*	5/7(71%)	3/6(50%)	1/3(33%)
TOTAL†	35/49(71%)	19/37(51%)	8/18(44%)

*Patients who had been treated previously.
†Nine patients were lost to follow-up or underwent biopsy less than three years ago.

TABLE 5.—Duration of Survival by Histological Features

Histological Type	No. of Patients	Median Yr.	3 Yr.	5 Yr.	10 Yr.
			SURVIVAL PERIOD		
Lymphocytic predominance	4	8.4	4/4(100%)	3/3(100%)	2/2(100%)
Nodular sclerosis	23	4.1	17/21(81%)	9/18(50%)	5/8(63%)
Mixed cellularity	19	3.3	12/17(70%)	6/12(50%)	1/5(20%)
Lymphocytic depletion	6	1.4	1/5(20%)	1/4(25%)	0/3(0%)
Unclassified	2	2.1	1/2(50%)	—	—
All groups	54*	3.9	35/49(71%)	19/37(51%)	8/18(44%)

*Four patients lost to follow-up.

apparently related to the larger number of patients in the younger age group who had clinical stage III disease on their admission to this hospital and the small number in the same age group who had the lymphocytic predominance type of Hodgkin's disease.

As illustrated in Table 6, the duration of survival and the sex of the patients also are related. Only one of the three Negro girls lived more than three years; she had the nodular sclerosis type of the disease and died three years and nine months after the diagnosis. The other two girls were the only females who died less than three years after diagnosis. Since all the girls in the younger group died within four years, it is apparent that only Caucasian girls in the older age group had a long period of survival.

Discussion

A comparison of various series of children with Hodgkin's disease is difficult because of: (1) the relatively small number of patients observed

TABLE 6.—Duration of Survival by Sex and Age

	No. of Patients	3	5	10
		YEARS OF SURVIVAL		
Female	14	12/14(86%)	6/11(55%)	3/4(75%)
Male	35	23/35(66%)	13/26(50%)	5/14(36%)
Total	49*	35/49(71%)	19/37(51%)	8/18(44%)
9 Years old or younger	21	12/21(57%)	4/14(29%)	2/8(25%)
10 Years old or older	28	23/28(82%)	15/23(65%)	6/10(60%)

*Nine patients were lost to follow-up or underwent biopsy less than three years ago.

in any one medical center, (2) the variation in age, sex, and race of the groups, (3) the upper age limit chosen for the studies, and (4) the clinical stage of the disease when the patients are first seen. As an example, among the five studies completed most recently, the age of 13 was chosen as the upper limit in one (Evans and Nyhan, 1964), 14 in two (Bailey, Burgert, and Dahlin, 1961; Kelly, 1965), 15 in one (Jenkin, Peters, and Darte, 1967), and 16 in one (Pitcock, Bauer, and McGavran, 1959). Each of the four difficulties enumerated above must be considered in an evaluation of the results of therapy and a comparison of survival rates. Differences such as those mentioned could explain the varied prognoses for children with Hodgkin's disease which have been observed by different authors. At one extreme is the series reported by Evans and Nyhan (1964) in which the upper age limit was 13 years; only two girls were included, and seven of the 23 patients were Negroes. In addition, although no analysis of clinical stage is reported, the descriptions given by the authors suggest that the majority of patients had generalized disease. It is not surprising that only two of their patients lived more than five years.

At the other extreme is the series reported from England by Kelly (1965) in which the upper age limit of the patients was 14 years. Of his patients, 33 per cent were girls, 64 per cent were 10 years of age or older, and 66 per cent were in clinical stage I of the disease. It was not stated whether any were Negroes. A three-year survival rate of 57 per cent and a five-year survival rate of 48 per cent of the group seem reasonable. With the exception of Kelly's series, the survival rate of children in the Anderson Hospital series is better than rates reported previously (Bailey, Burgert, and Dahlin, 1961; Evans and Nyhan, 1964; Jenkin, Peters, and Darte, 1967; Pitcock, Bauer, and McGavran, 1959). It is also better than the rates for adults reported by Peters and Middlemiss (1958), Lukes and Butler (1966), and Franssila, Kalima, and Voutilainen (1967).

One other feature that influences the duration of survival in patients with Hodgkin's disease and must be taken into account in a comparison of series is the histological subclassification. As mentioned earlier, this has been evaluated in only two of the five series of Hodgkin's disease in children most recently reported. In one of these two (Kelly, 1965), 39 of 42 tumors were classified as the granuloma type. As a result, the prognostic importance of the histological findings could not be determined. In the study of Pitcock, Bauer, and McGavran (1959), nine of 44 tumors were classified as paragranuloma and 35 as granuloma. The over-all five-year survival rate was 18 per cent; this included 56 per cent of the patients with the paragranuloma type and 9 per cent of those with the granuloma type. The authors found no examples of the nodular sclerosis subtype. This is surprising since their series included 11 girls, and the present study —as well as that of Franssila, Kalima, and Voutilainen (1967)—indicates that two thirds of females have this histological type.

In this series, the most meaningful data on prognosis were obtained from patients with the lymphocytic predominance, lymphocytic depletion, and nodular sclerosis types of Hodgkin's disease. All children with the lymphocytic predominance type had clinical stage I disease at initial observation; and all except one, who died 10.5 years after the diagnosis, are still alive four to 12 years after diagnosis. The children with the nodular sclerosis type exhibited all clinical stages of the disease at first observation; because of mediastinal involvement, over half the group was in stages I_2 and II. Patients in clinical stages II and III disease of this type survived longer than patients in these stages who had other types of Hodgkin's disease. Those in clinical stages I_1 and I_2 disease had a median survival period of 10.3 years. The majority of girls (64 per cent) had this histological type of disease; five have been alive from 3.5 to 12 years, one died 14.5 years after diagnosis, and three died 3.5 to four years after diagnosis. Five of the seven patients with the lymphocytic depletion type had clinical stage III disease. No lower limb lymphangiograms were made of the remaining two patients; since both died within six months, it seems reasonable to assume that both had stage III disease which could not be detected by physical examination, radiograms of the chest, or, in one, by an intravenous pyelogram. It was difficult to evaluate the duration of survival of patients with the mixed cellularity type of disease; six in this group had received treatment before admission to this hospital. Those who had clinical stage I_1 and stage I_2 disease at first observation had a median survival period of 4.9 years.

All of the small number of patients with clinical stage I_2 disease, in which tumor was confined to two contiguous areas of lymph nodes on the same side of the diaphragm, are living two to 13 years after diagnosis. It appears that this subgroup should be distinguished from stage II disease, as suggested at the Rye meeting on Hodgkin's disease (Rosenberg, 1966).

In addition to the characteristics already mentioned, the nodular sclerosis type of disease presented certain features which seemed to distinguish it from the other varieties. In the Anderson Hospital series, patients with this type of Hodgkin's disease had mediastinal involvement more often than those with all other types combined. The same observation has been reported by Franssila, Kalima, and Voutilainen (1967) and by

Lukes, Butler, and Hicks (1966). Also, of the peripheral lymph nodes, those of the supraclavicular group were affected most often. Only patients with this type of disease had tumor in the lung, chest wall, and other soft tissues, and compression of the spinal cord. That tumor at these sites did not indicate a disease in its terminal stage is evidenced by the fact that only three of seven patients with such lesions have died. One girl died 2.5 years after tumor appeared in the chest wall and 14 months after the lung became involved. Another girl died 10 months after the development of spinal cord compression and 14.5 years after diagnosis of the disease. A boy died 3.5 years after the lesions spread to the chest wall. Two other patients are alive five and seven years after the disease spread to the lung. The boy who had a mass in the knee region and compression of the spinal cord is alive and being treated with chemotherapy three years after the appearance of the mass and two years after manifestation of the compression. The third girl with tumor in the chest wall received treatment for this condition only one month ago.

Conclusions

1. Hodgkin's disease carries a poor prognosis for children who (1) are nine years old or younger, (2) are Negroes, (3) have clinical stages II and III disease, and (4) have disease which is histologically of the lymphocytic depletion type.

2. Hodgkin's disease carries a good prognosis for children who (1) are 10 years old or older, especially girls, (2) have clinical stages I_1 and I_2 disease, and (3) have disease which is histologically of the lymphocytic predominance type or, to a lesser extent, the nodular sclerosis type.

3. To enable other investigators to compare results, reports on childhood Hodgkin's disease should include a detailed analysis of the age, sex, and race of the patients and the clinical stage and histological type of the disease.

4. Of the present series of children, 71 per cent survived three years; 51 per cent, five years; and 44 per cent, 10 years. These are better survival rates than any previously reported for children or adults.

5. The nodular sclerosis type of Hodgkin's disease is characterized by many distinctive features. It was most common in girls and in older children, and was the type in which the mediastinum or the supraclavicular lymph nodes were most often involved at the patient's initial observation. The patients with clinical stages I_1 and I_2 disease had a median survival of 10.3 years. Those with the nodular sclerosis type in clinical stages II and III disease survived longer than patients in these stages with any

other type. In addition, children with the nodular sclerosis type were the only ones exhibiting involvement of lungs, soft tissues of the chest wall, and an extremity, and spinal cord compression.

REFERENCES

Bailey, R. J., Jr., Burgert, E. O., Jr., and Dahlin, D. C.: Malignant lymphoma in children. *Pediatrics,* 28:985-992, December 1961.

Evans, H. E., and Nyhan, W. L.: Hodgkin's disease in children. *Bulletin of the Johns Hopkins Hospital,* 114:237-248, April 1964.

Franssila, K. O., Kalima, T. V., and Voutilainen, A.: Histologic classification of Hodgkin's disease. *Cancer,* 20:1594-1601, October 1967.

Jackson, H., Jr., and Parker, F., Jr.: Hodgkin's disease; pathology. *New England Journal of Medicine,* 231:35-44, July 13, 1944.

Jenkin, R. D. T., Peters, M. V., and Darte, J. M. M.: Hodgkin's disease in children. *The American Journal of Roentgenology, Radium Therapy and Nuclear Medicine,* 100:222-226, May 1967.

Kelly, F.: Hodgkin's disease in children. *The American Journal of Roentgenology, Radium Therapy and Nuclear Medicine,* 95:48-51, September 1965.

Lukes, R. J., and Butler, J. J.: The pathology and nomenclature of Hodgkin's disease. *Cancer Research,* 26:1063-1083, June 1966.

Lukes, R. J., Butler, J. J., and Hicks, E. B.: Natural history of Hodgkin's disease as related to its pathologic picture. *Cancer,* 19:317-344, March 1966.

Lukes, R. J., Craver, L. F., Hall, T. C., Rappaport, H., and Ruben, P.: Report of the nomenclature committee. *Cancer Research,* 26:1311, June 1966.

Peters, M. V., and Middlemiss, K. C. H.: A study of Hodgkin's diesase treated by irradiation. *The American Journal of Roentgenology, Radium Therapy and Nuclear Medicine,* 79:114-121, January 1958.

Pitcock, J. A., Bauer, W. C., and McGavran, M. H.: Hodgkin's disease in children: A clinicopathological study of 46 cases. *Cancer,* 12:1043-1051, September-October 1959.

Rosenberg, S. A.: Report of the committee on the staging of Hodgkin's disease. *Cancer Research,* 26:1310, June 1966.

African (Burkitt's) Lymphoma: Characteristic Features of Response to Therapy

DENIS P. BURKITT, M.D., F.R.C.S. (ED.) AND
SEBASTIAN K. KYALWAZI, M.B.,
F.R.C.S. (ED.)

External Scientific Staff, Medical Research Council, London, England; and Ministry of Health, Kampala, Uganda

•

IT WAS PARTICULARLY FORTUNATE that cancer chemotherapeutic agents became available to some of us working in East Africa at the time when interest was first focused on the particular form of malignant lymphoma which subsequently became known as the African lymphoma or Burkitt's tumor.

In view of the rapidity with which this tumor causes death, any possibility of alleviation was grasped eagerly, and chemotherapy was tried in spite of a lack of personal experience or knowledge of drug action. This work was grafted onto an already full surgical program and the results of laboratory tests and clinical observations fell far short of what normally would be considered adequate for patients undergoing chemotherapeutic trials. As a result, patients were treated much less energetically than trained therapists would have considered necessary. With few exceptions, they were given much smaller doses than those required to produce toxic manifestations other than moderate marrow depression.

In retrospect, these "deficiencies" in treatment proved a blessing in disguise because they indicated not only that Burkitt's tumor is unusually responsive to chemotherapy, but also that small doses may be at least as good as, and possibly better than, treatment pressed to toxicity.

The observations on characteristics of response to therapy enumerated below are based on the treatment of 138 patients during the past six years.

The purpose of this paper is not to consider details of treatment or to evaluate the relative merits of different drugs, but merely to draw attention to the general features of response to therapy, many of which are believed to be characteristic of this tumor. Detailed descriptions of response to treatment with methotrexate (Oettgen, Burkitt, and Burchenal, 1963; Burkitt, Hutt, and Wright, 1965), cyclophosphamide (Burkitt, Hutt, and Wright, 1965), vincristine sulfate (Burkitt, 1966), nitrogen mustard, melphalan, Myleran, chlorambucil, orthomerphalan, and methylhydrazine (Clifford, 1966) have been published elsewhere.

Initial Response

The response to a wide range of chemotherapeutic agents is immediate and rapid. Significant and often considerable reduction in tumor size frequently is observed within a few days of drug administration. The breakdown of tumor tissue is so rapid that it results in a considerable rise in serum uric acid levels in the blood.

The response is demonstrated more easily in facial than in abdominal tumors; and as will be shown, sustained regression may be expected with superficial rather than deep-seated lesions.

Fig. 1.—A, a boy, age seven years, with tumors in his right mandible, maxilla, and orbit. B, the same patient one month after receiving a single injection of cyclophosphamide in a dose of 40 mg./kg.

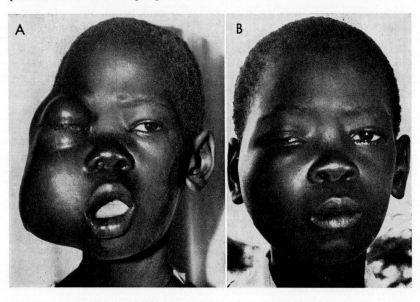

This rapid initial response resembles the remissions obtained in treating patients with acute leukemia, but here the similarity ends.

A boy, age seven years, was admitted with an advanced tumor involving his right maxilla and invading the orbit (Fig. 1A). He received a single injection of cyclophosphamide in a dose of 30 mg./kg. Significant tumor regression was observed within three days (Fig. 1B) and remission was almost complete in less than a month. His home is a long distance from the hospital, and he has not been traced since discharge.

Extent of Remission Related to Tumor Size

The prospect of obtaining total clinical remission appears to be related almost directly to tumor size. Advanced jaw tumors, for example, very rarely subside completely; although abdominal tumors may become nonpalpable, a prediction of complete remission is not possible.

Duration of Remission Related to Initial Response

Unless total clinical remission is obtained initially, recurrence is almost inevitable. The majority of Burkitt's tumors which had total clinical remission do not recur, although additional lesions may grow subsequently at other sites. Usually, only jaw tumors that are superficial and obvious are recognized early. Patients presenting with these lesions are those for whom there is hope of recovery. Unless clinical evidence of tumor has virtually disappeared within two to three weeks, the prospect of cure is slight.

Intracranial Involvement with Orbital and Maxillary Tumors

Patients with maxillary tumors, particularly those which invade the orbit, often develop intracranial complications weeks or months after successful treatment of the jaw lesion. These intracranial lesions, usually manifesting as cranial nerve palsies, have not responded to systemic chemotherapy. It appears, however, that tumor progress can be arrested with intrathecal therapy.

A girl, age four years, was admitted with a tumor of the right maxilla, which had invaded the orbit (Fig. 2A). She received a single injection of cyclophosphamide in a dose of 40 mg./kg. Almost total remission of the maxillary tumor was observed within two weeks, but some residual edema of the eyelids was still present (Fig. 2B).

Six months later, there was no evidence of the original orbital tumor

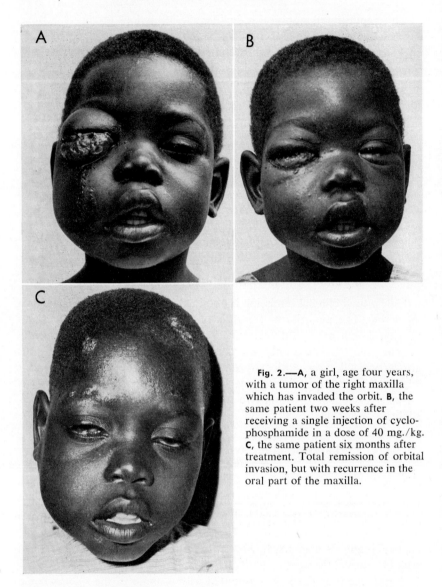

Fig. 2.—A, a girl, age four years, with a tumor of the right maxilla which has invaded the orbit. B, the same patient two weeks after receiving a single injection of cyclophosphamide in a dose of 40 mg./kg. C, the same patient six months after treatment. Total remission of orbital invasion, but with recurrence in the oral part of the maxilla.

(Fig. 2C), but there was evidence of tumor in the right upper alveolus and signs of intracranial involvement. The patient's symptoms subsided after systemic and intrathecal methotrexate; however, she is blind in her right eye, which shows optic atrophy. She remains well seven months after her relapse.

Response to Therapy Related to Tumor Characteristics rather than to Drug Characteristics

The Burkitt tumor has been shown to be sensitive to a wide variety of cytotoxic agents (Clifford, 1966). Although the efficacy of these agents varies, the tumor's sensitivity to chemotherapy in general is more significant than any variation in response to individual drugs.

Long-term Remissions after Short-term Therapy

Perhaps the most remarkable aspect of response to therapy observed in patients with this tumor is the relatively high proportion of long-term survivors (who may be considered potentially cured) after therapeutic doses in amounts far less than those required to produce toxic manifestations.

Fourteen patients are known to be well two to seven years after receiving no more than two doses of a cytotoxic agent (the term dose refers to a single injection or its equivalent given orally, either at once or spread over a few days). This suggests that the action of the chemotherapeutic agent has been supplemented by an immunologic response. Evidence for this has been recorded elsewhere (Burkitt, 1967a; Klein, 1968; Ngu, 1967a, b).

There is some evidence that long-term remissions are more likely if therapy is not pressed to toxicity.

This experience differs from that for patients with acute leukemia who require prolonged maintenance therapy, even to sustain remission.

A girl, age nine years, with a right maxillary tumor received 70 mg. of methotrexate orally over a period of four days. Further treatment was planned, but her mother removed her from the hospital. Six-and-a-half years later she remains well.

Reossification of Diseased Bone and Replacement of Dislodged Teeth

There is probably no other primary bone tumor in which the process of rapid bone destruction can be reversed so quickly with resulting reossification.

Adatia (1968) has drawn attention to a particular feature of this bone regeneration, which is the remarkable way in which partially dislodged teeth tend to become reimbedded in bone and then continue to grow.

A boy, age three years, was admitted with tumors in all four jaw quadrants. Radiograms showed gross bone destruction and partial dislodgment of teeth (Fig. 3A). Eight weeks after treatment with cyclophospha-

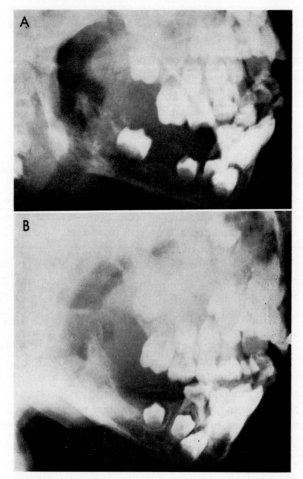

Fig. 3.—A, radiogram showing osteolytic lesion in right mandible of a boy, age three years, who presented with tumors in all four jaw quadrants. B, radiogram of the same patient taken 12 weeks after he received a single injection of cyclophosphamide in a dose of 30 mg./kg.; it shows bone reconstruction and reappearance of lamina dura.

mide, reossification of bone and reimplantation of teeth could be demonstrated radiologically (Fig. 3B).

Spontaneous Remission

Two Ugandan patients who had refused therapy after diagnostic biopsy made complete recoveries. One remains well three years after diagnosis, and the other one and a half years after diagnosis (Burkitt and Kyalwazi, 1967).

Remission Produced by Immune Plasma

In Nigeria (Ngu, 1967a, b) and Uganda (Burkitt, 1967b), temporary tumor remission has been observed after administration of plasma taken from patients who had been treated successfully for jaw tumors.

Subsequent Tumors

A characteristic of patients with Burkitt's lymphoma which is almost unique is the occurrence of "subsequent" tumors in other sites after successful eradication of the original lesion. Subsequent tumors arise in sites characteristically associated with the Burkitt's lymphoma and respond to therapy as readily as the tumor first managed. Moreover, with the exception of cervical lymph node involvement, which has been noted in two patients more than 18 months after successful eradication of a jaw tumor, we have not observed subsequent tumors in any patients in this series who have been symptom-free for over a year. On the grounds of this observation, patients surviving symptom-free for more than a year are considered potential cures.

Prognosis and Lymph Node Involvement

Although peripheral lymph node involvement is characteristically rare, its occurrence has grave prognostic significance. Response to therapy is better than with other forms of lymphoma, but total sustained remission is seldom obtained and any remission is usually temporary. No patient with Burkitt's tumor who had demonstrable involvement of the abdominal lymph nodes has survived; and the frequency of abdominal lymph gland involvement may be one reason for the poor prognosis associated with abdominal tumors. Klein (personal communication) has suggested that lymph node involvement reflects relative immunologic incompetence and that the reverse is also true. His suggestion is consistent with our clinical observations and their relation to prognosis.

A boy, age seven years, was admitted with a right maxillary tumor (Fig. 4A). He was treated with vincristine sulfate and cyclophosphamide and was discharged seven weeks later with incomplete remission (Fig. 4B). Nine months later he developed massive bilateral cervical involvement of lymph nodes and submandibular salivary glands (Fig. 4C) with dyspnea. The right maxillary tumor also recurred and the left maxilla

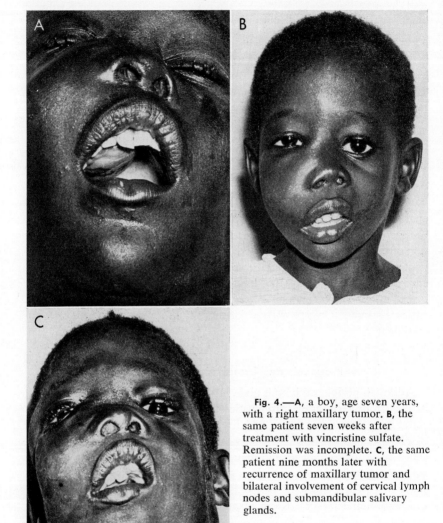

Fig. 4.—A, a boy, age seven years, with a right maxillary tumor. B, the same patient seven weeks after treatment with vincristine sulfate. Remission was incomplete. C, the same patient nine months later with recurrence of maxillary tumor and bilateral involvement of cervical lymph nodes and submandibular salivary glands.

subsequently became involved. Repeated therapy with both cyclophosphamide and vincristine resulted in a response of short duration. Eventually tracheotomy was necessary. The boy was discharged later at the request of his parents.

Prognosis and Central Nervous System Involvement

Central nervous system complications may take the form of paraplegia or intracranial involvement. Wright (1964a) believes the former is a vascular phenomenon caused by compression of nutrient cord vessels by retroperitoneal or paravertebral tumor. After paraplegia, even partial recovery has been observed in only two patients; and in both, therapy had been started for jaw lesions just before the onset of paraplegia. Intracranial tumors usually result from upward extension of a maxillary tumor and are most frequently seen after initially successful treatment for a jaw tumor. They are usually manifest as cranial nerve palsies, and no response to therapy has been observed. This complication may reflect the failure of systematically administered drugs to penetrate the intracranial cavity. An attempt now is being made to attack the tumors early by the administration of intrathecal methotrexate when tumor cells are found in the cerebrospinal fluid.

Effect of Age on Prognosis

Most long-term survivors are patients whose tumors developed at an early age. In large part, this is because the proportion of patients with jaw tumors is highest in young children and decreases in older age groups. It already has been noted that the prognosis is best in patients presenting with jaw lesions in early stages of development.

Discussion

Many aspects of the African lymphoma have been described as characteristic.

From an epidemiological standpoint, the endemic distribution is peculiar and follows a climatic pattern; the bizarre manifestations of the lesion attracted the first clinical attention. The gross pathology reflects the characteristic clinical pattern of tumor distribution.

Wright (1964b, 1965) has shown that the appearance of this lymphoma is histologically and cytologically distinct from those of other types.

Epstein and Achong (1965) and Epstein *et al.* (1966) have described the characteristic appearance of the cells under the electron microscope, and Pulvertaft (1965) has demonstrated their behavior in tissue culture.

A review of therapy response suggests that in this field, too, the tumor's behavior is different from that of other neoplasms.

From whatever angle the Burkitt's tumor is approached, it seems to declare itself as a distinct entity with a peculiar pattern of behavior. Examination of each aspect should produce a distinctive contribution to the knowledge now accumulated and thus forward progress toward the ultimate goal of understanding the cause and, hopefully, attaining prevention or cure.

Long-term remissions after minimal therapy suggest an immunologic mechanism. This in turn may suggest viral infection as the means whereby the cell membrane may be altered in nature and thus regarded by the host as foreign.

Summary

The characteristic features of response to chemotherapy observed in the African (Burkitt's) lymphoma have been described. It is suggested that the distinctive behavior supports clinical, pathological, and other evidence that this tumor is a separate entity distinguishable from other forms of malignant lymphoma.

Acknowledgments

We are grateful to Lederle Laboratories, Asta-Werke, and Eli Lilly and Company, who generously provided the methotrexate, cyclophosphamide, and vincristine used in the treatment of the majority of these patients.

For assistance in follow-up, we are grateful to the Kampala Cancer Registry.

Figures 1 and 2 have been provided by the Department of Medical Illustration, Makerere College Medical School, and Figure 3 by Kodak, London.

This work was made possible by financial assistance from the British Empire Cancer Campaign, the Medical Research Council, and the Ministry of Overseas Development.

We wish to thank Miss Christine Shenton for her general and secretarial assistance.

REFERENCES

Adatia, A. K.: Dental tissue and Burkitt's tumor. *Oral Surgery, Oral Medicine, and Oral Pathology*, 25:221-234, February 1968.

Burkitt, D.: Long-term remissions following one and two-dose chemotherapy for African lymphoma. *Cancer*, 20:756-759, May, 1967a.

————: Clinical evidence suggesting the development of an immunological response against African lymphoma. In Burchenal, J. H., and Burkitt, D. P., Eds.: *Treatment of Burkitt's Tumor* (UICC Monograph Series, Vol. 8). Berlin and Heidelberg, Germany, and New York, New York, Springer-Verlag, 1967b, pp. 197-203.

————: The African lymphoma. Observations on response to vincristine sulphate therapy. *Cancer*, 19:1131-1137, August 1966.

Burkitt, D. P., Hutt, M. S. R., and Wright, D. H.: The African lymphoma. Preliminary observations on response to therapy. *Cancer*, 18:399-410, April 1965.

Burkitt, D. P., and Kyalwazi, S. K.: Spontaneous remission of the African lymphoma. *The British Journal of Cancer*, 21:14-16, March 1967.

Clifford, P.: Further studies on the treatment of Burkitt's lymphoma. *East African Medical Journal*, 43:179-199, June 1966.

Epstein, M. A., and Achong, B. G.: Fine structural organization of human lymphoblasts of a tissue culture strain (EB1) from Burkitt's lymphoma. *Journal of the National Cancer Institute*, 34:241-254, February 1965.

Epstein, M. A., Achong, B. G., Barr, Y. M., Zajac, B., Henle, G., and Henle, W.: Morphological and virological investigations on cultured Burkitt tumor lymphoblasts (Strain Raji). *Journal of the National Cancer Institute*, 37:547-559, October 1966.

Klein, G.: Personal communication.

Klein, G., Clifford, P., Klein, E., and Stjernswärd, J.: Search for tumour specific immune reactions in Burkitt lymphoma patients by the membrane immunofluorescence reaction. In Burchenal, J. H., and Burkitt, D. P., Eds.: *Treatment of Burkitt's Tumour* (UICC Monograph Series, Vol. 8). Berlin and Heidelberg, Germany, and New York, New York, Springer-Verlag, 1967, pp. 209-232.

Klein, G., Klein, E., and Clifford, P.: Host defenses in leukemia and Burkitt's tumor. *Cancer*, 21:587-594, April 1968.

Ngu, V. A.: Clinical evidence of host defenses in Burkitt's tumor. In Burchenal, J. H., and Burkitt, D. P., Eds.: *Treatment of Burkitt's Tumour* (UICC Monograph Series, Vol. 8). Berlin and Heidelberg, Germany, and New York, New York, Springer-Verlag, 1967a, pp. 204-208.

————: Host defences to Burkitt tumour. *British Medical Journal*, 1:345-347, February 1967b.

Oettgen, H. F., Burkitt, D., and Burchenal, J. H.: Malignant lymphoma involving the jaw in African children: Treatment with methotrexate. *Cancer*, 16:616-623, May 1963.

Pulvertaft, R. J. V.: A study of malignant tumours in Nigeria by short-term tissue culture. *Journal of Clinical Pathology*, 18:261-273, May 1965.

Wright, D. H.: Burkitt's tumour. A post mortem study of 50 cases. *British Journal of Surgery*, 51:245-251, April 1964a.

————: Cytology and histochemistry of the malignant lymphomas seen in Uganda. In Roulet, F. C., Ed.: *The Lymphoreticular Tumours in Africa* (UICC Monograph Series, Vol. 3). Basel, Switzerland, S. Karger, 1964b, pp. 291-304.

————: Lymphoma in Africa. *Israel Journal of Medical Sciences*, 1:177-179, March 1965.

Present Status of Research on Burkitt's Tumor*

JOSEPH H. BURCHENAL, M.D., AND

NORMA WOLLNER, M.D.

Sloan-Kettering Institute for Cancer Research, Memorial Hospital for Cancer and Allied Diseases, and Cornell University Medical College, New York City, New York

BURKITT'S TUMOR is the most common form of cancer in African children; indeed, in some areas it accounts for 70 per cent of all childhood tumors (Edington and Maclean, 1964). The peculiar geographical distribution of the lesion, its possible viral etiology, and its remarkable response to chemotherapy have excited the interest of investigators in many parts of the world. A conference on Burkitt's tumor and acute leukemia was held under the auspices of the American Cancer Society and the National Cancer Institute at Rye, New York, in May 1967, and a large portion of the new data mentioned in this review comes from that conference (ACS-NCI Conference on Acute Leukemia and Burkitt's Tumor [Rye 1967], 1967).

Burkitt's tumor apparently has existed in Africa for an indefinite period of time, as ancient statuettes showing children with tumors of the jaw suggest (Ngu, 1967). Sketches of a child with a jaw tumor were found in the journal of Sir Albert Cook, a medical missionary in the Ugandan area in the early 1900's. The disease, which Burkitt recognized as a multicentric lymphoma in 1958 (Burkitt, 1958), is endemic in certain areas of Africa and New Guinea (Ten Seldam, Cooke, and Atkinson, 1966). However, it also occurs sporadically in many other parts of the world, such as Brazil (Luisi, de Padua Bertelli, Machado, and Ache de Freitas, 1965), Colombia (Beltran, Baez, and Correa, 1966), India (Desai, personal communication), England (Wright, personal communication), and

---

*This study was supported in part by National Cancer Institute grants CA-08748 and CA-05826 and by American Cancer Society grant T-45.

the United States (O'Conor, Rappaport, and Smith, 1965; Dorfman, 1965). In Africa, Burkitt's tumor is characterized by a definite anatomic distribution, *i.e.,* a high incidence of jaw tumors in young children and involvement of abdominal lymph nodes, ovaries, kidneys, adrenal glands, and breasts. Characteristically, the peripheral nodes, lungs, and spleen are spared (O'Conor and Davies, 1960; Burkitt, 1967b). It is of interest that in areas of Africa where the tumor is common, the average patient is younger and the percentage of jaw tumors is higher. In areas where the tumor is less common, the average patient is older, the percentage of jaw tumors is considerably less, and there is a great increase in abdominal tumors (Burkitt, 1967b).

O'Conor and Davies (1960) classified Burkitt's tumor histologically as a malignant lymphoma of the poorly differentiated lymphocytic type. They noted the presence of large foamy histiocytes between the lymphoid cells, giving the tumor a "starry-sky" pattern. Wright (1967) described the cytological imprint preparations stained with May-Grünwald-Giemsa or Wright's stain as follows: "The lymphoid cells are 20–30 μ in diameter: although they vary in size they do not vary in apparent maturity. Their nuclei are round, oval, or deeply cleft and have a stippled chromatin pattern. Nuclei number two to five but are not conspicuous in Giemsa-stained preparations. The cytoplasm forms a well-defined rim around the nucleus. It is intensely basophilic, apart from a pale staining area adjacent to the nuclear indentation. Cytoplasmic vacuoles are always present in at least some of the cells but their number varies widely. Detached fragments of vacuolated cytoplasm can usually be seen between the lymphoid cells." Pulvertaft (1967) stated that the granules which stain with osmic acid and lack of cell motility are the main diagnostic criteria under phase microscopy.

The geographical distribution of this tumor has excited considerable interest. The careful studies of Burkitt (1967a, c) have shown that the lesion is endemic in most of the areas of equatorial Africa under 5,000 ft. of altitude, except those in which rainfall is limited. As one proceeds down the east coast of Africa, Burkitt's lymphoma usually is not seen in elevations over 3,000 ft. in the Rhodesias or over 1,000 ft. in Portuguese East Africa. These facts suggest that a mean minimum temperature above 60° F. and a rainfall of more than 20 inches are required for the endemic distribution of this disease. This temperature- and humidity-dependent distribution holds for Africa and New Guinea, but does not appear to obtain in the United Kingdom, the United States, or Canada, where the disease is sporadic rather than endemic (MacMahon, 1968). The relation of temperature and humidity to the distribution of the disease in

South America and Mexico has not been worked out completely, but Aguirre (1967) mentioned that most of the patients with extranodal lymphoma whom he had seen in Mexico City came from the small villages in the lowlands rather than from the city proper, which is located at an altitude of 7,000 ft. This temperature and humidity dependence suggests an arthropod vector.

The painstaking studies of Haddow (1961), Williams (1967), and Barnley (1967) have shown that the only vectors consistent with this distribution in Africa are mosquitoes of the *Anopheles* and *Mansonia* genera. Since these mosquitoes also carry malaria, the incidence of Burkitt's tumor seems to vary according to the areas in which malaria is hyperendemic. Other than this circumstantial evidence, however, there has been nothing to implicate the mosquito as a vector of this disease. That Burkitt's tumor does not occur during the first year of life and that, of 545 cases reported from Uganda, only one occurred in a child under two years of age suggest an infectious agent and some protection from maternal antibodies (Burkitt, 1967c). Similarly, the occurrence of this disease in adult migrants from the highly elevated, nontumorous area of Rwanda 18 months to three years after arriving in endemic areas in Uganda points to an infectious etiology (Burkitt, 1967c).

In areas where Burkitt's tumor is common, acute leukemia previously was considered to be extremely rare, and vice versa. Recent studies have suggested that the incidence of acute leukemia in these areas may be considerably higher than originally reported (Hutt, 1967). In the United States, where leukemia accounts for 40 to 50 per cent of all childhood cancer, lymphosarcoma and reticulum cell sarcoma together represent less than 10 per cent of the total (Murphy, 1959). What fraction of this figure constitutes true Burkitt's tumor has not been determined as yet. At the conference held in Rye, New York, in May 1967, Rappaport, Wright, and Dorfman (1967) made the following statement about the diagnosis of Burkitt's tumor: "Although it has been agreed that Burkitt's tumor is a malignant lymphoreticular neoplasm that is composed of primitive cells, the identification of this tumor, on the basis of purely morphologic criteria, has met with difficulty, particularly outside the geographic areas where it is endemic. For this reason, the diagnosis of Burkitt's tumor must be based on a combination of histologic, cytologic, clinical, and gross anatomic features until such time when agreement will have been reached as to the precise identity of its component cells, and as to the method or methods by which these cells can be identified. No single feature can be considered as diagnostic by itself." In the United States, because of the difficulty in making a clearcut pathological diagnosis and the rare occurrence of jaw tumors, all abdominal lymphomas of children and young adults (except Hodgkin's disease), regardless of whether they have been diagnosed pathologically as reticulum cell sarcoma or as lymphosarcoma, should be managed chemotherapeutically as if they were variants of Burkitt's tumor (Burchenal, 1967, 1968).

As far as viruses—etiological or passenger—are concerned, reovirus 3 has been isolated from a few patients with Burkitt's tumor; and antibodies to the virus have been found in 73 per cent of the lymphoma patients and 18 per cent of the controls in a study reported from Uganda by Bell (1967). Reovirus 3 has been shown to infect mosquitoes in Australia and to produce a runting syndrome in mice. Stanley (1967) has reported that isologous mice injected with spleens from these runted mice also develop runting and some also develop lymphoma. Herpes-simplex virus and *Mycoplasma* (Dalldorf and Bergamini, 1964) also have been isolated from biopsy specimens of Burkitt's tumor on several occasions.

After the original success of Epstein and Barr (1964) in growing the EB_1 culture line, a large number of continuous cell cultures have been isolated from Burkitt's tumor (Pulvertaft, 1964; Osunkoya, 1965; Epstein, Achong, and Pope, 1967; Epstein and Barr, 1965; Stewart, Lovelace, Whang, and Landon, 1965; Minowada *et al.*, 1967; O'Conor and Rabson, 1965). When they examined the lymphoblast-like cells of these cultures with the electron microscope, Epstein and Barr (1965) demonstrated that a small proportion of the cells harbor virus particles which are morphologically indistinguishable from members of the herpes group of viruses. Since 1965, these herpes-like virus particles (EB virus) have been found in a number of cell culture lines grown in many different laboratories; and they have been derived from patients from Uganda, and also from Kenya (Minowada *et al.*, 1967), Nigeria (Pulvertaft, 1964; Osunkoya, 1965), New Guinea (Epstein, Achong, and Pope, 1967), England, and the United States (O'Conor and Rabson, 1965). Griffin, Wright, Bell, and Ross (1966) have found such herpes-like particles in biopsy specimens taken directly from patients.

Henle (1968) recently has reported on the status of these virus-like particles in Burkitt's tumor. Using an indirect immunofluorescence test and fixed cells Henle and Henle (1966a, b), Levy and Henle (1966), and Grace (personal communication) showed that the sera of patients with Burkitt's tumor produced a brilliant fluorescence in a small proportion of cultured Burkitt cells of various EB virus-positive lines. These sera, even when diluted 100 to 1,000 times, still caused detectable immunofluorescence. Relatively low concentrations of such antibodies also were found in African and American control sera. Henle (1968) states:

"The age distribution of reactive sera among American children conforms to that of antibodies to several common viruses. The incidence of positive sera was high at age 0–3 months, reflecting presumably maternal antibodies; it declined to about 10% at age 4–24 months and rose again to about 50% by 4 years of age. It remained at this level until adolescence, but then increased gradually to greater than 80% after 40 years of age." Henle's immunofluorescence technique appears to detect those cells which contain the virus particles, since the percentage of fluorescent cells and the percentage of cells containing the virus particles were approximately equal under electron microscopic examination (Henle and Henle, 1966a). Strongly immunofluorescent human sera produced electron microscopic evidence of antibody coating and agglutination of virus particles extracted and concentrated from Burkitt cell cultures (Henle, Hummeler, and Henle, 1966). Antibodies which were produced in rabbits by immunization with concentrated suspensions of virus particles and then conjugated with fluorescein produced fluorescence indistinguishable from that obtained with positive human sera (Epstein, personal communication). Individually picked immunofluorescent cells, after they were embedded and thin-sectioned, were demonstrated to contain many virus particles, whereas nonstaining cells prepared by the same technique contained no particles (Henle, 1968). An increase in the percentage of viral particles in cultured cells with the use of preincubated media or media deficient in arginine caused an increase in the immunofluorescence (Henle, 1968). A decrease in virus particles produced by 5-methylamino-2'-deoxyuridine was accompanied by a decline in the number of fluorescent cells (Henle, 1968). When a short pulse of tritiated thymidine was used in cultured Burkitt cells, both cellular and viral deoxyribonucleic acid (DNA) became labeled (zur Hausen et al., 1967). In nonfluorescent cells, the label was demonstrable only in the cellular DNA of the nucleus; whereas in the majority of immunofluorescent cells, the label was also demonstrable in the viral DNA of the cytoplasm. Thus, it seems clear that the immunofluorescence technique described by Henle (1968) clearly detects the EB virus-producing cells. These reactions differed from those of Old et al. (1966) and Oettgen et al. (1967) who used an immunodiffusion technique and an antigen extracted from Jijoye cells; they also differ from those of the Kleins (Klein, Clifford, Klein, and Stjernswärd, 1966; Klein, Klein, and Clifford, 1967; Klein, 1968), who used living Burkitt's tumor cells from either fresh biopsy specimens or the Jijoye cell line and sera of patients with Burkitt's tumor for their immunofluorescence studies. A different antigen presumably is involved in this membrane fluorescence which, however, might be induced by the EB virus.

The immunodiffusion test reported by Old *et al.* (1966) and Oettgen *et al.* (1967) has shown positive sera in 59 per cent of 70 patients with Burkitt's tumor from East and West Africa, 83 per cent of 29 patients with nasopharyngeal carcinoma from Kenya, and 82 per cent of 33 patients with nasopharyngeal cancer from the United States. In addition, 44 per cent of 28 American patients with lymphosarcoma and 25 per cent of 100 American patients with acute leukemia had positive sera. In all other groups, including healthy individuals and patients with other carcinomas of the head and neck and other types of neoplastic and nonneoplastic disease, sera showed approximately 14 per cent positive reactions.

Klein, Clifford, Klein, and Stjernswärd (1966), Klein, Klein, and Clifford (1967), and Klein (1968) have shown that the sera of patients with Burkitt's tumor who are responding well to chemotherapy produce a positive reaction in the indirect membrane immunofluorescence tests with allogenic and autochthonous Burkitt's tumor cells, but do not produce a similar reaction with normal marrow cells. The reaction is much less noticeable with the sera of patients who have only partially regressing or unresponsive tumors. Using the cell culture lines Jijoye, EB_3, B35M, and SL_1, Klein, Clifford, Klein, and Stjernswärd (1966), Klein, Klein, and Clifford (1967), and Klein (1968) demonstrated an indirect membrane immunofluorescence reaction with a somewhat broader spectrum of Burkitt sera. The results were negative when Burkitt cell lines Ogun, Kudi, and Raji and eight different cell lines of human acute leukemia were employed (Klein, 1968).

Henle *et al.* (1967) also have been able to show that irradiated Jijoye cells incubated with leukocytes from female children would cause the leukocytes to grow in permanent culture lines, whereas neither leukocytes nor irradiated Jijoye cells would grow when incubated alone. They also demonstrated that these leukocytes became positive in the immunofluorescence test and that when examined under the electron microscope, they contained the herpes-like virus particles. In a somewhat similar experiment, Klein (personal communication) was able to transfer the membrane immunofluorescence from irradiated Jijoye cells to various permanent cell cultures of Burkitt's tumor and acute leukemia, which normally were negative by his immunofluorescence study.

The remarkable response of Burkitt's tumor to chemotherapy also has excited great interest among many investigators. This tumor responds to a variety of agents such as methotrexate, cyclophosphamide, orthomerphalan, mechlorethamine, vincristine sulfate, and actinomycin D; but long-term, permanent regressions have been seen mainly with methotrexate, cyclophosphamide, and orthomerphalan. As reported at the Conference on Acute Leukemia and Burkitt's Tumor at Rye, New York, in May 1967 (ACS-NCI Conference on Acute Leukemia and Burkitt's Tumor [Rye 1967], 1967) the results of 245 patients treated by Clifford, Singh, Stjernswärd, and Klein (1967), Ngu (personal communication), and Burkitt (1967c) showed that 38, or 15 per cent, had been in remission without further maintenance therapy for over a year (Burchenal, 1967). Since of all the patients treated so far, only one of those who remained in unmaintained remission for over a year ever relapsed, these remissions may be considered as fairly permanent. Thus this disease would appear to have the highest incidence of prolonged remissions of any disseminated tumor in human beings with the exception of choriocarcinoma in females.

Of the drugs employed, cyclophosphamide and orthomerphalan appear to be the best. Methotrexate, when given in doses of 25 mg./day by mouth for four to eight days, produced regressions in patients with jaw tumors in early stages (Oettgen, Burkitt, and Burchenal, 1963; Burkitt, 1967). At least two long-term survivors (who have now lived more than seven years) have been recorded. However, lengthy survival was achieved only in patients with small tumors—not in those with large lesions. In contrast, Burkitt (1967c) and Clifford, Singh, Stjernswärd, and Klein (1967), concluded that the size of the tumor was much less important with cyclophosphamide or orthomerphalan, and that good regressions occasionally could be achieved in large tumors. They did agree, however, that the staging is extremely important. In other words, stage I disease in which the lesion is localized to one area, even though it may be large, is more likely to respond and produce long-term survivors than stage II disease in which the lesion is in two contiguous areas or stage III disease in which it is both above and below the diaphragm. Burkitt (1967c) and Clifford, Singh, Stjernswärd, and Klein (1967) believe that abdominal disease generally responds less well than jaw tumors, although they have reported long-term survivors who previously had widespread abdominal disease. They suggest administering 40 mg./kg. of cyclophosphamide intravenously, and repeating the dose in two to three weeks. If complete regression is achieved with these two doses, no further therapy is given. If the regression is not complete, a third or fourth dose may be given, although Burkitt believes strongly that if an almost complete regression is not seen with the first two doses, the chances of achieving any permanent regressions are very small. The study of these long-term survivors shows, however, that in some the tumor regressed temporarily, returned in one to six months, and then responded with a permanent regression after further therapy. For this reason, one should not become discouraged if the tumor returns after the initial two doses of cyclophosphamide, but should continue with the drug.

In the United States, Carbone (personal communication) and Frei (personal communication) have recommended that the dose of 40 mg./kg. of cyclophosphamide be repeated every three to four weeks for six doses even though complete regression is achieved with the first two doses, on the assumption that six doses would be more likely to produce total tumor cell kill. Such a regimen is now being tested in Uganda by Ziegler (personal communication). All patients with Burkitt's tumor are treated initially with one injection of cyclophosphamide; those who go into complete remission are being randomized into two series—one to get no further therapy and the other to get another five doses. Such a study should determine whether there is any advantage in more protracted treatment of patients with Burkitt's tumor in Africa. These results may not be valid for the United States, though, because less host defense may be present than in Africa and six doses may be necessary to eradicate all the tumor cells.

Since such excellent results have been achieved with the management of this disease in Africa, it is suggested (Burchenal, 1968) that in the United States, all abdominal and extranodal lymphomas (except Hodgkin's disease) in children be managed in the same way that the typical Burkitt's tumor is managed in Africa, with 40 mg./kg. of cyclophosphamide given intravenously. Since very little evidence of host defenses has been observed so far in American patients with Burkitt's tumor, it is recommended that the 40 mg./kg. of cyclophosphamide be given every three to four weeks for six doses. In addition, if the tumor appears to be localized and is accessible to radiotherapy, a total of 3,000 to 3,500 rads in three weeks should be given with the hope of producing complete obliteration of the localized tumor. In this way, the physician presumably is giving a curative treatment for the localized disease with irradiation while guarding against the likelihood of occult disseminated disease with chemotherapy.

REFERENCES

ACS-NCI Conference on Acute Leukemia and Burkitt's Tumor (Rye 1967). *Cancer Research*, 27:2414-2660, December 1967.

Aguirre, A.: Discussion. In Burchenal, J. H., Chairman: Panel 20. Advances in the management of leukaemias and lymphomas. In Harris, R. J. C., Ed.: *Proceedings of the 9th International Cancer Congress* (UICC Monograph Series, Vol. 10). Berlin and Heidelberg, Germany, and New York, New York, Springer-Verlag, 1967, p. 245.

Barnley, G. R.: Discussion: Williams, M. C.: Implications of the geographical distribution of Burkitt's lymphoma. In Burchenal, J. H., and Burkitt, D. P., Eds.: *Treatment of Burkitt's Tumour* (UICC Monograph Series, Vol. 8). Berlin and Heidelberg, Germany and New York, New York, Springer-Verlag, 1967, pp. 48-51.

Bell, T. M.: Review of the evidence for a viral aetiology for Burkitt's lymphoma. In Burchenal, J. H., and Burkitt, D. P., Eds.: *Treatment of Burkitt's Tumour* (UICC Monograph Series, Vol. 8). Berlin and Heidelberg, Germany, and New York, New York, Springer-Verlag, 1967, pp. 52-58.

Beltran, G., Baez, A., and Correa, P.: Burkitt's lymphoma in Colombia. *The American Journal of Medicine,* 40:211-216, February 1966.

Burchenal, J. H.: Formal Discussion: Long-term survival in Burkitt's tumor and in acute leukemia. *Cancer Research,* 27:2616-2618, December 1967.

————: Long-term survivors in acute leukemia and Burkitt's tumor. *Cancer,* 21: 595-599, April 1968.

Burkitt, D.: Chemotherapy of jaw tumours. In Burchenal, J. H., and Burkitt, D. P., Eds.: *Treatment of Burkitt's Tumour* (UICC Monograph Series, Vol. 8). Berlin and Heidelberg, Germany, and New York, New York, Springer-Verlag, 1967, pp. 94-101.

————: Long-term survivors in acute leukemia. In Zarafonetis, C. J. D., Ed.: *Proceedings of the International Conference on Leukemia-Lymphoma.* Philadelphia, Pennsylvania, Lea & Febiger, 1968, pp. 469-474.

————: Recent developments in geographical distribution. In Burchenal, J. H., and Burkitt, D. P., Eds.: *Treatment of Burkitt's Tumour* (UICC Monograph Series, Vol. 8). Berlin and Heidelberg, Germany, and New York, New York, Springer-Verlag, 1967a, pp. 36-41.

————: A sarcoma involving the jaws in African children. *British Journal of Surgery,* 46:218-223, November 1958.

————: Some clinical features. In Burchenal, J. H., and Burkitt, D. P., Eds.: *Treatment of Burkitt's Tumour* (UICC Monograph Series, Vol. 8). Berlin and Heidelberg, Germany, and New York, New York, Springer-Verlag, 1967b, pp. 2-6.

Burkitt, D. P.: *Possible Relationships Between the African Lymphoma and Acute Leukaemia.* London, England, The Queen Anne Press Ltd., 1967c, 28 pp.

Carbone, P.: Personal communication.

Clifford, P., Singh, S., Stjernswärd, J., and Klein, G.: Long-term survival of patients with Burkitt's lymphoma: An assessment of treatment and other factors which may relate to survival. *Cancer Research,* 27:2578-2615, December 1967.

Dalldorf, G., and Bergamini, F.: Unidentified, filtrable agents isolated from African children with malignant lymphomas. *Proceedings of the National Academy of Sciences of the U. S. A.,* 51:263-265, February 1964.

Desai, P. B.: Personal communication.

Dorfman, R. F.: Childhood lymphosarcoma in St. Louis, Missouri, clinically and histologically resembling Burkitt's tumor. *Cancer,* 18:418-430, April 1965.

Edington, G. M., and Maclean, C. M.: Incidence of the Burkitt tumour in Ibadan, Western Nigeria. *British Medical Journal,* 1:264-266, February 1, 1964.

Epstein, M. A.: Personal communication.

Epstein, M. A., Achong, B. G., and Pope, J. H.: Virus in cultured lymphoblasts from a New Guinea Burkitt lymphoma. *British Medical Journal,* 2:290-291, April 29, 1967.

Epstein, M. A., and Barr, Y. M.: Characteristics and mode of growth of a tissue culture strain (EB1) of human lymphoblasts from Burkitt's lymphoma. *Journal of the National Cancer Institute,* 34:231-240, February 1965.

————: Cultivation in vitro of human lymphoblasts from Burkitt's malignant lymphoma. *Lancet,* 1:252-253, February 1, 1964.

Frei, E., III: Personal communication.

Grace, J.: Personal communication.

Griffin, E. R., Wright, D. H., Bell, T. M., and Ross, M. G. R.: Demonstration of virus particles in biopsy material from cases of Burkitt's tumour. *European Journal of Cancer,* 2:353-358, December 1966.

Haddow, A. J.: Malignant lymphoma in African children. Bioclimatic distribution. *East African Virus Research Institute Annual Report for 1960-1961,* No. 11, 30 (1961).

Henle, G., and Henle, W.: Immunofluorescence in cells derived from Burkitt's lymphoma. *Journal of Bacteriology,* 91:1248-1256, March 1966a.

————: Studies on cell lines derived from Burkitt's lymphoma. *Transactions of the New York Academy of Sciences,* 29:71-79, November 1966b.

Henle, W.: Evidence for viruses in acute leukemia and Burkitt's tumor. *Cancer,* 21: 580-586, April 1968.

Henle, W., Diehl, V., Kohn, G., zur Hausen, H., and Henle, G.: Herpes-type virus and chromosome marker in normal leukocytes after growth with irradiated Burkitt cells. *Science,* 157: 1064-1065, September 1, 1967.

Henle, W., Hummeler, K., and Henle, G.: Antibody coating and agglutination of virus particles separated from the EB3 line of Burkitt lymphoma cells. *Journal of Bacteriology,* 92:269-271, July 1966.

Hutt, M. S. R.: The pathology of Burkitt's tumour in the context of lymphomas and leukaemias. In Burchenal, J. H., and Burkitt, D. P., Eds.: *Treatment of Burkitt's Tumour* (UICC Monograph Series, Vol. 8). Berlin and Heidelberg, Germany, and New York, New York, Springer-Verlag, 1967, pp. 11-13.

Klein, G.: Personal communication.

Klein, G., Clifford, P., Klein, E., and Stjernswärd, J.: Search for tumor-specific immune reactions in Burkitt lymphoma patients by the membrane immunofluorescence reaction. *Proceedings of the National Academy of Sciences of the U. S. A.,* 55:1628-1636, June 1966.

Klein, G., Klein, E., and Clifford, P.: Host defenses in leukemia and Burkitt's tumor. *Cancer,* 21:587-594, April 1968.

————: Search for host defenses in Burkitt lymphoma: Membrane immunofluorescence tests in biopsies and tissue culture lines. *Cancer Research,* 27:2510-2520, December 1967.

Levy, J. A., and Henle, G.: Indirect immunofluorescence tests with sera from African children and cultured Burkitt lymphoma cells. *Journal of Bacteriology,* 92:275-276, July 1966.

Luisi, A., de Padua Bertelli, A., Machado, J. C., and Ache de Freitas, J. P.: "Linfoma Africano" em criancas brasileiras. *Revista Brasileira de Cirurgia,* 49:280-295, May 1965.

MacMahon, B.: Epidemiologic aspects of acute leukemia and Burkitt's tumor. *Cancer,* 21:558-562, April 1968.

Minowada, J., Klein, G., Clifford, P., Klein, E., and Moore, G. E.: Studies of Burkitt lymphoma cells. I. Establishment of a cell line (B35M) and its characteristics. *Cancer,* 20:1430-1437, September 1967.

Murphy, M. L.: Leukemia and lymphoma in children. *Pediatric Clinics of North America,* 6:611-638, May 1959.

Ngu, V. A.: The Burkitt tumour. In Harris, R. J. C., Ed.: *Proceedings of the 9th International Cancer Congress* (UICC Monograph Series, Vol. 10). Berlin and Heidelberg, Germany, and New York, New York, Springer-Verlag, 1967, pp. 232-244.

————: Personal communication.

O'Conor, G. T., and Davies, J. N. P.: Malignant tumors in African children. With special reference to malignant lymphoma. *The Journal of Pediatrics,* 56:526-535, April 1960.

O'Conor, G. T., and Rabson, A. S.: Herpes-like particles in an American lymphoma: Preliminary note. *Journal of the National Cancer Institute,* 35:899-903, November 1965.

O'Conor, G. T., Rappaport, H., and Smith, E. B.: Childhood lymphoma resembling "Burkitt Tumor" in the United States. *Cancer,* 18:411-417, April 1965.

Oettgen, H. F., Aoki, T., Geering, G., Boyse, E. A., and Old, L. J.: Definition of an antigenic system associated with Burkitt's lymphoma. *Cancer Research,* 27:2532-2534, December 1967.

Oettgen, H. F., Burkitt, D., and Burchenal, J. H.: Malignant lymphoma involving the jaw in African children: Treatment with methotrexate. *Cancer,* 16:616-623, May 1963.

Old, L. J., Boyse, E. A., Oettgen, H. F., de Harven, E., Geering, G., Williamson, B., and Clifford, P.: Precipitating antibody in human serum to an antigen present in cultured Burkitt's lymphoma cells. *Proceedings of the National Academy of Sciences of the U. S. A.,* 56:1699-1704, December 1966.

Osunkoya, B. O.: The preservation of Burkitt tumour cells at moderately low temperature. *The British Journal of Cancer,* 19:749-753, December 1965.

Pulvertaft, R. J. V.: Cytology of Burkitt's tumour (African lymphoma). *Lancet,* 1:238-240, February 1, 1964.

———: The use of tissue culture in the diagnosis of Burkitt's tumour. In Burchenal, J. H., and Burkitt, D. P., Eds.: *Treatment of Burkitt's Tumour* (UICC Monograph Series, Vol. 8). Berlin and Heidelberg, Germany, and New York, New York, Springer-Verlag, 1967, pp. 24-28.

Rappaport, H., Wright, D. H., and Dorfman, R. F.: Suggested criteria for the diagnosis of Burkitt's tumor. *Cancer Research,* 27:2632, December 1967.

Stanley, N. F.: Reovirus type 3 and the etiology of Burkitt's lymphoma: A discussion of Dr. Bell's paper. In Burchanel, J. H., and Burkitt, D. P., Eds.: *Treatment of Burkitt's Tumour* (UICC Monograph Series, Vol. 8). Berlin and Heidelberg, Germany, and New York, New York, Springer-Verlag, 1967, pp. 59-63.

Stewart, S. E., Lovelace, E., Whang, J., and Landon, J.: A herpes-like virus in lymphoma cells in culture. (Abstract) *Proceedings of the American Association for Cancer Research,* 6:62, March 1965.

Ten Seldam, R. E., Cooke, R., and Atkinson, L.: Childhood lymphoma in the territories of Papua and New Guinea. *Cancer,* 19:437-446, March 1966.

Williams, M. C.: Implications of the geographical distribution of Burkitt's lymphoma. In Burchenal, J. H., and Burkitt, D. P., Eds.: *Treatment of Burkitt's Tumour* (UICC Monograph Series, Vol. 8). Berlin and Heidelberg, Germany, and New York, New York, Springer-Verlag, 1967, pp. 42-48.

Wright, D. H.: The gross and microscopic pathology of Burkitt's tumour. In Burchenal, J. H., and Burkitt, D. P., Eds.: *Treatment of Burkitt's Tumour* (UICC Monograph Series, Vol. 8). Berlin and Heidelberg, Germany, and New York, New York, Springer-Verlag, 1967, pp. 14-23.

———: Personal communication.

Ziegler, J. L.: Personal communication.

zur Hausen, H., Henle, W., Hummeler, K., Diehl, V., and Henle, G.: Comparative study of cultured Burkitt tumor cells by immunofluorescence, autoradiography, and electron microscopy. *Journal of Virology,* 1:830-837, August 1967.

The Management of Malignant Lymphoma in Childhood

R. D. T. JENKIN, M.B., F.R.C.P. (C), F.F.R.,
AND M. J. SONLEY, M.D., F.R.C.P. (C)

The Princess Margaret Hospital, Toronto, Ontario, Canada

DURING THE PERIOD 1930 TO 1965, 75 children with Hodgkin's disease who were less than 16 years old presented at the Hospital for Sick Children, the Department of Radiotherapy at Toronto General Hospital, or The Princess Margaret Hospital, Toronto. This group of patients was reviewed recently (Jenkin, Peters, and Darte, 1967) and is excluded from the present discussion.

In the same period, approximately twice as many children presented with other malignant lymphomas. This paper is an initial review of 121 of these children, with special attention to their response to treatment.

Pattern of Clinical Presentation

In these 121 children, the primary sites of involvement were the gastrointestinal tract (40), the upper gastrointestinal or respiratory tract (12), and elsewhere within the abdomen or retroperitoneum (16). Twenty-six had lesions originating in the mediastinum. Fourteen presented with one or more lymph node regions involved, but without other clinical evidence of spread. Thirteen children presented with a mixture of these types (Table 1). This pattern of presentation differs significantly from that of children with Hodgkin's disease, two thirds of whom can be expected to present with involvement of lymph node regions only, with the concentration in sites above the diaphragm.

TABLE 1.—PRIMARY SITES OF INVOLVEMENT IN CHILDREN
WITH LYMPHOSARCOMA AND RETICULUM CELL SARCOMA

ANATOMICAL SITE	NUMBER OF PATIENTS
G.I. tract	40
Upper G.I. and respiratory tracts	12
Other sites in abdomen and retroperitoneum	16
SUBTOTAL	68
Mediastinum	26
Lymph node region	14
Mixed	13
TOTAL	121

Abbreviation: G.I., gastrointestinal.

Gastrointestinal Tract

When lymphosarcoma or reticulum cell sarcoma arises in the gastrointestinal tract—as it did in 40 of the children in this series—it does so predominantly in the region of the terminal ileum, cecum, appendix, or ascending colon. Only eight of 40 lesions occurred at other sites: four in the midileum, one in the upper ileum, one in the jejunum, one in the duodenum, and one in the stomach.

Most of these children, among whom boys outnumbered girls in the ratio of nine to one, presented with an acute abdomen. Fifteen are known to have presented with intussusception, one with a perforated viscus, and one with a gastrointestinal hemorrhage. All 40 of the patients with gastrointestinal tract lesions were diagnosed at laparotomy, at a time when the surgeon was not often expecting to find a malignant tumor. Appendicitis or appendiceal abscess was a common preoperative diagnosis. The surgeon excised the involved segment with its mesentery if possible. Commonly, this included the terminal ileum, cecum, appendix, and ascending colon.

Only one of 16 children who did not receive postoperative irradiation survives, compared with nine of 24 who did receive it (Table 2). These are crude figures which ignore differences in extent of disease between the two groups. There were no survivors when only part of the primary tumor was excised, when macroscopic evidence of infiltration of the adjacent structures by the primary lesion was present, or when peritoneal or mesenteric implants of tumor tissue were present. When children who fulfill

TABLE 2.—PRIMARY LYMPHOMA IN THE GASTROINTESTINAL TRACT: NUMBER SURVIVING RELATED TO TREATMENT METHOD

TREATMENT	ALL STAGES		ADVANCED STAGES EXCLUDED	
	Total	Total Alive	Total	Total Alive
Surgical excision	16	1	9	1
Surgical excision and postoperative irradiation	24	9	15	9
TOTAL	40	10	24	10

Ratio of males to females: nine to one.

one or more of these criteria are excluded, nine of 15 irradiated patients survived (60 per cent) compared with one of nine unirradiated (11 per cent). The one survivor in the unirradiated group had a local resection of appendix and base of cecum without further exploration. He clearly presented with very early disease.

Involvement of regional lymph nodes does not appear to be a major factor in length of survival when postoperative irradiation is used. Of 11 children with histologically positive nodes, five are alive and well. For only six of 40 patients was a definite statement made by the surgeon that no abnormal nodes were present. Frequently enlarged nodes were not biopsied or the sample sent was negative.

The length of survival in patients who have died is of interest. All were dead within nine months; 25 of 29 were dead within 18 weeks of operation (Fig. 1). Any child who remained free of disease for nine months continues alive and well without recurrence.

The histological type of the malignant lymphoma did not influence the operation or irradiation. Of the 10 survivors, five were classified as having reticulum cell sarcoma, four as having lymphosarcoma, and one as having malignant lymphoma of an unspecified type. For the whole group, the histological types were as follows: reticulum cell sarcoma, 10; lymphosarcoma, 27; and unspecified malignant lymphoma, three. No child with Hodgkin's disease presented with a primary lesion of the gastrointestinal tract.

In summary, for patients with primary lymphoma of the gastrointestinal tract and spread limited to mesenteric nodes who are treated by surgical excision and postoperative irradiation (2,500-3,000 rads/28 days, whole abdomen), the prognosis can be favorable; but when the disease is advanced at diagnosis or if it recurs, a fatal outcome is both inevitable

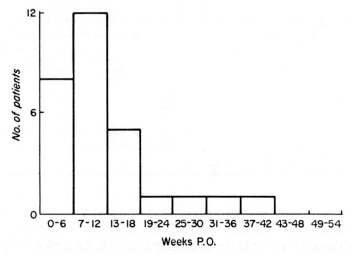

and rapid. Response to irradiation or chemotherapeutic agents is then at best transient.

Upper Gastrointestinal and Respiratory Tract

Twelve children presented with the primary site of involvement in the upper gastrointestinal or respiratory tract (tonsillar region, seven; nasopharynx, one; jaw, two; and antrum, two) (Table 3).

In the seven children with a primary lesion in the tonsillar region and in the child with a primary lesion in the nasopharynx, the cervical lymph

TABLE 3.—Upper Gastrointestinal and Respiratory Tract
Lymphosarcoma and Reticulum Cell Sarcoma:
Primary Site by Anatomical Region

Anatomical Site	Number
Tonsillar region	7
Nasopharynx	1
Antrum	2
Jaw	2
Total	12

Ratio of males to females: five to one.

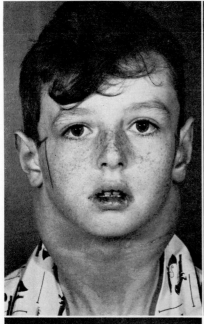
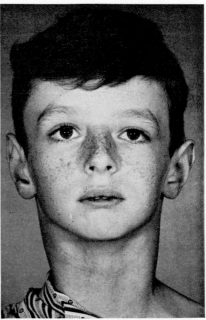
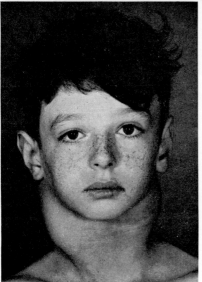

Fig. 2 (above left).—G. W., age nine years, was photographed on June 13, 1961. At that time he gave a six-week history of nasal obstruction and cervical adenopathy. His disease was diagnosed as lymphosarcoma, and he was given regional irradiation (2,640 rads/22 days) with no response.

Fig. 3 (above right).—G. W., photographed on June 30, 1961, three days after a 10-mg. dose of vinblastine given intravenously in 10 fractions at hourly intervals. He showed a rapid and significant response to chemotherapy.

Fig. 4 (left).—G. W., photographed on July 18, 1961. Lymphoma showed rapid regrowth despite weekly doses of vinblastine and later cyclophosphamide.

nodes were clinically involved. In four of the eight children in these two groups, the liver was palpable and probably abnormal. In one, the inguinal glands were suspicious. The clinical suspicion that all eight of the children had widespread lymphoma at diagnosis was confirmed by the response to regional irradiation. In four, the primary and secondary nodes disappeared rapidly during irradiation; but length of survival from the time of diagnosis was 6, 7, and 20 weeks with one patient lost to followup. Dissemination to the abdomen and to the skin and bone was quickly dominant in the first two children and the pattern of recurrence is unknown in the third. In two of the other four patients, the primary lesion and nodes regressed only partially during irradiation; in the third, they were static and in the fourth they progressed. The dose range was 2,500 to 4,000 rads in three to four weeks. One of the patients had a dramatic but brief response to vinblastine (Figs. 2, 3, 4), but later he did not respond to cyclophosphamide. These patients survived 22, 12, 20, and 8 weeks from diagnosis, with rapid dissemination.

Although the two children with antral tumors and one of the children with a jaw tumor had slowly progressing disease and achieved more useful remission with local irradiation, they survived only 35, 74, and 82 weeks. The other child with a jaw tumor was treated with nitrogen mustard and survived 15 weeks.

None of the 12 children in this group survived. Whether the primary tumor responded to local irradiation or not, distant tumor became apparent during or shortly after primary treatment.

Abdomen

In addition to the 40 children with primary gastrointestinal tract lymphomas, another 16 presented with abdominal symptoms and signs; 15 of these required laparotomy to establish a diagnosis. The remaining patient demonstrated lymphosarcoma-type cells in ascitic fluid and was spared laparotomy. In four of these children, there was modest evidence of intrathoracic involvement, but superficial lymph node areas were negative (Table 4).

In 11, there was retroperitoneal tumor with or without widespread intra-abdominal disease. There was no strong evidence in any that the primary site was in the gastrointestinal tract, but this could have been obscured in a few by the extent of disease. In one, a mass of lymphosarcoma nodes was present in the ileocecal mesentery without definite evidence of disease elsewhere.

TABLE 4.—LYMPHOSARCOMA AND RETICULUM CELL SARCOMA ELSEWHERE
IN THE ABDOMEN OR RETROPERITONEUM: CLASSIFICATION BY DOMINANT
ANATOMICAL SITE (PRIMARY GASTROINTESTINAL INVOLVEMENT EXCLUDED)

ANATOMICAL SITE	NUMBER OF PATIENTS
Retroperitoneum ± extensive intra-abdomen	11
Localized mesenteric	1
Ovary (possibly) + retroperitoneum + intra-abdomen	3
Kidney	1
TOTAL	16

Ratio of males to females: three to one.

Two girls had large bilateral pelvic masses and one had a single large pelvic mass, together with more extensive intra-abdominal disease, which suggested the possibility of ovarian origin. Girls comprised four of the 16 patients in this group, and three of the four had tumors which were possibly ovarian in origin. One boy had a primary lymphosarcoma of the kidney without definite evidence of lymphatic spread.

Two children in this group of 16 survive. A 12-year-old boy with a renal primary lesion was treated by nephrectomy and postoperative radiation to the whole abdomen (2,500 rads/25 days). He has been alive and well for three years, but required local excision and irradiation for scar recurrence 11 weeks after the original procedure; an eight-year-old boy with a lymphosarcomatous group of nodes in the ileocecal mesentery underwent a local excision of nodes and whole abdomen irradiation (3,000 rads/29 days). He is alive seven years and six months after treatment without further trouble.

The remaining 14 children did poorly and behaved in a fashion similar to the patients with advanced primary gastrointestinal lymphoma. Six were essentially untreated after laparotomy and survived a maximum of three weeks.

Five children received irradiation to the whole abdomen. Two had a complete remission and survived 48 and 55 weeks. Three had partial remissions and survived 11, 20, and 20 weeks.

One received adrenocorticotropic hormone for 17 days without remission and survived four weeks. One received prednisone followed by intermittent vinblastine, had a partial remission of eight weeks attributed to vinblastine, and survived 12 weeks. One received prednisone without effect followed by vincristine sulfate and maintenance 6-mercaptopurine; there was complete remission of five weeks, and 25 weeks' survival. Vincristine was thought to have induced the remission.

When disease is not known to be present outside the abdomen, abdominal irradiation is favored as the first treatment measure.

Mediastinum

Twenty-six children had predominantly mediastinal disease (19 boys and seven girls). In only one was disease confined to the mediastinum at diagnosis. Anatomical sites of involvement at diagnosis are shown in Table 5. There was no evidence of acute leukemia in bone marrow and peripheral blood studies.

In this group, a tissue diagnosis was obtained in only 14; a cytological diagnosis was made after examination of pleural fluid in eight and the diagnosis was made on clinical grounds and then borne out fully by subsequent progress in four. Of the 14 patients with a tissue diagnosis, two had reticulum cell sarcoma and 12 had lymphosarcoma.

This group of patients responded to initial treatment, whether with prednisone or irradiation, with rapidity and often with apparent completeness (Figs. 5, 6, 7, 8, 9).

The duration of first remission is known for only 20 children (Table 6). When induced by whole-chest irradiation, the duration of remission in six patients varied from one to 27 weeks; two of the six had periods of remission longer than three months. In five patients in whom remission was induced by prednisone (three then receiving irradiation), the range was 0 to 22 weeks (one patient did not go into remission); two of five patients had a remission of longer than three months. Four of the 11

TABLE 5.—ANATOMICAL SITES OF INVOLVEMENT AT PRESENTATION IN 26 CHILDREN IN WHOM MEDIASTINAL DISEASE DOMINATED THE CLINICAL PICTURE

ANATOMICAL SITE		NUMBER OF PATIENTS
Nodes	cervical	15
	axillary	7
	inguinal	2
Liver		13
Spleen		8
Pleural effusion		9
Abdominal mass		2
Testis		1

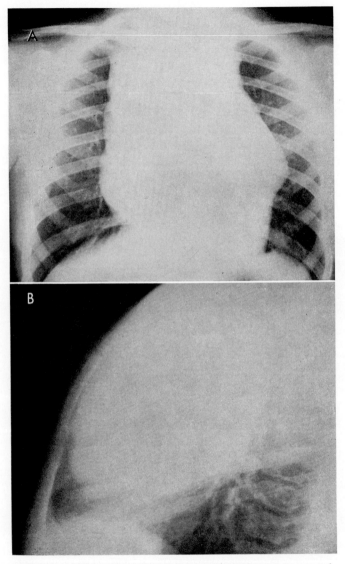

Fig. 5.—N. H., an eight-year-old boy with a two-week history of progressive wheezing and orthopnea. **A,** a very large mediastinal mass was present, along with moderate hepatosplenomegaly. Oral prednisolone (50 mg./day) was started. **B,** four days later, his chest x-ray film appeared nearly normal. Mediastinal irradiation then was given (3,000 rads/20 days). Maintenance 6-mercaptopurine was started. The boy was in remission for six months before the onset of acute leukemia. A further complete remission was induced by prednisone and maintained with methotrexate.

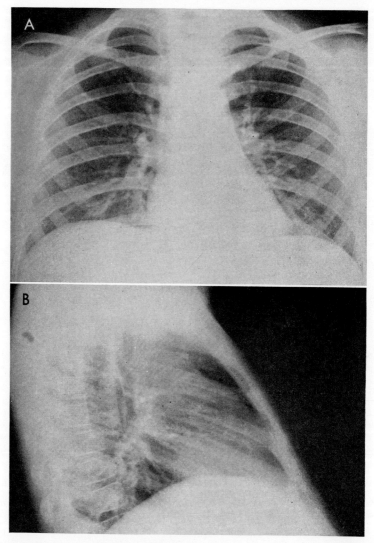

Fig. 6.—N. H. A and B, essentially normal chest x-ray films one month before death. No further intrathoracic problem during illness after initial control was achieved.

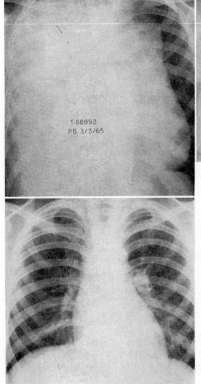
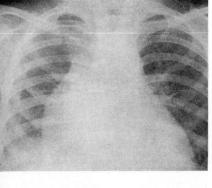

T.66992
P.B. 3/3/65

Fig. 7 (above left).—P. B., a seven-year-old boy with lymphosarcoma. At diagnosis, a large mediastinal mass and gross right pleural effusion were present.
Fig. 8 (above right).—P. B., five days after whole-chest irradiation was started (350 rads/5 days). Significant radiological and symptomatic improvement had occurred.
Fig. 9 (left).—P. B., two weeks after completion of radiotherapy (2,000 rads/28 days). He remains in remission at 136 plus weeks on maintenance doses of 6-mercaptopurine.

patients in these two treatment categories had a remission longer than three months.

When maintenance oral 6-mercaptopurine or methotrexate was added after induction of a remission, the remission was prolonged. Thus, of nine patients who had a remission induced by prednisone or prednisone plus radiation and then received maintenance therapy, six remained in remission longer than three months (range four to 136 plus weeks, median 19 weeks).

One boy, who had a large mediastinal mass and massive pleural effusion responded to whole-chest irradiation (Figs. 7, 8, 9) and remains in remission on 2.5 mg./kg. of 6-mercaptopurine daily 136 weeks later. There was no evidence of extrathoracic disease at diagnosis.

In general, when there is gross extrathoracic disease, we induce a remission with 2 mg./kg./day of prednisone and maintain it with 2.5

TABLE 6.—MEDIASTINAL LYMPHOSARCOMA AND RETICULUM
CELL SARCOMA: DURATION OF FIRST REMISSION
RELATED TO TREATMENT METHOD

INITIAL TREATMENT	No. PTS.	REMISSION		
		No. > 3 Months	Range (Wk.)	Median (Wk.)
R or P ± R	11	4	0–27	4
P ± R + M	9	6	4–136	19

Abbreviations: R, radiation; P, prednisone; M, oral maintenance therapy.

mg./kg./day of 6-mercaptopurine. When disease is predominantly intra-thoracic, chest irradiation is added to give additional control at this site. When the disease is entirely intrathoracic, we feel that full-chest irradiation is obligatory, for under these circumstances there may be a small chance of cure.

Response to chemotherapy or irradiation is more likely in disseminated lymphosarcoma when it arises within the mediastinum than when it arises at an abdominal site, and it is always worth a further attempt to induce remission after relapse.

Eleven patients treated during the years 1940 to 1959 had a median survival period of 13 weeks compared with 37.5 weeks for 11 treated since 1960. This improvement is believed to stem mainly from the introduction of maintenance therapy after induction of a remission.

Lymph Node Region

Ten children presented with nodal involvement in one lymphatic region only. Seven had cervical involvement, one had axillary, one had pre-auricular, and one had post-auricular. Biopsy demonstrated lymphosarcoma in eight and malignant lymphoma of an unspecified type in two.

Nine patients received regional irradiation, two for post-surgical recurrence. Two are alive and well 13 and 14 years later without recurrence. Seven had recurrences; five of the first recurrences were at distant sites, e.g., abdomen, bone, and brain. One had a recurrence elsewhere in the neck and one had recurrence at an unknown site. More often than not a regional nodal presentation of lymphosarcoma is only one manifestation of disseminated disease. This is demonstrated by the fate of four children presenting with two or more nodal areas involved. Three had involvement of neck and axilla, two on one side only; and one had involvement of multiple areas above the diaphragm. Response to initial radiation was limited to three to four weeks because of disease appearing at distant sites. These four patients did no better than those with wide dissemination at onset, surviving for 13, 13, 16, and 23 weeks.

Mixed Presentation

Thirteen children presented with a mixed picture, mainly involvement of nodes in the neck or axilla combined with the presence of liver, spleen, or moderate intrathoracic disease or effusion. None of these children survived. The pattern of their transient response to radiation or chemotherapy followed that of children with advanced mediastinal disease.

Acute Leukemia

Twenty of the 121 children developed acute leukemia during their illness (16.5 per cent) (Table 7). When the disease process arose in the mediastinum, 12 of 26 (46 per cent) developed leukemia. Conversely, for origin in the gastrointestinal tract, abdomen, or retroperitoneum, the incidence drops to three of 68 (4.4 per cent). None of the long-term survivors developed leukemia.

These are strictly minimum incidence figures. We cannot state with certainty that a patient died with acute leukemia unless we followed him closely until the time of death. Many of our earlier patients were not followed closely in the terminal phase of their illness.

The time from diagnosis to onset of acute leukemia is in the range of three to 106 weeks, with a median of 14.5 weeks.

TABLE 7.—INCIDENCE OF ACUTE LEUKEMIA IN CHILDREN WITH LYMPHOSARCOMA AND RETICULUM CELL SARCOMA

ANATOMICAL SITE	NO. PTS.	NO. WITH ACUTE LEUKEMIA
G.I. tract ⎫		
Upper G.I. + ⎪		
respiratory tract ⎬	68	3
Abdomen ⎭		
Mediastinum	26	12
Lymph node region ⎫		
Mixed ⎬	27	5
TOTAL	121	20

Incidence of acute leukemia 16.5%

Abbreviation: G.I., gastrointestinal.

Of 12 patients with adequately managed acute leukemia, eight achieved a complete remission.

Central Nervous System Involvement

Thirteen children developed central nervous system involvement during the course of their disease. One child presented with initial involvement of the floor of the fourth ventricle, which was controlled for a year by irradiation; she then developed disseminated disease and later leukemia.

Of these 13 children, five developed central nervous system involvement during the leukemic phase of their disease; two later developed leukemia and six did not.

All presented with intracranial rather than spinal symptoms. Indeed, the cord was clinically involved at a later time in only one patient.

In seven patients, the primary site was mediastinal. Five of these had previously developed leukemia and one did so later. The association of leukemia with a mediastinal site of origin probably accounts for the association of central nervous system complications with this site.

The time of onset was in the range of 11 to 82 weeks from diagnosis, with a median of 27 weeks. Central nervous system involvement was thus a complication in long-term survivors.

Remissions were obtained with intrathecal methotrexate or cerebral irradiation. Both methods gave good remissions and in general it was possible to solve the central nervous system problem with appropriate repetition of either treatment until death from another cause.

Summary

The end result of this retrospective review is that 12 per cent (14/121) of our children with lymphosarcoma and reticulum cell sarcoma appear to be cured. Twelve had surgical excision of an abdominal primary lesion followed by wide-field irradiation. Two nodal primary tumors responded to irradiation alone. In addition, one child presenting with mediastinal involvement remains in remission at 136 weeks on maintenance 6-mercaptopurine.

It is apparent that the majority of these children presented with disseminated disease with little or no hope for permanent cure by the methods employed. This contrasts sharply with the results in children with Hodgkin's disease; in recent years, about two thirds presented with stages

I or II disease and had an even chance of being alive and well 10 years later.

REFERENCE

Jenkin, R. D. T., Peters, M. V., and Darte, J. M. M.: Hodgkin's disease in children. *American Journal of Roentgenology, Radium Therapy and Nuclear Medicine,* 100:222-226, May 1967.

The Guy H. Heath and Dan C. Heath Memorial Lecture: The Control of Cancer in Children

SIDNEY FARBER, M.D.

*The Children's Cancer Research Foundation, Harvard Medical School,
and The Children's Hospital Medical Center, Boston, Massachusetts*

May I express my thanks to you, Dr. Grant Taylor, and to the director and staff of The University of Texas M. D. Anderson Hospital and Tumor Institute at Houston for the honor you have conferred upon me. I accept the Guy H. and Dan C. Heath Award in the name of the many colleagues, associates, and pupils with whom I have had the privilege of working in the field of pediatric oncology. Sir Stanford Cade, I am honored by your presence today.

I am particularly happy to have this opportunity to speak of my warm feelings for those responsible for the great growth of this cancer institute. Shortly after the end of World War II, I came to the city of Houston as a voluntary consultant to discuss some of the proposals then being considered for the development of pediatrics in Texas. At that time, I heard about plans for a cancer hospital and research institute from Dr. R. Lee Clark, who was then working in a wooden shack. I am certain he would not be offended if I call the building a shack, because it was one. The important point is that he and his colleagues were already taking care of patients, even in totally inadequate facilities. I remember the jungle which they pointed out to me as a place where great medical developments were to be made. Not even in my wildest dreams could I have imagined what would happen here in little more than 20 years. The jungle now is covered by beautiful buildings dedicated to medical education and research and to many different kinds of patient care. There is a world-renowned cancer institute housing patient care, research, and educational ventures on a level never before known in this part of the world.

A magnificent medical school, splendid hospitals, and other institutions devoted to medicine surround us. This is a great accomplishment and one to which I pay tribute.

I am particularly happy, too, that this is an occasion when I can speak of the developments in pediatric oncology under Dr. Grant Taylor. Children with cancer are being cared for at Anderson Hospital with humane consideration and in the highest traditions of medicine. I salute you, Dr. Taylor, and your colleagues, Dr. Margaret Sullivan and Dr. Waturu Sutow.

The meetings which you have held yesterday and today in pediatric oncology could not have been held 20 or even 10 years ago. There were not enough people who were expert in the various phases of childhood cancer to meet and discuss results of such importance. It was a lonely experience 40 years ago when I first became deeply interested in pediatric oncology. I wish that Dr. Harold Dargeon, the pioneer in pediatric oncology at Memorial Hospital in New York City, were here today, because he, too, must have felt quite lonely in that big cancer hospital where there were so many experts in adult cancer and so few in childhood cancer. Forty years ago pediatricians were not very involved with cancer in children, nor were surgeons. The feeling of hopelessness was widespread; it was generally believed that very little or nothing of importance could be done for children with cancer. This feeling of hopelessness had its origins in what was known about cancer in adulthood and especially in the belief that if a patient could not be cured immediately by the techniques of surgery and radiotherapy, the outlook was hopeless. There was no hope at all for the treatment of children with acute leukemia and related disorders. I have wondered at times about what might be called the "obstacles" to greater progress in pediatric oncology. For many years, no beds in pediatric divisions of general hospitals or in children's hospitals were set aside for children with cancer; nor was there financial support for research or clinical investigation until the programs of the National Cancer Institute and the American Cancer Society reached a suitable size and that has only happened in the last 10 to 15 years. Until recently, techniques in pediatric surgery were not well developed and diagnostic tests, still badly needed, were lacking. Radiotherapy in early life is not exploited completely even today, and the number of experts in radiotherapy of cancer in children is still woefully inadequate.

From the teaching of men who preceded me and from the conceptions expressed by my own teacher, the late S. Burt Wolbach, I established— more than 35 years ago—a generalization to alert doctors, residents, and students to the possibility of earlier diagnoses of solid tumors in the young. It has also been of aid in the education of parents. May I repeat its words:

> Every solid, or semisolid, semicystic mass in an infant
> or child should be regarded as a malignant tumor until
> its exact nature is determined by histological examina-
> tion of the removed tumor.

This generalization is still useful. The words not only indicate the most reliable means of early recognition of a malignant tumor but also imply the ideal treatment. When a solid mass is found in a patient, the surgeon, the radiotherapist, the chemotherapist, the pathologist, the hematologist, and any other experts whose opinions might be of value in determining the nature of the tumor and the ideal form of treatment should conduct a rapid study. The ideal treatment for any patient with cancer, and particularly the child with a malignant tumor, should be selected after discussion by a group of experts in a number of different disciplines. It follows from this that the best treatment for a given patient will be mapped out from the moment of recognition of the tumor and subsequent therapeutic procedures will depend on the response to treatment. Optional methods should be recorded far in advance of need. This approach, which is embodied in the "total care" of the patient with cancer, makes use of all available knowledge from the very beginning and brings together in a logical and coordinated program the talents and knowledge of representatives of many different disciplines. Such an approach replaces the traditional one which is unfortunately still in wide use, *i.e.,* sequential, uncoordinated treatment first by the surgeon; later, possibly, by the radiotherapist; and finally, after metastases have occurred, by the chemotherapist.

The recent increase in interest in pediatric oncology and the many accomplishments growing out of that interest had to wait for two important developments. The first was the recognition after World War II of what was already apparent in the 1930's, that the great reduction in death from infectious disease, brought about by improvements in public health, sanitation, and use of antimicrobial agents, unmasked the importance of cancer in the young. By the end of World War II, cancer was found to be the leading cause of death from disease in children between the ages of one and 15 years. The second important development was the opening of the era of cancer chemotherapy at the end of World War II with the discovery of the nitrogen mustards and other alkylating agents and the demonstration that folic acid antagonists could produce remissions in patients with acute leukemia. Progress in cancer chemotherapy was very slow at first, not only because important advances in medicine are traditionally given proper recognition after a long lag period, but also because beds, manpower, facilities, and resources were lacking in most institutions in this country concerned with children. Not until after the inauguration of the Cancer Chemotherapy National Program in 1955 and the striking increases in support for research from the National Cancer Institute (which went from less than a million dollars in 1945 to 175 million in 1967) could programs of effective size be undertaken in the chemotherapy of leukemia and solid tumors in children. It is heartwarming to see the evidence at this conference of such high caliber work in the clinical investigation of childhood cancer and such advanced programs of patient care.

However, I would like to emphasize, at the same time, that only a small percentage of all children with cancer are receiving the benefit of everything that is known today about care and treatment. Sophisticated patient care and research programs are costly, particularly if the patient is to be given the benefit of the most advanced supportive care, including blood platelets for the prevention and treatment of hemorrhage, white cells for the prevention and treatment of sepsis associated with leukopenia, and antibiotics and other antimicrobial agents when indicated for the good of the patient. There is no question that much better results in the prolongation of life, and even the saving of life, can be achieved if the child is treated in a center where sufficient resources are available to support the work of trained pediatric oncologists. The relationship between the doctor in private practice and the pediatric oncology center that we at The Children's Cancer Research Foundation have developed over the last 21 years may be employed as a prototype for the regional medical programs established by the President's Commission on Heart Disease, Cancer, and Stroke. From its inception, our program has been described to the doctors in our region of the country as one designed to assist them in the care of their patients. The expensive and difficult diagnostic tests, follow-up studies, and specialized treatments are carried out in our institution. The home care is provided by the doctor. Our institution's purpose is to join with the doctor in doing everything that is possible for the child and for his family. This has worked so effectively that there has been no complaint in more than 21 years of operation from any doctor in our region. Special resources must still be obtained for this program of total care.

Fundamental knowledge about the biochemical differences between the normal cell and the cancer cell is still lacking. None of the sciences basic to cancer research has produced the information which would enable us to construct the ideal anticancer agent on a perfectly rational basis. The empirical method is not regarded highly by scientists, but the history of medicine is replete with examples of great discoveries in medicine made on an empirical basis. The discovery in 1954 of the effectiveness of the antibiotic, actinomycin D, in the treatment for Wilms' tumor was made more than six years *before* the first studies on the drug's mechanism of action. Physicians are able now to eradicate pulmonary metastases when they use actinomycin D and small doses of radiotherapy. The discovery of the site of action of the drug on deoxyribonucleic acid-related ribonucleic acid (RNA) has inspired a vast amount of research in biochemistry and molecular biology. There is still no explanation, however, for the striking effect on the Wilms' tumor cell and the relative lack of effect at the same dose on the normal cell. Progress in research on the structure of RNA and the recent synthesis of actinomycin D give hope for more sophisticated clinical research programs. Some recent discussions in cancer chemotherapy have produced the pessimistic prediction that no more important anticancer agents will be discovered. It seems unreasonable to believe that the few antibiotics which are now in use in the treatment for cancer represent the total yield which can be recovered from the earth, nor does it seem logical to assume that the few chemical compounds proved to be carcinolytic represent the total number of possibilities which can be devised by the mind of man.

A final word concerning clinical investigation. The scientific criteria applied to clinical investigation should be as strict as can be carried out within the framework of moral control in studies on man. The statistical method and even the random selection pattern do not represent the only methods of discovery or evaluation of the anticancer effects of new drugs. The striking effect of actinomycin D on a Wilms' tumor which had spread to many parts of the body of a girl with advanced disease before initial chemotherapy was administered was demonstrated by clinical examination and postmortem studies. Knowledge of the history and biological behavior of the tumor gained from studies over a period of many years provided a background for the appraisal of a new treatment method for a tumor which is relatively rare, in comparison with solid tumors in adults. Of greatest importance in clinical investigation is the formulation of the questions which should be answered by the experimental design chosen.

In 1945, I included in the plans for clinical investigation in pediatric oncology at the Boston Children's Hospital a proposal that as soon as effective chemicals were available, an attempt should be made to prevent metastases in addition to destroying those already established. This attempt had to be based on knowledge of the life history and biological behavior of the tumor and its response to the most effective methods of therapy. Because of long familiarity with the Wilms' tumor and the total experience of my colleagues, we chose this lesion as our first test project. The most expert use of the techniques of surgery and radiotherapy yielded cure rates of no more than 40 per cent. We reasoned that if any chemical agent were added at the time of diagnosis and initial treatment and utilized as effectively as possible, it would not take long to determine whether metastases could be prevented. Our target was the 60 per cent of children with Wilms' tumor who died when only surgical procedures and radiotherapy were employed. Experiments were carried out for every anticancer agent that became available, but without success until 1954. In that year, the carcinolytic and toxic effects of actinomycin D were studied, and an important and seemingly specific effect on Wilms' tumor was found in the management of metastases and also in the prevention of spread from the primary source. It was noted when the antibiotic was used from the time of diagnosis and initial treatment, and at intervals of eight to 10 weeks over the next two years. The percentage of children who survived for periods of two to 13 years, with no demonstrable evidence of metastases, rose from 40 per cent before actinomycin D was used to more than 80 per cent. Not all forms of cancer in the child or the adult can be evaluated so easily. However, the principle of attempting to prevent metastases from tumors about which much knowledge concerning life history, biological behavior, and response to the most effective forms of treatment is available is one that deserves careful application in the hands of experts in oncology. It is clear that in many patients so treated, no metastases would have developed if chemotherapy had been used. One should be aware, however, that the more widespread use of chemical agents in an attempt to prevent metastases may result in harm if the chemicals are not employed by experts. Programs for the prevention of metastases can be instituted today against a number of forms of cancer in patients of all ages if the experimental conditions are sharply defined and proper care is instituted to prevent complications.

The greatest obstacle to rapid progress in clinical investigation in cancer is the fact that we are dealing with human beings who are sick. Basic requirements for such studies, which we have followed for many years, include the following:

The patient is not to be deprived of any treatment of proved value merely to permit trial of a new and unproved remedy; nothing should be done to the patient that is not primarily for his good. A new treatment must not cause toxic effects that are worse than the changes in the body produced by the untreated tumor, except for short periods of time when intensive treatment may possibly save life.

The present era of chemotherapy of cancer has not yet come to an end. It is likely that new hormone analogues, chemical agents, and antibiotics will be discovered which will be much more effective than those presently in use. The developments in immunology now being made in the laboratory and, to a small extent, in the clinic probably will lead to combined immunological and chemotherapeutic approaches. These, in turn, will make possible far greater utilization of the techniques of surgery and radiotherapy. Ultimately, the therapy for cancer will be much more sophisticated and subtle than anything presently available, or within our immediate reach. When a diagnostic test is perfected that can be carried out on the population as a whole—rapidly, inexpensively, and with great simplicity and accuracy, we shall be able to use it to recognize the change or transformation of a normal cell into a cancer cell before the cancer cells have increased to such an extent as to produce a tumor. On the basis of such a diagnostic test, the discovery of the biochemical disorder responsible for the transformation of the normal cell to a cancer cell will permit the use of the ultimate in chemotherapy. This therapy can be described in terms of neutralization or correction of the biochemical abnormality which is cancer. When that day comes, the problem of cancer in children, as well as in adults, will be in the hands of the doctor thoroughly skilled in oncology, molecular biology, and preventive medicine.

The treatment for cancer *before* it becomes a tumor which destroys organs or parts of the body is the ultimate goal for which we must strive. Until we reach that goal, the application of all that medicine and science can offer, *i.e.,* utilization of the total care treatment program, will prolong good life and increase the number of cures in infants and children suffering from many forms of cancer.

Index

329